Sustenance
for the Body
& Soul

Sustenance for the Body & Soul

Food & Drink in Amerindian, Spanish and Latin American Worlds

Edited by
Debra D. Andrist

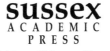

sussex
ACADEMIC
PRESS
Brighton • Chicago • Toronto

2 4 6 8 10 9 7 5 3 1

First published in Great Britain in 2022 by
SUSSEX ACADEMIC PRESS
PO Box 139, Eastbourne BN24 9BP

Distributed in North America by
SUSSEX ACADEMIC PRESS
Independent Publishers Group
814 N. Franklin Street
Chicago, IL 60610

British Library Cataloguing in Publication Data
A CIP catalogue record for this book is available from the British Library.

Library of Congress Cataloging-in-Publication Data
To be applied for.

Hardcover ISBN 978-1-78976-130-6

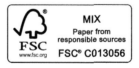

Typeset & designed by Sussex Academic Press, Brighton & Eastbourne.
Printed by TJ Books Limited, Padstow, Cornwall.

Contents

Preface

The sixth book in the Hispanic Worlds series, *Death & Dying in Hispanic Worlds: The Nexus of Religions, Cultural Traditions, and the Arts* (details of which are available on the Sussex Press website), was in preparation at the beginning and appeared at the height of the COVID-19 Pandemic, 2020. This book, *Sustenance for the Body & Soul: Food & Drink,* seventh in the series, was prepared and came to fruition fully during the Pandemic worldwide, even as the vaccines appeared, as well as being marked/marred by the human rights protests and divisive political atmosphere in the U.S., late 2020–late 2021. Both collections' general titles and themes feel somewhat ironic or at least, uncomfortable, reminders of the suffering and challenges associated with said timing, although neither book directly addresses the climates (not to mention the additional worsening actual climate change on the Earth) which surrounded them. In comparison, the chapters in each book focus on issues at psychological, intellectual distance, making them more palatable than the titles might imply, almost allowing mental escape from reality into the philosophical and interpretive spaces of scholarship. Yet, the distressing personal and social realities outside scholarship were never far from the daily experience of either the collaborators or the editor . . . whether we had been lucky enough previously to be able to be "foodies" and/or denizens of the restaurant scenarios in our pre-pandemic lives or not.

This collection recognizes that the food-secure and/or privileged worldwide no longer eat and drink simply to maintain life itself. They have had the advantage and choice to regard "sustenance" not just as fuel for the body/machine but as a source of pleasure and entertainment for the mind/intellect. This enhanced concept of "sustenance" embraces all the senses: visual, auditory, olfactory, gustatory and tactile, thus including not just food & drink but ceremonies & art forms dealing with them. Food & drink start with the physical, morph into nutrition, the most basic requirements for organic life, but progress from the beginning of physical process to ceremony and expression. The result and the experience highlight physiological and sensual concepts, and indeed, preference. Food & drink staples are determined by geographic availability and cuisine & beverage are closely associated with culture & ethnicity.

Therefore, this book explores the substantive ways that food & drink impact and have impacted human existence, focusing on indigenous, Latin American Hispanic & Iberian areas. The work is comprised of five main parts with sub-foci dividing the chapters among them. As each is proceeded by an introduction with segues from one to the next, this Preface is necessarily somewhat truncated in order avoid repetition. **Part I, Sustenance & Socio-Political Spaces: Intents & Agendas,** includes chapters on (proto) socio-political issues, advertising and teaching associated with food and drink; **Part II, Sustenance & Physical Space,** addresses architecture & food preparation & presentation; **Part III, Sustenance for the Body & Soul: Applications & Interpretations,** encompasses the role of food and drink preparations in medicine & healing & ceremony & religion; **Part IV, Sustenance & the Soul: Representation via the Visual Arts,** consists of observations about visual representations of food and drink, both studio art & cinema; and **Part V, Sustenance & the Soul: Representation via the Literary Arts,** incorporates chapters on writers of, writing in, the genres of poetry, fiction & essay, about food and drink, as well as a previously-unpublished essay itself after the chapter on the works of the writer herself.

Even though ever-increasing degrees of physical sequester and/or actual physical distancing characterized the experience of most of us who took the situation as seriously as scientists recommended, necessitating dramatic changes in personal lifestyle and careers, (relatively new activities for those of us born and educated pre-internet), scholarly pursuits continued. Techniques like zoom, texting, email, etc., allowed some respite socially and professionally, even as the efforts exhausted. In fact, reliance on the electronic media actually provided an even wider range of research possibilities, from on-line libraries to on-line sources (the arduousness of verifying on-line content aside) and more. Not for lack of options but due to appropriateness, this seventh book features not only a majority of new articles specifically written for this collection but several reprints of thematically relevant chapters from earlier books in the series to round-out the overview of the topic(s).

More specific preface-like information about the why of each of the five parts, their sub-parts and the chapters therein appears in the introductions to each part.

Acknowledgments

All reprints featured in this volume are from previous books in the Hispanic Worlds series, published by Sussex, and approved by the authors themselves. Chapter 4 (reprint from *S/HE: Sex & Gender in Hispanic Cultures*); *Chapter 6* (reprint from *Crossroads: Time & Space/Tradition & Modernity in Hispanic Worlds*); Chapter 8 (reprint from *The Body: Subject & Subjected: The Representation of the Body Itself, Illness, Injury, Treatment & Death in Spain and Indigenous and Hispanic American Art & Literature*); Chapter 15 (reprint from *Family, Friends & Foes: Human Dynamics in Hispanic Worlds*).

Chapter 10 is a reprint of "Transformation, Code, and Mimesis: Healing the Family in *Like Water for Chocolate*," in *Laura Esquivel's Mexican Fictions*, edited by Elizabeth Willingham (Sussex Academic Press, 2010).

All translations are by the chapter authors themselves unless otherwise indicated. The whole chapter translation of Jorge Chavarro's chapter is by Debra D. Andrist. See original volumes for translations in reprints.

All photographs accompanying chapters are by the chapter authors themselves unless otherwise indicated and/or are not under copyright. See original volumes for acknowledgements for photos accompanying reprints.

All references to illustrations of artworks and/or literature by Picasso in the two chapters by Enrique Mallén are from *The On-Line Picasso Project* founded and edited by Mallén, authorized by the Picasso Foundation. Request a password at https://picasso.shsu.edu/

Indigenous & Hispanic Worlds

The thus-far published seven-volume series of *Hispanic Worlds* morphed from a single first volume published by Sussex in 2016, *The Body: Subject & Subjected: The Representation of the Body Itself, Illness, Injury, Treatment & Death in Spain and Indigenous and Hispanic American Art & Literature*. Twenty years as a university department chair whose administrative duties necessitated reduced time for publication scholarship, as well as personal & professional interests in Hispanic worlds and medical fields over-all (detailed in the *Preface* of the first volume), led to the realization that I was far more enthused about, and inspired by, collaborative work, not just for efficacy of content. Certainly, I had plenty of unpublished material for several published volumes on my own. However, my continuing professional conference participation, thus hearing—and later read-ing of—colleagues' work, convinced me to not only publish my own works on particular themes as chapters in books but to undertake the organization, coordination, editing, and sometimes translating, of colleagues' works in a series of collaborative volumes.

The forenamed first volume combined material from the art & literature components of many of my medical (and gender-related) Spanish classes over the years (focused on practical, almost "hands-on" medical content in Spanish with much role-play, etc., not the traditional vocabulary-acquisition type of class). Like-minded works on related topics from pre-Conquest Aztec worlds by former Baylor University colleague, Jeanne Gillespie, PhD, now at University of Mississippi; the content of the monumental *Online Picasso Project* and related works on topics from Spain by current Sam Houston State University (SHSU) colleagues, Enrique Mallén, PhD and Montse Feu, PhD; an MFA thesis by my former graduate student at University of St. Thomas/Houston (UST), later founder and publisher of *Literal: Voces Latinoamericanas*, Rose Mary Salum, MFA; papers by my graduate students, Norma Mouton, MFA, at UST and Jorge Chavarro, MD, MA, at SHSU; and a presentation at the South Central Modern Language Association (SCMLA) conference by University of Texas graduate student, Lauren M.P. Derby, MA, fit together for broad, yet focused, insights into so many Hispanic worlds and the "selfies," the hominid body obsession, the metaphor I chose as the overarching theme of the first volume.

The second and third volumes, *Insult to Injury: Violence in Spanish, Hispanic American and Latino Art & Literature* (2017) and *S/HE: Sex & Gender in Hispanic Cultures* (2018), also highlighted and followed up on my scholarly interests and works on gender and related issues, as well as those of the same mind. My Argentine friend from even before a co-post-graduate Mellon fellowship at Rice University, University of St. Mary professor emerita, Gwendolyn Díaz; my former colleague at UST, Elizabeth Coscio, PhD; one of Rose Mary Salum's Mexican writer-colleagues, Eduardo Cerdán; several SCMLA colleagues: Smith College professor, Colombian Patricia González Gómes Cásseres, PhD; independent scholar, Michelle Sharp, PhD; Texas A&M professor, Stephen Miller, PhD; plus my former Baylor colleague, now chair at Regis University (who happens to be my sister-in-law), Kimberly Habegger, PhD, joined several of the collaborators from *The Body* to be featured in these volumes. Patterns of focus in, and segues between, subsequent chapters submitted emerged with the continuing collaborations, leading to the next theme and the applicability of some reprints of chapters from former volumes.

The fourth and fifth volumes, *Family, Friends & Foes: Human Dynamics in Hispanic Worlds* (2019) and *Crossroads: Time & Space/Tradition & Modernity in Hispanic Worlds (2020)*, followed suit. New and a few reprints of chapters by continuing collaborators were joined by chapters which added more breadth to the *Hispanic Worlds* series' themes. For example, political scientist working in *mestizaje*, John Francis Burke, PhD, a former UST fellow chair now at Trinity University, and Haiqing Sun, PhD, Texas Southern University professor, whose work with culturally comparative aspects, especially in film, expanded the collaborator group.

The inspiration for the next book's theme comes from the last book published and the planning and the editing process for each following book begins almost as soon as the last volume has been submitted to Sussex each year. The latest published, the seventh volume, *Sustenance for the Body & Soul: Food & Drink in Amerindian, Spanish and Latin American Worlds*, appears in 2022. Like its 2021 predecessor, *Death & Dying: The Nexus of Religions, Cultural Traditions & the Arts in Hispanic Worlds* was in progress when the COVID-19 pandemic changed all worlds as we knew them across cultures in early 2020. Even so—or perhaps even more so in continuing self-preserving sequester—food & drink play a, if not the, central role in the lives of everyone, food-secure and food-insecure. Always fuel for the body/machine but a source of pleasure and entertainment for the mind/intellect when experience & mental stimulation is limited, the enhanced concept of "sustenance" embraces all the senses: visual, auditory, olfactory, gustatory and tactile, thus including not just food & drink but ceremonies & art forms dealing with them. This book explores the substantive ways food & drink have impacted and impact human existence.

Volume number eight, *Rites, Rituals & Religions in Amerindian, Iberian & Latin American Worlds* (to appear 2023), is already "in the works" and will feature some appropriate reprints but much new material by the faithful cadre of collaborators, plus some insights and studies by new participants!

PART I

Sustenance & Socio-Political Spaces: Intents & Agendas

Introduction to Sustenance & Socio-Political Spaces: Intents & Agendas

A. (Proto) political (Perhaps Unintended) Cultural Influences

While culinary issues are seldom considered even *proto* socio-political, at least in my personal and professional preparation and experience, the influence of American-continents-origin foodstuff plants on European cuisine is undeniable! As a practical matter, I have taught university classes on (mostly Hispanic with sections on various Amerindian) cultures and civilizations for decades and always utilized food and drink topics and content as not only historical aspects but as attention-grabbers-and-maintainers for U.S. students, whatever their ethnic or cultural background. Many, if not most, save perhaps botany majors, are simply not aware of the intercontinental exchange of these basic components of life, let alone which items or their origin. And, scheduled tasting-samples-days generally feature no-absence attendance. Of course, I emphasize the iconic European dishes which would not have been but for the conquest of the Americas by the Spanish (and Portuguese and French et al.), particularly utilizing the best-known ingredients in European dishes with which the students are most familiar, potatoes, tomatoes and chocolate.

Yet, even so, I myself had not necessarily considered the even more far-reaching effects of American-origin food plants throughout the entire world until beginning to write the/my first chapter of *Sustenance for the Body & Soul*, intending simply to introduce said foodstuffs per se to the collection! I did plan to posit the culinary counter-conquest as unintended rather than an agenda but found more and more justification for characterizing the influence as a counter-conquest as I researched. Thus, I am indebted to those whose work I have extensively quoted for broadening my own culinary—and socio-political—horizons. The huge difference between the Conquest of the Americas and the culinary conquest, specifically of Europe, is, of course, the contrast, truly antonyms, between destruction in the first case and enhancement in the second.

Continuing in the same vein, though not necessarily as long-term historical, the next three sub-parts, whether teaching students and influencing the public, whether via formal schooling or by way of informal socialization in the family or by shaping public consumption through advertising follow a similar pattern.

B. TEACHING & INFLUENCING THE STUDENT(S) AS AN AGENDA: FORMAL
    EDUCATION

As a segue, literary critic, Elizabeth Coscio highlights her "take" on food & drink as syllabus themes and students' reactions in such classes and the linguistic theories on why in the second focus of this section, education, both formal and familial. She details the incredibly involved linguistics behind vocabulary choices, etc., to explain/justify teaching acquisition of the language via foodstuffs/cuisine.

While both of the chapters by Michelle Sharp in Part I B & C could have appeared in Part III B The Kitchen & Dining Room, since the first also addresses formal education, it seemed more appropriate after Coscio's chapter on course themes of food & drink. Sharp's chapter, written initially as a food-conference presentation, addresses food and contemporary home economics classes in Spain (and the U.S.). And, the socio-political influences of the 19th century cookbooks in Spanish in Sharp's reprinted chapter tied not only to her first (new) chapter in Part I B but also to the concept of, if not advertising per se, at least attempts to influence familial formation and socialization via food preparation. Sharp's specialties include not only literary topics but food science. She has contributed two chapters to this collection, both of which directly tie food to socialization and socio-political influences in Spain.

C. TEACHING & INFLUENCING THE FAMILY AS AN AGENDA:
    SOCIALIZATION & NATIONAL POLITICS

Sharp's second chapter, "Family Responsibilities: A Recipe for the Modern Spanish Nation: Carmen de Burgos' and Emilia Pardo Bazán's Cookbook Discourses," is a reprint of her contribution to *S/he: Sex & Gender in Hispanic Cultures*. Cookbooks, and their role in shaping the family and the public, provide a segue to the formidable role that commercial advertising plays in shaping—and basically, deter-mining—all aspects of food and drink consumption, as so many other studies have statistically documented about consumers' choices.

D. TEACHING & INFLUENCING THE PUBLIC AS AN AGENDA:
    COMMERCIAL ADVERTISING

Addressing not just art-based merchandizing and identification of a beverage, Kimberly Habegger's chapter on wine labels in Spain, written specifically for this collection, is a direct tie-in to her reprinted chapter from the fifth book in the series, *Crossroads: Time &*

Space/Tradition & Modernity in Hispanic Worlds in Part II, which highlights the architecture of the wineries and their wine museums. Since the chapters dovetail, as the labels very frequently graphically represent the wineries themselves, the labels function as visual advertisements/attractions for the buyer of the wine. This chapter could easily have appeared in Part IV on visual art dealing with food/drink— but felt more logical as an "agenda" chapter due to the marketing strategies the labels employ, as well as being a logical segue to Habegger's reprinted chapter on the wineries and their wine museums which follows it.

1

A (Culinary) Counter-Conquest: Imports from the Americas that Conquered European Cuisine

Debra D. Andrist

As many have observed over time, history is invariably interpreted and written by the powerful from their perspective.[1] For example, reams of information about the Spanish so-called "discovery of the New World(s)"[2] from 1492 & beyond establish the enforced imposition of every aspect of Spanish and/or Latin[3] culture from language to religion to daily life itself upon the indigenous worlds in the Americas. Yet, the reverse, a culinary counter-conquest via the importation of arguably up to a couple dozen foodstuff plants native to the Americas into Europe, directly transformed the latter's cultures and food via their use in now-characteristic European dishes especially attributed to almost every Western European country, not to mention other areas of the globe.

Admittedly, and it's vital to emphasize, the importation and dissemination of these foodstuffs from the Americas to Spain/Europe represents an enhancement-type cultural "conquest" of European cuisine, a kind of "taking/giving," contrasted with the horrific long-term imposition on/extermination of multiple peoples and cultures in the Western Hemisphere over centuries, as was that enacted by the *conquistadores* in the Americas. That was "taking" in every sense of the word. The roles of "take," when actually imposed, as in extract, versus "give," are relative terms in these contexts.[4]

Because I am not a specialist in food-related studies per se, though over my entire career, I've taught culture courses enumerating which items originated in the Americas, this chapter relies far more than usually advisable, or maybe even desirable, on quotes from various sites and works by trained professionals in the appropriate fields. Yet, the combination of these sources provides a unique look at the phenomenon I posit. Furthermore, the applicability of this chapter as an introduction to the themed collection of articles that is *Sustenance for the Body & Soul: Food & Drink in Indigenous, Spanish & Latin American Worlds* undeniably justifies the heavy reliance on quotations, in my opinion.

In addition to consulting too many cookbooks in several languages, which also feature historic aspects of ingredients and dishes, to cite in this essay, most of these foodstuff plants have dedicated websites which have been great sources of information. Among the most complete, well-documented and helpful of general sources, the article on the Colombian Exchange by Nathan Nunn and Nancy Qian focuses on not only the effect of American-origin foodstuff plants on the cuisines and nutrition of other countries but also on the effects of other consumables like tobacco, cocaine and quinine, since the authors detail the exchange of diseases and plants of other uses, on the economies of European countries and the rest of the entire globe. Being economists, they document further the effects on European population growth, urbanization, world currencies, agriculture and even how the Exchange facilitated colonization of other world places by the European powers. Clearly, though not the focus of this chapter in this collection, the "counter-conquest" by American-origin foodstuff plants and other consumables is much wider than simply European cuisine! They quote

> Historian Alfred Crosby (1989, 666) [who] describes the significance of the transfer of food crops between the continents, writing: 'The coming together of the continents was a prerequisite for the population explosion of the past two centuries, and certainly played an important role in the Industrial Revolution. The transfer across the ocean of the staple food crops of the Old and New Worlds made possible the former.'[5]

Moreover, Nunn & Qian also observe that

> There are two channels through which the Columbian Exchange expanded the global supply of agricultural goods. First, it introduced previously unknown species to the Old World. Many of these species . . . resulted in caloric and nutritional improvements over previously existing staples. Other crops . . . not by themselves especially rich in calories but complemented existing foods by increasing vitamin intake and improving taste. In many instances, the New World foods had an important effect on the evolution of local cuisines. . . . Second, the discovery of the Americas provided the Old World with vast

quantities of relatively unpopulated land well-suited for the cultivation of certain crops that were in high demand in Old World markets.
Crops such as sugar, coffee, soybeans, oranges, and bananas were all
introduced to the New World and the Americas quickly became the
main suppliers of these crops globally . . . Among oils, the fourth most
consumed oil, sunflower oil, is derived from sunflowers, a New World
crop . . . a number of additional New World foods . . . such as chili
peppers and cacao, which despite not being consumed in large
quantities, are of central importance to the cuisines of many countries
. . . The primary benefit of the New World staples was that they could
be grown in Old World climats that were unsuitable for the cultivation of Old-World staples. Crosby (2003, 177) writes 'The great
advantage of the American food plants is that they make different
demands of soils, weather and cultivation than Old World crops and
are different in the growing seasons in which they make these
demands. In many cases the American crops do not compete with Old
World crops but complement them. The American plants enable the
farmer to produce food from soils that, prior to 1492, were rated as
useless because of their sandiness, altitude, aridity, and other factors.'[6]

Reiterating Nunn and Qian's claim about the effect of the potato
on European culture, not just cuisine, who can imagine Spain without
the ubiquitous Spanish tortilla (potato omelet), possibly as a
tapa/appetizer, possibly in a sandwich, or any number of other iterations? This is not to mention the potato's omnipresent role in nearly
every other Western European cuisine post-Conquest. Perhaps the
most notable, so very many of Ireland's dietary items, signature dishes,
are dependent on potatoes, like colcannon (potatoes, cabbage &
cream), all of which led to the Great Famine of 1845–49 due to late
(potato) blight, thus resulting in much of the Irish diaspora, especially
to the Americas, in the mid-19th century. However, the potato had a
rather vacillating introduction to European cuisine, as Kimberly
E.A.U. traces in her blog:

> Europeans first came in contact with the potatoes in 1532 when
> Spaniard Francisco Pizarro landed in Peru, learning of it from local
> Amerindians. Within three decades, the vegetable had spread
> throughout Spain's American holdings, and by 1573, we have the first
> evidence of the potato in Europe, when a hospital in Seville, Spain
> bought some for their garden. From Spain, it then migrated to the
> Spanish controlled regions of Italy by 1586, England by 1596, and
> Germany by 1601. It's important to mention here that the early
> adoption of the potato was not as a food staple but rather as an object

of curiosity for botanists and the earliest use of the potato was for decoration rather than cuisine.

There were three key factors which led to a general unease towards the potato as a food item. First, was that the potato was miscategorized as a species related to the nightshade family which was notoriously poisonous. This misconception was made due to the dominant school of botanist thought in the period, which was deeply rooted in the old (Roman and Greek) ways of thinking. This meant that there were a lot of issues when trying to reconcile new-world plant species into the old systems of thinking, with many being wrongfully compared to old-world species. Second, the appearance of the potato created an unfortunate association between the plant and the skin of lepers. Lastly, the newness and foreignness of the species create a general suspicion and apprehension towards the plant. One trait which was met with a great degree of suspicion was the fact that potatoes didn't require seeds to be grown, a first for European agriculture.

This suspicion was eventually overcome towards the end of the 17th century, but even into the 18th century, there was a great deal of controversy and criticism leveled at the potato. In Denis Diderot's *Encyclopedias* (1751–65), he describes the potato as something that . . . 'cannot be regarded as an enjoyable food, but it provides abundant, reasonably healthy food for men w[h]o want no[th]ing but sustenance' . . . Another critic of the potato was England, where it was denounced as an agent of Roman Catholicism, with the slogan 'No Potatoes, No Popery!' being used in 1765. However, even with its critics, the adoption of the potato as a food item could not be stopped. As early as the late 17th century, there is evidence of widespread cultivation and eating of potatoes in Ireland, Spanish Netherlands, and the Alsace region of France. By the early 18th century, it had been adopted within England and Scotland, and by the mid-18th century had arrived in Scandinavia.

By 1744, we have the first widespread adoption of the potato in Germany, when Frederick the Great of Prussia ordered his peasantry to eat it in order to alleviate a famine at the time. In France, the adoption of the potato was spearheaded by a single gentleman by the name of Antoine-Augustin Parmentier. Parmentier was a veteran of the Seven Years' War (1756–1763) and during the conflict was captured by the Prussians, who fed him little beside potatoes. After the war, he dedicated his life to the vegetable, doing everything in his power to promote it. Some of his most high-profile publicity stunts included: An all-potato banquet for an international gathering of high society; persuading the king and queen of France to wear potato blossoms on their outfits; and planting 40 acres of potatoes on the edge of Paris in order to encourage the poor to steal them and plant them for themselves. By 1775, France was in the perfect position to adopt the potato, as this was the year when the price controls on grain were lifted, leading to the rapid increase of bread prices, leaving room for the potato to really shine as an alternative staple in French diets. From Europe, the potato was then spread across the rest of the old world via colonial trade networks and mariners. It arrived in China by the 17th century via the Dutch, it was introduced to India by the 17th century by the Portuguese and British and had reached Ethiopia by 1858 via the Germans. By the end of the 18th century, the potato was a well-established staple of European diets with anywhere between 10–30% of the population solely consisting [rather, subsisting] on them within the Netherlands, Belgium, Prussia, and Poland, and 40% of the population in Ireland.[7]

For details on why the potato had such a pivotal role in European cuisine after its introduction from the Americas, again Nunn and Qian not only describe the nutritional reasons behind the Irish diaspora post-blight but the changes in population growth and urbanization that the potato occasioned.

Because it provides an abundant supply of calories and nutrients, the potato is able to sustain life better than any other food when consumed as the sole article of diet (Davidson and Passmore, 1965, 285). Humans can actually subsist healthily on a diet of potatoes, supplemented with only milk or butter, which contain the two vitamins not provided by potatoes, vitamins A and D (Connell, 1962; Davidson and Passmore, 1965). This, in fact, was the typical Irish diet, which although monotonous, was able to provide sufficient amounts of all vitamins and nutrients (Connell, 1962). The potato was also adopted as a core staple in many other parts of the World (Connell, 1962) . . . We find that the potato had a significant positive impact on population growth, explaining 12 percent of the increase in average population after the adoption of the potato. We also estimate the effect the potato had on urbanization, a measure that is closely correlated with GDP. We find that that 47 percent of the post-adoption increase in urbanization is explained by the potato.[8]

The use of the tomato, too, as omnipresent as it is today in most of European cuisines, evolved over time. As Maríaluz López-Terrada notes in her study of the arrival of the tomato, arguably the second most influential import to Europe from the Americas, though it certainly applies in nearly all the cases of foodstuff plants which originated in the Western Hemisphere, these foodstuff plants thoroughly changed the culinary scene in Europe post-Conquest.

> Food plants have a fundamental place in human life. The introduction of the new world of American plants into Europe was therefore a process that gave rise to profound social and cultural changes. The encounter between Europe and America was perhaps the most important act of globalization in history: two different cultural and natural worlds came into contact, and the results of that contact had a huge impact on the landscape, as well as on everyday experience and intellectual life. The arrival of American plants changed cooking and eating habits, medicinal products, drugs, poisons, gardens, but also wood types, pigments, solvents and many other materials with practical applications. This complex process of dissemination and assimilation is the historical context [for this study of food and drink].[9]

A member of the belladonna family and first considered poisonous, the tomato now is nearly everywhere in European kitchens, perhaps best-known in Italian sauces, not to mention in other dishes beyond count in that and other cultures, notably the Spanish. López-Terrada goes on to say that

> Leaving aside the origin of the plant, Europeans first came into contact with the domesticated tomato in Mesoamerica after the capture in 1521, by Hernán Cortés, of the [Aztec] city of Tenochtitlan [today's Mexico City], where it was an integral part of the Nahua diet and culture in the sixteenth century . . . . There are many other well-known references to the tomato in the Chronicles of the Indies . . . which describe the ways in which tomatoes were consumed by native Americans, but also reveal their assimilation into the cuisine of the Spaniards living in what was by now called New Spain. In 1571, for example, the Franciscan friar and priest Alonso de Molina, in the second edition of his Nahuatl–Spanish dictionary, *Vocabulario en lengua mexicana y castellana*/Vocabulary of the Mexican and Castilian Languages, translated the Nahuatl term *tomatl* as 'a certain fruit used to add a sour flavour to stews and sauces,' and indicated that *xaltomatl* was 'a certain fruit like tomatoes,' whilst *xitomatl* was translated as 'large red, yellow and white tomatoes.' In the Spanish–Nahuatl section, the 'fruit added to stews instead of sour grapes' was '*tomatl, xaltomatl* or *xitomatl*.' In other words, Spaniards had already

adopted the plant that the Nahuas termed *xitomalt*, and that groups further south called *tomati*, to add acidity to sauces and stews cooked in the New World, and they appropriated the latter name, as there was no fruit like it in Europe. American pumpkin and beans were similar to species grown in Europe [but] they were called by the Spanish term. [The author notes elsewhere in her article that recipe examples were found early on which called dishes using tomatoes as *alla Spagnuola*/in the Spanish style.] Thus, it is the Mesoamerican name [for tomato] that survives in almost all languages, despite the French and Italians who from the outset called it "apple of love" (*pomme d'amour*) or "golden apple" (*pomodoro*) . . . Botanists believe that approximately 1,000 years before the Spanish arrived in the Americas, an unidentified wild ancestor of the tomato made its way and came to be cultivated in South and Central America (Smith, 1994, 17). The tomato is first mentioned in European texts in 1544. Mathiolus described how tomatoes, *pomi d'oro* (golden apple), were eaten in Italy with oil, salt, and pepper, suggesting tomatoes in Europe were yellow and not red (Gould, 1983, 30–53) . . . The first documented authentic recipe in Italy appeared in 1692 in an early Italian cookbook, *Lo scalco alla moderna*, by Antonio Latini. Tomatoes were brought to Asia by Spaniards who visited the Philippines in 1564. However, in China, where they were regarded as foods of the "southern barbarians," they were not cultivated until the twentieth century (Anderson, 1988, 94). In North Africa, English travelers reported that Spanish tomatoes were in fields of North Barbary as early as 1671 (McCue, 1952, 330). One of the difficulties in consuming tomatoes was that that they did not preserve well. Ripe tomatoes can become putrid within days in hot climates. The canning process helped increase the shelf life of the tomato to several months, but prior to 1890, it was a costly manual process. The mechanization of canning at the turn of the twentieth century significantly lowered the cost of this process and resulted in a significant increase in tomato consumption (Gould, 1983, 30–53). Tomatoes have truly become a global food . . . nine of the top ten tomato-consuming countries are Old World countries. Greece consumes the most tomatoes per capita, followed by other Mediterranean and Middle Eastern countries. Italy, known for its use of tomato sauces with pasta and on pizza, ranks [only] sixth on the list.[10]

On the other hand, the integral role of chocolate (cacao) began immediately! Especially well-known in Europe in terms of the world-famous Austrian, German, Swiss and Belgian confections of all sorts, chocolate eventually also necessitated specific dishware like chocolate pots and cups and led to enhanced social interactions and commerce in chocolate cafes and shops. The love-affair history of the cacao bean in Europe was not nearly so fraught with mixed reception as the tomato and potato or even corn.

Mayans grew cacao trees in their backyards and used the seeds to brew ceremonial drinks. In the fifth century, Aztecs consumed *xocoatl* (bitter water) flavored with vanilla and chili pepper. The highly valued bean served as currency in Aztec society. One turkey, for example, cost 100 cacao beans. As far back as 1504, Christopher Columbus may have brought cacao beans toSaion from his fourth and final voyage to the Americas. Hernán Cortés, the Spanish conquistador who subdued Mexico with luck and pluck (and guns, germs and steel), wrote in 1519 that chocolate is 'the divine drink which builds up resistance and fights fatigue. A cup of this precious drink permits a man to walk for a whole day without food.' Cortés brought cacao beans and chocolate-brewing apparatus back to Spain when he returned in 1528. And Dominican friars, who introduced native peoples to Spanish royalty in 1544, also gave chocolate to their majesties. Yet for all this, the great onrush of the continental cocoa craze is often traced to July 7, 1550, and July 7 is even gaining currency as Chocolate Day. . . . Whatever its original date of introduction in Spain, chocolate did not stay there. Spanish friars spread the gospel of *Theobroma cacao* throughout Europe as they traveled from monastery to monastery. Hot chocolate became a hit with French royalty after cocoa enthusiast Marie Therese married Louis XIV in 1660. At the Palace of Versailles, courtiers regarded the drink as an aphrodisiac. London's first chocolate house opened in 1657. English café society believed the drink to be a cure-all medicine capable of treating tuberculosis. Initially flavored with coffee, wine and pepper, hot chocolate finally achieved liftoff in the early 1700s when English and Dutch impresarios hit on the idea of adding milk and sugar. It was only a matter of time before mass-production technologies would transform bean-based treats from luxury to everyman staple. A century later, chocolate assumed solid form, courtesy of Fry and Sons. The British confectioners [other histories cite the Austrians as the source of the addition of sugar for a more palatable hot chocolate drink for their chocolate houses] figured out how to add sugar and cocoa butter to create a malleable paste that could then be packaged as 'eating chocolate.'[11]

Additionally, Nunn and Qian tell us about

The Codex Mendoza—an Aztec record of administration and description daily life, written approximately 20 years after the Spanish conquest of Mexico [which] documents that by the time Cortes arrived, chocolate was being cultivated by farmers in the Yucatan and was traded in large quantities throughout the Empire armers in the Yucatan (Prescott, 1843,11; West, 1992, 108). Historical records indicate that Columbus first brought back specimens of cacao pods to King Ferdinand I after his voyage to the New World. Outside of the Americas, cacao was first cultivated in 1590 by the Spanish off the coast of Africa on the island of Fernando Po (West, 1992, 110–111). At first, it was used in expensive chocolate drinks, mainly confined to aristocratic courts.[12] From Spain, it spread to Italy, and then to France via the royal aristocratic courts via the royal marriage of Philip III's daughter, Ana of Austria, with Louis XIII. In England, Samuel Pepys, the renowned seventeenth century diarist, records that chocolate drinks changed from being novelty drinks to a regular luncheon beverage of the middle class during his lifetime (McLeod 2001). The Spanish held a monopoly on production and trade of cacao up the seventeenth century when the French began cacao production in Martinique. The Dutch also began production of cacao in Indonesia, which was the Dutch East Indies at the time . . . While chocolate is most popularly consumed as a condiment, candy or dessert, cacao is also a high energy food known for lifting psychological effects. Pure chocolate, which is more than half cocoa butter, has a higher energy output per unit of weight than most other carbohydrate- or protein-rich foods. This has made it an important food for physically taxing expeditions where travelers needed to minimize the food carried.[13]

Grains like corn (and amaranth and quinoa in South America), which characterized every aspect of the pre-Colombian Mesoamerican diet, have not had so overwhelming influence on European cuisine as the tomato and potato and chocolate. Though, in fact, corn, too, had a spotty introduction to, and less-profuse effect on, the so-called Old-World cuisine. *Food Reference* observes that

Corn's journey to the Old World began with Christopher Columbus who ferried it back to Spain. By 1500 it was under cultivation in Spain and by the 17th century it was a major crop for a number of European countries . . . Interestingly, the early Spanish invaders of Mesoamerica were aversive to corn. Some of the Indian tribes practiced human sacrifice and grisly rituals which involved corn. The conquistadors thus correlated corn with internecine paganism and considered its consumption unchristian. [While the Europeans did not know the scientific side but only the physical results] Corn consumption was also associated with pellagra, a deficiency disease of niacin in conjunction with the amino acid tryptophan. Corn is barren of niacin. Tryptophan can be converted to niacin in the body thus attenuating the depletion of niacin. A diet dominated by corn with little other vegetables or sources of tryptophan can result in pellagra. Pellagra causes dermatological, gastrointestinal and neurological symptoms and ultimately death. Eventually of course, the Europeans transcended their initial prejudices against corn.[14]

One of the "three sisters" of Mesoamerican cuisine (corn, beans and squash), "new" legumes (more than corn) particularly transformed European cooking (e.g., where would the French be without the particular American varieties of beans for *cassoulet*?), though not to the extent of the aforementioned Western Hemisphere-origin foodstuff plants. The fact that other varieties of beans were known and consumed in Europe also eased the introduction of the American varieties.

The discovery of the New World bean and its many forms revolutionized world agriculture, yet for several centuries the scientific approach to this body of plants has been chaotic at best. At the very outset, Europeans began calling them *fasiolius*, the name previously used for cowpeas by the Greeks and Romans. This led to heated debates about the origin of the bean and whether or not it was from the Old World or the New. As long as Europeans thought American Indians were the Lost Tribes of Israel—an idea that survived into the nineteenth century—it was logical to conclude that their foodstuffs also originated in the Middle East. The oldest depiction of the common garden bean in a European work is thought to be a 1543 woodcut of a bush bean in the German herbal of Leonhart Fuchs. Later in the same century, in 1553, another German herbalist by the name of Georg Oelinger made a watercolor of a red pole bean that is probably related to the variety known today as *frijoles rojos*, or Montezuma Red. While this is a bush variety, it can also appear as a pole bean. One of the important lessons in understanding beans and their evolution is to discard the myth that pole beans and bush beans represent different species. Botanically speaking, the two are only extreme forms of the same thing.[15]

As to the importation of the American varieties to Europe, "scholarly research indicates that beans were domesticated in two places: the Andes mountains of Peru, and the Lerma-Santiago basin of Mexico."[16]

Before Columbus, the Old World was familiar with numerous kinds of beans, but neither [the American-origin] common bean, *Phaseolus vulgaris*, nor the lima bean, P. *lunatus*, was known. Their American origin is fixed by descriptions and references to finding them at many widely scattered points over the Americas about 1500 and soon after . . . The English first used the name "kidney bean" in 1551 to distinguish our American common bean from Old World types . . . Not long ago, Brazil was believed to be the country of origin of lima beans, but new evidence points to Guatemala. Wild primitive lima beans have been found there, along with a remarkable diversity of cultivated forms. Their distribution from Guatemala has been traced by the various "prehistoric varieties" left along Indian trade routes . . . Another course extended down through Central America into Peru, where the large-seeded, large-podded types were developed in the warm coastal areas. The name "lima bean" obviously came from Lima, Peru, one point at which the species was found by early European explorers . . . Since dry common and lima beans are highly concentrated foods and are easily carried and stored for long periods, the explorers and slavers of the early 1500's found them ideal for replenishing their ships' stores. Supplies were obtained from Indians in numerous places in the Americas and incidentally carried to the farthest parts of the earth—Europe, Africa, the East Indies, India, the Philippines. By the late 1700's, there were many records of the lima bean in all those places. Apparently, it was first recorded in Europe about 1591. It is far less important in most of Europe than is the common bean [known in Europe prior to the Conquest], since it requires warm weather for good growth.[17]

Like beans, Europe had varieties of native squashes but the imported American-origin squashes had similar, though lesser, effect on European cuisine.

Squash (genus Cucurbita), including squashes, pumpkins, and gourds, is one of the earliest and most important of plants domesticated in the Americas, along with maize and common bean. The genus includes 12–14 species, at least six of which were domesticated independently in South America, Mesoamerica, and Eastern North America, long before European contact.[18]

Peanuts, pineapple, avocado and additional American-origin food-stuff plants have also affected European cuisine, particularly peanuts as additives to chocolate candy and in desserts—and the cuisines of countries they colonized.[19] But, arguably, the peanut did not so dramatically and daily transform those cultures' cuisines as it did eventually that of the U.S., dedicated as that country is to, e.g., PB & J (peanut butter & jelly being perhaps the sandwich most known to U.S. mothers and children), among other concoctions.

> The peanut . . . is a native South American legume . . . At the time of the discovery of the American and European expansion into the New World, this cultivated species was known and grown widely throughout the tropical and subtropical areas of this hemisphere. The early Spanish and Portuguese explorers found the Indians cultivating the peanut in several of the West Indian Islands, in Mexico, on the northeast and east coasts of Brazil, in the warm land of the Río de la Plata basin (Argentina, Paraguay, Bolivia, extreme southwest Brazil), and extensively in Peru. From these regions the peanut was disseminated to Europe, to the coasts of Africa, Asia, and the Pacific Islands.[20]

Certain crops which provide less nutritive or fewer calories, known more as flavoring additives, but are now no less important to Old World cuisines, and three less-healthy New World crops consumed in different ways, tobacco, coca and quinine, are notable in their long-term effect on European, if not cuisine, consumption. Among those entities better known for flavoring value,

> The capsicum pepper originated in the areas that today are and southern Brazil. By the arrival of the Europeans, the plant had migrated to Mesoamerica and the Caribbean. Mesoamerica and the Caribbean. Capsicum annuum, which was domesticated in which was Mesoamerica, is the ancestor to most of the peppers commonly consumed today: the cayenne pepper, bell peppers, and the jalapeño pepper. A second variety, *Capsicum frutescens*, first cultivated in the Amazon basin, gives us the tabasco pepper (Andrews, 1992, 82–83). By 1493, capsicum peppers had arrived in Spain and Africa. They then reached the East Indies by 1540 and India by 1542 (Andrews, 1993a, 1993b). In Hungary, paprika, the spice made from grinding dried fruits of the capsicum pepperis, was first mentioned in 1569. Paprika has since been widely adopted in a variety of Hungarian dishes, including goulash, and today is the country's national spice (Halasz, 1963). The capsicum has also had a significant impact on the cuisine

of many other countries [colonized, or at least influenced, by Europeans]. In South and South East Asia, some form of pepper is used in the base of almost every dish (for example, curries. In China, cuisine in the southwest (like Sichuan, Guizhou, and Hunan) are defined by uses of certain chili peppers. In Korea, a side dish of spicy kimchi is consumed with every meal.[21]

Another flavoring,

> Vanilla was completely unknown to the Old World prior to 1492, but despite having little nutritional importance, it has become so widespread and so common that in English its name is used as an adjective to refer to anything that is "plain, ordinary, or conventional.' Vanilla comes from the tropical forests of eastern and southern Mexico, Central America, and northern South America . . . It is unclear whether vanilla was first brought back to Spain by a Spanish traveler. In any case, it achieved popularity quickly in Spain, where factories were using it to flavor chocolate by the second half of the sixteenth century. Like chocolate, it was considered a luxury for the wealthy. King Phillip II was known to have drunk vanilla-flavored chocolate as a nightcap. It was also quickly adopted by aristocratic circles in other parts of Europe. Queen Elizabeth I of England was also known to have been a frequent user of vanilla products (Rain, 1992, p. 40). In the eighteenth century, the French began to use it widely as a flavoring for confectionaries and ice, and also as a scent for perfumes and tobacco.[22]

Not only plants but animals of American origin became parts of European cuisine as well. For example,

> the earliest signs of domesticated turkeys found to date appear in Maya sites such as Cobá beginning about 100 BCE–100 CE. All modern turkeys are descended from M. *gallapavo*, the wild turkey having been exported from the Americas to Europe during the 16th century.[23]

As a linguistic aside, though the Nahuatl word for turkey is *huehxolotl*, the Spanish word for the bird, probably from Greek for peacock, *pavo*, is reportedly one of the only common vernacular words shared by the two members of the Fino-Ugric family of languages. Neither Finnish nor Hungarian features that word formally as a name for turkey but acquaintances from both cultures have assured me that *pavo* is the word they use in informal situations.[24]

Though not a foodstuff plant but a consumable of considerable influence on European (and other) cultures, Nunn and Qian highlight that tobacco, another New World crop,

> was so universally adopted in Europe that it came to be used as a substitute for currency in many parts of the world. It is believed that Native Americans began to use tobacco around the first century BCE. There is no evidence that Native Americans ever consumed tobacco recreationally. It was instead used as a hallucinogen during religious ceremonies and as a painkiller. Ramon Pane, a monk who accompanied Columbus on his second voyage, gave lengthy descriptions about the custom of smoking tobacco He described how natives inhaled smoke through a Y-shaped tube. The two ends were placed in the nostrils and the third end over a pastille of burning leaves . . . Tobacco was quickly adopted by Europeans. At first tobacco was regarded and consumed only as a medicine. In 1560, the French ambassador to Portugal, Jean Nicot de Villemain (from whom the term "nicotine" originates) proclaimed that tobacco had a panacea of medicinal properties. In 1561, Nicot sent tobacco leaves to Catherine de Medici, the Queen of France. She was so impressed with the plant that she decreed that tobacco be called *Herba Regina* (the Queen's Herb). In England, tobacco was first introduced by Sir John Hawkins and his crew in the 1580s. It was chiefly used by sailors, including those employed by Sir Francis Drake. By the beginning of the seventeenth century, tobacco had spread to all parts of Europe (Brooks, 1952, 16). Besides being consumed—but not swallowed per se, tobacco has also been used as currency at various times.[25]

The equally infamous effects of tobacco and cocaine versus the positive value of quinine in Europe are due to importation from the Americas as well, as Nunn & Qian document:

> Coca leaves are grown from bushes native to the Andes. The leaves contain alkaloids that can be extracted to produce commercial cocaine. The use of coca leaves has a long history. During the Incan Empire, they were chewed during religious rituals. Early Spanish settlers adopted this practice and brought it back to Europe . . . Quinine, an important medicinal 'gift. from the New World, had significant consequences for the relationship between Europe and its tropical Old-World colonies, particularly its African colonies. Quinine and related anti-malarial alkaloids (quinidine, cinchonine, cinchonidine) are derived from the bark of cinchona trees native to the Andes. The trees grow in scattered clumps in the eastern mountainous forests of Colombia, Ecuador, Peru, and Bolivia . . . Quinine

was the first effective treatment of malaria . . . The British government, amidst the expansion of its empire into many malaria-ridden regions, and seeing the potential benefits of quinine, encouraged the Royal Society to research the properties of quinine and explore the possibilities of farming it outside of the Andes . . . the evidence suggests that it was an important 'tool of empire' and significantly enhanced Europe's ability to colonize tropical regions of the globe . . . it is fair to assume that the medical reforms of the 1840's reduced European mortality on shore by at least half and perhaps more.' Curtin concludes that 'the history of tropical Africa would certainly have been very different if European mortality had continued at the old rate' [before quinine].[26]

In every case, accompanying preparation utensils and presentation vessels, possibly also imported or invented later for the purposes, were occasioned by the importation/inclusion of the aforementioned American-origin items, as detailed in Chapter 7 in this collection.

And, not only did these foodstuff/ingredients conquer cuisine in general, "home-cooking" as it were, but likewise, contributed to the modern proliferation of so-called "ethnic" restaurants, particularly those serving interpretations of "Mexican" cuisine, and in "fast-food" style, especially in 20th century Spain, which underlines the eventual overwhelming culinary counter-effect I posit. For example, the entire first page of a cursory Google search for just "Mexican restaurants in Spain" shows photos of about three dozen and lists multiple specific sites for the "ten top" in Madrid, along with at least one in each of Seville and Málaga. Comparable multiple sites for such food exist in Italy, Ireland, Germany and more.

Thus, perhaps an "insidious" counter-conquest, and certainly a positive one for worldwide cuisine rather than negative one, Western Hemisphere-origin entities have transformed cuisine world-wide! Not really so much an after-thought to the historical tracing of the food items as much as additional commentary, the enormous irony of the culinary counter-conquest is that the initial and long-time discriminatory and prejudicial view of the Spanish towards these *New World* origin foods was actually resistance! A major source of the historical so-called reasoning behind the Spanish food attitudes, Linda Álvarez, observes several key concepts, food xenophobia on the part of the Spaniards in terms of "genetic superiority," socio-economic class, religious alignment:

Columbus himself was convinced that Spaniards [during the Conquest] were dying because they lacked 'healthful European foods.' Herein began the colonial discourse of 'right foods' (superior European foods) vs. 'wrong foods' (inferior Indigenous foods). The Spaniards considered that without the 'right foods,' they would die or, even worse, in their minds, they would become like Indigenous people. Europeans believed that food shaped the colonial body. In other words, the European constitution differed from that of Indigenous people because the Spanish diet differed from the Indigenous diet. Further, bodies could be altered by diets—thus the fear that by consuming 'inferior' Indigenous foods, Spaniards would eventually become 'like them.' Only proper European foods would maintain the superior nature of European bodies, and only these 'right foods' would be able to protect colonizers from the challenges posed by the "new world" and its unfamiliar environments. In the minds of Europeans, food not only functioned to maintain the bodily superiority of Spaniards, it also played a role in the formation of social identity.[27] For example, in Spain, elites generally consumed bread, "meat," and wine. The poor in Spain, however, could not afford such luxuries and instead ate such things as barley, oats, rye, and vegetable stew. Even vegetables were classified based on social status; for example, in some cases rooted vegetables were not considered suitable for elite consumption because they grew underground. Elites preferred to consume food that came from trees, elevated from the filth of the common world. Thus, food served as an indicator of class.

In addition, at the time of conquest, Spain was facing internal divisions of its own. In an effort to expel Spanish Muslims, as well as Jewish people, from Spain, King Ferdinand V and Queen Isabella I relaunched what was known as the *Reconquista*, the re-conquest of Spain. As a strong Spanish identity formed around the idea of the *Reconquista*, food became a powerful symbol of Spanish culture. For instance, consider 'pork:' among Muslim, Jewish, and Catholic people, only Catholics could eat 'pork,' since for Muslim and Jewish people, the consumption of 'pork' was forbidden. During the re-conquest, as individuals were being forced to prove that they were pureblooded Spaniards, they would often be offered 'pork' to eat. Any refusal to consume 'pork' would be taken as a sign that such people were not true Catholic Spaniards and would subsequently be expelled from Spain, persecuted, or even killed.

As the Spanish arrived in the 'new world' and initiated the European colonization of the Americas, they also brought with them the notion of cultural and class-based distinctions that were founded on the types of food people ate. For example, upon their arrival, the Spaniards determined that guinea pig 'meat' was a fundamentally

'Indian' food, thus anyone who consumed guinea pig was considered 'Indian.' The same was true for other staple Indigenous foods, such as maize and beans. The Spanish considered such Indigenous fare 'famine foods,' fit for consumption only if all other 'right foods' had been thoroughly exhausted.

The symbolic nature of food was also seen in the imposition of religion, another destructive aspect of the conquest. The Eucharist, the holiest rite among Catholics, was composed of a wafer made of wheat, which signified the body of Christ, and wine, which signified the blood of Christ. Initially, before wheat was harvested in the Americas, it was difficult to obtain wheat from abroad, since much of it spoiled in transit. The wafers that were necessary for this rite could easily have been made from the native maize, but Spaniards believed that this inferior Indigenous plant could not be transformed into the literal body of Christ, as could European wheat. Similarly, only wine made from grapes was acceptable for the sacrament. Any potential substitute was considered blasphemy.

If Spaniards and their culture were to survive in these foreign lands, they would need to have readily available sources of the 'right food.' Often, as Spanish officials reported back to the Crown on the suitability of newly conquered lands, the 'lack of Spanish food' was mentioned. Frustrated with what the 'new world' had to offer, Tomás López Medel, a Spanish official, reported that, 'there was neither wheat, nor grapevines, nor any proper animal . . .' present in the new colonies. Hearing this, the Crown commissioned a number of reports that were to elaborate on which European plants grew well in the colonized lands, as well as details as to where they grew best. It was soon determined that the most suitable arrangement would be for colonists to grow their own foods, and it was not long before Spaniards began to rearrange agriculture to meet their own needs. Although wheat, wine, and olives only thrived in certain regions of Latin America, the Spaniards considered this a success. Colonists were elated that their own foods were successfully growing in foreign lands, and while crops were important, the Europeans' most significant success was with farmed animals, which thrived in ways that were unparalleled.[28]

One dramatic difference had to do with the attitudes about domesticated animals and the consumption of meat were present when Europeans arrived in what is now known as Latin America. Among them were dogs, llamas and alpacas, guinea pigs, turkeys, Muscovy ducks, and a type of chicken. In Mesoamerica, any "meat" and leather that was consumed or utilized usually came from wild game, and generally, there were no animals exploited for labor, with the exception of dogs, who were at times used for hauling. Europeans considered this lack of proper animals for work and consumption unacceptable. Thus, the first contingent of horses, dogs, pigs, cows, sheep, and goats arrived with Columbus' second voyage in 1493 . . . By the 17th century, herds of cows, pigs, sheep, and goats numbered in the hundreds of thousands and roamed throughout the entire continent. As a result, "meat" prices plummeted and the consumption of "meat" exponentially increased. In Spain, the consumption of "meat" was a luxury, but in the "new world," the sheer availability of these animals made this luxury accessible to all . . .

Although resistance to European culture was not uncommon, in time, Indigenous people went on to adopt many European foods into their diet. Similarly, many colonists eventually went on to incorporate Indigenous foods into their daily eating. [Eventually] the Crown demanded that Iberian women be sent to join their husbands in order to civilize society in the 'new world.' As these women arrived, Spanish households were reunified and Iberian women began to solidify the role of the Spanish family in the colonies. This reunification of Spanish families paralleled the destruction of the Indigenous household, as many Indigenous women were forced into working as domestic workers, cooks, nannies, and wet-nurses in Spanish homes. Part of the role of these Indigenous women was to learn to cook European foods and reproduce colonial practices in the home; Iberian women were present to make sure it was done properly. The presence of Spanish women was meant to provide an example of how a 'civilized' woman looked and behaved, and much of this "civilization" took place in the kitchen. If Indigenous women were to reproduce Spanish cooking—the source of superior Spanish bodies—they would need to be instructed by a Spanish woman who could teach them how to make 'civilized' food. Thus, many Indigenous women began reproducing Spanish cuisine as a result of their new role in the European household. However, there is also documentation of the introduction of Indigenous foods and cooking practices into European diets. This was a consequence not only of Indigenous women working in Spanish households, but also a result of *mestizas* who married Spanish men and began integrating aspects of their mixed heritage into these mixed households . . . we see Indigenous variations in cooking with, for instance, the use of chili. Europeans accepted the use of chili in their food since it was similar to pepper. This similarity allowed for its widespread acceptance among Europeans. Alterations to Spanish diets were most common during times of famine, where famine meant a lack of Spanish foods. During these times, Indigenous cooks would prepare indigenous foods, which Spaniards would be forced to consume . . .

Colonization is a violent process that fundamentally alters the ways of life of the colonized. Food has always been a fundamental tool in the process of colonization. Through food, social and cultural norms are conveyed, and also violated . . . Understanding the history of food and eating practices in different contexts can help us understand that the practice of eating is inherently complex. Food choices are influenced and constrained by cultural values and are an important part of the construction and maintenance of social identity. In that sense, food has never merely been about the simple act of pleasurable consumption—food is history, it is culturally transmitted, it is identity. Food is power.[29]

Notes

1   A quote from many in various forms but notably in his 2003 novel in English, *The Da Vinci Code*, Dan Brown writes "When two cultures clash, the loser is obliterated, and the winner writes the history books— books which glorify their own cause and disparage the conquered foe."

2   Now characterized as *The Encounter*, while better than *Discovery*, this takeover was a violent conquest of multiple indigenous cultures by European ones.

3   Post-conquest, the Western Hemisphere has been known as the Americas, the very name being another European imposition. Particularly Central and South America and the Caribbean are commonly referred to as Spanish America and/or Latin America, ignoring the heritage of the sophisticated indigenous cultures.

4   This study does not parse the difference between food history (foodstuff plants and their socio-cultural effects) and cuisine history (ingredients & recipes themselves), as do purists in the fields.

5   Nunn, Nathan and Qian, Nancy. "The Colombian Exchange: A History of Disease, Food, and Ideas." *Journal of Economic Perspectives.* Vol. 24, No. 2, Spring 2010, pp. 163–188. Web.

6   Nunn & Qian. Web.

7   Kimberly e.a.b. "The Impact of the Potato and Tomato on European Demographics and Culture." June 8, 2019. Web.

8   Nunn & Qian.

9   López-Terrada, Maríaluz. "European Tomato project TRADITOM." Jurate Straseviciene, *History of Tomatoes in Europe*. World Tomato Society. Web.

10 López-Terrada, Maríaluz.

11 "Europeans Discover Chocolate. July 7, 1550." WIRED. July 7, 1550.

12 Nunn & Qian. The Aztecs also restricted cacao consumption to the privileged classes, priests & royals, in mostly ceremonial situations, as documented by their surviving documents. Web.

13 Nunn & Qian. Web.

14 "Corn: The A-Maize-ing History of Corn." *Food Reference*. Web.

15 "Heirloom Spotlight: The History of Beans." *MOTHER EARTH NEWS*. Web.

16 "The History of the Common Beans." *Thoughtco.com*. Web.

17 "Two New Beans from America." *Archives. Aggie Horticulture. Tamu.edu*. Web.

18 Hurst, K. Kris. "The Domestication History of Squashes." Oct. 8, 2019. *Cucurbita spp. Thoughtco.com*. Web.

19 Hammons, Ray O., Herman, Danielle and Stalker, H. Thomas. "Chapter 1—Origin and Early History of the Peanut." *Peanuts: Genetics, Processing and Utilization*. AOCS Press: 2016. Web. The U.S. is, however, only the fourth greatest consumer of peanuts, behind China (also the largest producer), India and Nigeria.

20 Hammons, Herman & Stalker. Web.

21 Nunn & Qian. Web.

22 Nunn & Qian. Web.

23 *Turkey (Meleagris gallapavo) History*. thoughtco.com. Web.

24 Much anecdotal evidence supports that Finnish, particularly, is not only so challenging for learners due to the 16 declinations, including of nouns, but because formal vocabulary is so frequently supplanted by vernacular usage words.

25 Nunn & Qian. Web.

26 Nunn & Qian. Web.

27 The later chapter in this collection on the works of Rose Mary Salum underlines this supposition about maintenance of social identity.

28 Álvarez, Linda. "Colonization, Food and the Practice of Eating." *Food Empowerment Project*. Web.

29 Álvarez. Web.

Bibliography

Álvarez, Linda. "Colonization, Food and the Practice of Eating." *Food Empowerment Project*. Web.

"American Indian Health & Diet: Food Indigenous to the Western Hemisphere." *American Indian Health World Health* (ku.edu.) Web.

"Peanuts: A Brief History." *American Peanut Council*. Peanutsusa.com. Web.

"Corn: The A-Maize-ing History of Corn." *foodreference*.com. Web.

Prado, Daisy. "10 Foods Native to the Americas." CUESA. Web.

"Europeans Discover Chocolate." *WIRED*. Web.

Hammons, Ray O., Herman, Danielle and Stalker, H. Thomas. "Chapter 1—Origin and Early History of the Peanut." *Peanuts: Genetics, Processing and Utilization*. AOCS, 2016. Web.

"The History of Corn." *Rlrouse.com*. Web.

"The History of the Common Bean." *Thoughtco.com*. Web.

"The History of San Antonio's Chili Queens." *San Antonio Magazine*. Web.

"How Did Potatoes Adapt to Europe?" *Potato News Today*. Web.

"How the Potato Changed the World." History. *Smithsonian Magazine*. Web.

Hurst, K. Kris. "Domestication History of Squashes." *Cucurbita.spp. thoughtco.com.* Oct. 8, 2019.

Kimberly E.A.B. "The Impact of the Potato and Tomato on European Demographics and Culture." June 8, 2019. Web.

"List of Food Plants Native to the Americas." *Wikipedia.* Web.

López-Terrada, Maríaluz. "European Tomato project TRADITOM" in *Jurate Straseviciene, History of Tomatoes in Europe.* World Tomato Society. Web.

Nunn, Nathan and Qian, Nancy. "The Colombian Exchange: A History of Disease, Food, and Ideas." *Journal of Economic Perspectives.* Vol. 24, No. 2, Spring 2010, 163–188. Web.

Science Direct.com. Web.

"Top Peanut (Groundnut)-Consuming Countries." *World Atlas.* Web.

"Two New Beans from America." *Archives. Aggie Horticulture* (tamu.edu). Web.

Weaver, William Woys. "Heirloom Spotlight: The History of Beans. *MOTHER EARTH NEWS.* Web.

2

Food Culture in Higher Education Spanish Courses: Political Allegory in *Lazarillo de Tormes*

Elizabeth Coscio

A very old newspaper comic with a visual of mom and daughter speaking goes something like this:
"Is it green eggs and green ham or green eggs and regular ham, I'm easily confused?
Mom: "How about we read this one?
Daughter: "Sam. Green eggs. Ham. Breaking down our reluctance to try new things. The end."
"<next frame> I read the Cliff Notes"[1]

This cartoon is revealing of another time, but still relevant to how students in American universities tend to break down any reading assignment to importance in their own everyday life. As they say, why study this if I cannot relate it to my own life? The teaching of advanced Spanish courses often involves precisely this type of breaking-down process to the very essence of the assignment for that student at that moment. The area of food as a cultural topic has always been part of any level of Spanish learning from the very beginning courses to advanced courses in a variety of areas in applied language courses for medical professions with nutrition, business, culture, linguistics, and literature courses. Although the overall goal of this writing begins as a documentation of the ever-changing, but still prevailing presence of food culture in Spanish college courses and student interest, the end will include a specific analysis of how food culture, and specifically hunger, is used as political allegory in the iconic Spanish picaresque satirical novella, *Lazarillo de Tormes*.

With the age of the smart screen and pandemic online preparations of all courses, more and more the Internet has provided the delicious visual sources that served the purpose in the past for those variety of classes where we used to sample real foods after guest speakers, student and teacher presentations. One of the more revelatory finds in researching food and higher education included a number of special topics courses in various programs at different universities with Hispanic food as the main focus. As part of ongoing research to update and improve Spanish classes at the higher education level, I have found a variety of projects created for all levels of learning such as those usually a part of any interesting field trip or study abroad course, prior to the pandemic where students experienced food culture in a home-stay situation, where the housemother would be introducing local cuisine every day as part of meal preparation. Professors also took students to restaurant kitchens to watch chefs prepare and explain in Spanish the meal they were about to try. Students in Spain viewing octopus or other local food items in an outdoor market or in a home or restaurant kitchen in study-abroad situations provided living experiences for food culture. Learning about food and culture at the real source is the ideal for real time places, sources and people. There are, of course, many videos and travel ads that serve in the online environment to replace these real experiences. The proposal here is to view Spanish food culture in relationship with the development of the literary allegory and specifically of a political nature.

The following suggestions for use in learning and teaching a variety of advanced Spanish language classes probably already exists in a myriad of places in a variety of formats but the investigation involved in this undertaking allowed insights into new and openly available resources on the internet for industrious, busy teachers and learners to extrapolate materials.

First, for students planning on teaching Spanish at the middle and elementary level, a good resource for designing other projects located was the "Foods of Latin America Project," presently used in Arizona ISD, authored by Sam Heywood at the Center for Latin American Studies at University of Arizona. This resource includes pdf sources where students can access information about a variety of typical dishes served in Hispanic America. From these sources, the students can work in groups to create simple presentations on the elementary and high school levels and even the novice learning that happens in beginning Spanish classes at the higher academic level. These are mainly cultural lessons to be used in Spanish language classes, the site says and mentions the adaptability for Language Arts and Social Studies classes as well. Foods in the Caribbean/African Latin America, Mexico,

Central and South American regions are covered in the appropriate grade-level approaches. The focus is Mexico but Venezuela/Colombia, Argentina, El Salvador, and Ecuador of the Spanish-speaking countries are included. The proficiency level matches the American Council of Teachers of Foreign Language (ACTFL) description of a novice speaker of any age with a specific description. This food project is also a good resource for a beginning Spanish course on the higher-education level due to the modern language learning continuum and the very broad general language proficiency markers used. Also, quite simply, students could improve on the template and create the same research for other countries.

The ACTFL website is still of value in judging language materials, providing the following about the descriptors used that can help instructors create a teaching/learning map targeted to the appropriate performance desired, while still challenging students to continue to improve, similar to improvement from keyboarding skills on the beginning level. The novice learners practice and even memorize collocations (chunks of words) within very structured parameters. Some features of these speakers' performance include producing words and phrases learned by communicating in repeating conversation partner's words with a different intonation or a memorized response. Here is where the experienced teacher can guide the process by considering the cognitive and developmental appropriateness of all learning activities to provide for multiple ways to practice language skills and appropriately assess adult learners in higher education for career readiness.

> Language learners in instructional settings from prekindergarten through graduate studies are in a continuous process of cognitive development that influences their ability to perform language tasks. Learning targets need to consider the age appropriateness and cognitive development of the language learners and may require varying amounts of time to achieve. The description of three ranges of performance (Novice, Intermediate, and Advanced) allows users of these Performance Descriptors to identify appropriate learning targets for language learners who begin at any age or grade level (prekindergarten, elementary school, middle school, high school, or postsecondary institutions) and whose language learning continues for varying amounts of time.[2]

The "Foods of Latin America Project" site suggests using additional apps and games to get the most out of the group assignments and individual research. Vocabulary is incorporated and the grammar points are well-chosen, including the conditional tense, the verb *"pedir"* (to ask for) in learning to order food in a restaurant, making comparisons and superlatives with a "basic comparison recipe." The final finished project is presented by students to facilitate the "cultural significance of food in Latin America." Suggested research materials on the five different Hispanic national dishes: *mole, arepa, empanada, pupusa,* and the *encebollado* dishes are provided, as well as a soup from French-Creole-speaking Haiti. Questions include asking about the origin, history, importance, ingredients and sources, as well as cultural traditions and holidays associated, regional differences and adaptations made to the meal for the U.S. Hispanic population.[3]

The following course offerings at various U.S. universities serve as a reminder of the constant interest in Hispanic food culture. Following are just a few university special topics courses focused on this very area:

The first one is "332 Food and Identity in Latin America and Spain," a course taught by Professor Infante at Amherst College. The course description rightly notes that food is sometimes revealing of culture and very related to the cultural and literary food story of Spain and Latin America. Relating what we eat to our self-definition, the approach to the topic is interwoven into areas such as gender, race, religions, and social identification.[4] Seeing that cookbooks were added to normal literary texts, historical accounts, movies and paintings in this course made sense to this researcher since my culture and literature courses have included several different ones as well, including the cookbooks of the list of banned spices in Isabel Allende's *Aphrodite*, Carmen de Burgos' and Emilia Pardo Bazán's early cookbooks in Spain, revealing of what Michelle M. Sharp refers to as "subversive versions in 'low' literature . . . to reach new audiences and to pull Spanish society towards the modern era" (Sharp 20), as well as many different genres of literary works, including Laura Esquivel's *Como agua para chocolate.* Other kinds of studies including sustainable gastronomy, the food industry and distribution, etc., are included as part of cultural heritage for culture and business Spanish classes.

Also, as a reference book on life in Cuba, the 2005 *Food in Cuba* by Hanna Garth, an anthropology professor, is another source that talks about the social and emotional meaning of food in post-Soviet Cuba. She points out that sourcing ingredients for even a decent meal, much less the traditional recipes, is not only time-consuming but often futile. These foods are so much of the Cuban cultural identity that the very notion of not being able to prepare them results in drastic character change similar to an existential crisis. Free time is spent simply trying to hunt down basic food staples, once plentiful and part of the Cuban diet, such as corn. This causes stress and anxiety on a daily basis and often causes Cubans to abandon family recipes handed down for generations.

Another similar course offering by Professor Mariselle Meléndez, is conducted in Spanish at the University of Illinois Urbana-Champaign Department of Spanish and Portuguese, Fall 2020, SPAN 324 Why We Eat What We Eat: Food and Culture in Latin America. This course begins with the colonial period and takes students to the U.S. Hispanic world. Wisely, the course returns to European, indigenous and African cultures and what is called "the result of subsequent centuries of social interaction." Since discussion includes a "variety of written and visual texts from the colonial period (15th to 18th century)" and more current materials, there is the cultural triangulation rightly presented in relationship to Hispanic food culture that includes the European. Spanish cuisine also includes an amalgam of ancient cuisines not mentioned in this short course description since it begins with the colonial period: Roman, Jewish and Arabic traditions of Spain, as well as other European influences.

A few other examples include even more specific topics within the food culture. Instructor Daniela Gutiérrez Flores offered in the 2020–2021 catalog at the University of Chicago "ACS 28622 SPAN 26822 Women and Food in Latin America." Looking at a variety of "cultural artifacts" from the sixteenth century to now, the course includes readings by Sor Juana Inés de la Cruz, some chronicles regarding the Mexica and food, cookbooks and baroque, colonial and Latinx art. On the foodscape scene, the gastronomic questions provided would provoke curiosity on the part of most college students having to do with more contemporary women's culinary topics as well. The focus is on motherhood, femininity and sexuality in relation to the food culture and the kitchen space.

And not because it is the only other, but just one other very specific topic course of interest, is offered on an advanced level with hands-on, in the community learning with a blog project about their experiences. The University of Southern California Latin American and Iberian Cultures department offers "SPAN 385 The Culture of Food in Hispanic Los Angeles" by Sarah Portnoy, which is cross-listed for credit in a number of areas such as nutrition, geography and other areas. The course-learning goals provide a detailed explanation of how student blogs will be evaluated with action verbs: identify diet components, recognize food ingredients and cultural importance, describe trends and historical production, distinguish cooking methods, identify cooking objects and utensils and recognize and use associated Spanish vocabulary. She uses the *taquerías, pupuserías,* and *panaderías* close to the campus for student engagement and exploration of the injustices in the South LA food system by imagining life as a low-income Latino immigrant trying to feed a family a healthy diet. Projects also involve other national or regional cuisines by visiting food trucks or restaurants specialized in those areas. Assignments also include interviews with chefs and employees with a video for the class documenting their experiences. She reveals on her blog, lataco.com how some of her students have gone on to be food critics or travel writers.

To document the interest here in the U. S. academy in the last fifteen to twenty years, outside of the food and beverage studies that have always included food production, storage transportation and consumption for students entering those areas, we can look to any number of areas for past and growing interest in food culture and its importance: general humanities, social sciences, anthropology, history, nutrition, and political science, as well as the literary and cultural areas.

Here, although it is not a Spanish course offering, I would add a rather interesting 2015 dissertation, *Eating Spain: National Cuisine Since 1900* by Matthew J. Wild, as reflective of other recent research on the area of cookbooks, gastronomic guides, literature and film for more information from the Food and Cultural Studies area and primary works. This work provides a relatively recent bibliography on Food Studies in general and information on the development of a Spanish national cuisine from the early twentieth century. The author studies the works of Carmen de Burgos, Emilia Pardo Bazán, Dionisio Pérez, Ana María Herrera, Juan Mari Arzak and Ferrán Adrià and others who wrote cookbooks and gastronomic guides.

The discussion of the creation of nationalist discourse with common and recurring themes in the historical and cultural evolution of Spanish food includes cookbooks, culinary manifestos, the *Michelin Guidebook* and others. There are comments from historians, anthropologists and sociologists like Stanley Mintz, Mary Douglas, Jack Goody and Stephen Mennell, who have furthered the study of food in academic investigation.

Mintz, who wrote prolifically on the same topic, traced the story of sugar and relationship to social and economic power, all the while showing the importance of that staple in modern cuisines. Douglas' article *Deciphering a Meal* (1972) analyzed food from the structural, symbolic function and the act of eating. Her *Food and Culture: A Reader in 1997* quickly became the food studies bible. Her anthology shows food's universal but different cultures with a series of articles covering race and gender, globalization, post colonialism, nationalism, ecology, nutrition, as well as a host of sociopolitical and economic topics. West African food and social structures are the topic covered by Goody in his seminal *Cooking, Cuisine and Class: A Study in Comparative Sociology* (1982), which explores the link between food and social structures in his study of West Africa. *In All Manner of Food: Eating and Taste in England and France from the Middle Ages to the Present* (1985). Mennell also dealt with sugar in modern history as a sociocultural process in literature, art or music. Even more in-depth analyses appear pushing toward a kind of theoretical base to consider food culture. New definitions such as the one in Ashley et al relate to five major cultural processes: "1) production; 2) regulation; 3) representation; 4) identity and 5) consumption" (vii). It must be noted that the study of food is not unique to any one of these cultural processes and that it is most often defined by an exchange between two or more of these processes simultaneously (1975). Around the same time, Roland Barthes looks at the deep underlying structures in food choice and representation in *Toward a Psychosociology of Food Consumption* (1975). Another well-known name in literary criticism, Claude Levi-Strauss, has dealt with the anthropology of the "Culinary Triangle," which stressed the relationship of culture and food by way of the transformative processes from raw to cooked, then rotten. This influenced other studies on how food can contribute to civilization and culture.

Wild's work also cites specific research about Spain: Rebecca Ingram's *Spain on the Table: Cookbooks, Women, and Modernization, 1905–1933* (2009), with a view of cookbooks through the lens of gender in the early twentieth century. Alison Atkins' *Authorship and the fogones: Gastronomy and the Artist in Post-Transition Spain* (2012) provides invaluable knowledge on the rise of the Spanish *alta cocina* movement of the 1980s and 90s. María Paz Moreno's *De la página al plato: El libro de cocina en España* (2012), for example, serves as a foundational work in the examina-tion of cookbooks as literature in Spain.

The following comes from the abstract for Wild's dissertation:

With an analysis of nationalism through the perspective of gastronomy as a cultural practice that contributes to individual and collective identity building this dissertation concludes that Spanish national cuisine has been defined as a unique, pluralistic blend of regional cuisines since the early twentieth century. While early authors such as Pardo Bazán admit to heavy French influence and the central-ized hegemony of Madrid due to its privileged status as economic and political capital of Spain, most subsequent authors acknowledge that Spanish national cuisine is a construction of various regional influ- ences and by the 1960s, this regional view of national cuisine is universally accepted. Shaped during the twentieth century by civil war, Francoism and globalization, Spanish cuisine today continues to be a blend of regional cuisines that mutually influence each other while also exhibiting the effects of a globalized world by incorpo- rating non-Spanish ingredients and techniques into nationally accepted dishes. (iv)

The work by Wild, with its focus on twentieth century, can be used when discussing the literary canon regarding cultural and gastronomic works not usually covered in an advanced literature or culture course. This defense of food studies certainly explains the list of relatively new courses with food culture as the specific special topic and defends the food culture as a viable field of study in Hispanic and Spanish Cultural Studies. It recognizes the relationship among food, nation and culture as an interdisciplinary field so important in these times of waning enrollments in advanced Spanish classes of any sort as an interesting hook. Hispanists have generally written more about Latin America and Mexican food and cooking specifically. The notion of studying both lived practices and artefacts or performances as symbolic systems is also important, as performance effectively ties various categories together with signification produced for an audience. Food intersects life everywhere. Cookbooks, menus, dishes, etc., all become fair game (5). Gastronomic ideas are affected by "modernization, war, famine, migration" (23) and others. The collective, as well as the individual is represented by national, regional and more local trends. The questions of this dissertation are pertinent to students: "What does eating say about us? Do foods reflect personal views? Does how we eat comment on who we are and what we stand for as humans?"

From the very earliest works of Spanish literature, including the allegorical depictions of scripture passages about the Lord's supper in the *auto sacramental, Lazarillo de Tormes.* the *Quijote* and other Golden Age Spanish works, we see the relationship of food to the narrator and the characters. Many books and articles have been written examining the role of food within canonical works by Cervantes, Pérez Galdós and Emilia Pardo Bazán—and many others as well.[5] Food imagery and symbols have always been important in literary criticism especially when we employ historiography to look back at history. We consider Spain as a major crossing point for conquerors bringing their own foods with new modes of production and cooking in early times in culture classes, there are the original wild pigs and goats to consider that lived on the Peninsula, which have little to do with the special breeds consumed today (Gázques Ortiz 10 and Almódovar, *Hambre* 23). There was also the wild rabbit, which has an interesting relationship with Spain's very name then, *Hispania*. A linguistic food culture notes that this word comes from the same root as a Phoenician and Hebrew word for cliff terrier but at a coin history site, only the Phoenicians were credited for naming Iberia the land of the hyrax (a North African animal). [6] Later this was incorrectly rendered as the word "rabbit" by Martin Luther in his Bible translation. The latinized version also described what we know of as the rabbit today. Since they do adapt and multiply, these rabbits became a very common food source. That certainly rings true. Even the early Roman coin had a picture of the rabbit. This gastronomic novelty begat "the land of the rabbit," so even Spain's very nomenclature is related to its own food culture.

Susanne Muhleisen speaks of globalized tongues and of how gastronomic vocabulary and food etymology serve as "lexical food history" (71). From studying food etymology, we can derive from where and when foods come. There was also a traditional seafood diet of limpets, oysters, clams, mussels, sea urchins and razor clams. Grains cultivated included wheat, rye and barley, according to the history cited by Dionisio Pérez (23). Native fruits and vegetables were there but the most Spanish of foods, olives and garlic, were not there originally. There is the paradox of today's amazing pork products from a nation that was a Caliphate from 711 to 1492. The Arabs brought lemon, grapefruit and the bitter orange (D. Pérez 16). Pérez notes that the sweet orange, a product of China, was introduced via the Portuguese. In addition to staple fruits and vegetables, the Muslims were responsible for bringing all types of spices ranging from saffron, nutmeg, black pepper and sugar (D. Pérez 16).

In popular culture, Spanish food became *paella, tortilla española* and *gazpacho*. Microsoft Word includes both *paella* and *gazpacho* within their English vocabulary. Even if we include olive oil and wine, other European countries, such as France, are better known. Wild mentions an increase in well-known Spanish chefs arriving on the world scene and regional hams such as *jamón ibérico* and *queso manchego*, as reasons for more notice of Spanish food globally.

First things first would be a simple definition of allegory but since that is really not possible, the following is a summary from the excellent source always recommended to literature students: *The Princeton Encyclopedia of Poetry and Poetics: Fourth Edition*. Included are original sources from that source, so that students can follow the original writings. The term "allegory" itself in Western literary terminology eludes a strict definition. It has been applied since ancient times to such diverse forms as a literary trope, a sustained metaphor or simply ironic discourse. Some critics even apply the term to any reformulation in altered terminology. It is possible to conceive the term as a concept, as part of history, a reflection of conscience or as a literary structure. To interweave food culture and the development of the allegory, the notion of conquest after conquest comes to mind in Spain. The issue could be authenticity when looking at the diverse and highly developed gastronomic culture that is the Spain of today. Much of the diversity merely reflects conquest after conquest through the Golden Age, which resulted in food varieties from all corners of the globe, including the importance of the seven-hundred-year Arabic traditions, to offerings sent back to Spain from the New World of the Americas during that period.

The Moors introduced many new crops including the orange, lemon, peach, apricot, fig, dates, ginger and pomegranate, as well as saffron, sugar cane and rice, which remain some of Spain's main products today. It is fairly common knowledge today that Spain benefitted from the Americas; the explorers not only brought gold and silver but also corn, potatoes, pineapples, tomatoes, tobacco, beans, vanilla and chocolate. It is interesting that typical Spanish dishes using potatoes are considered indigenous although they were unknown in that area prior to the fifteenth century.

The New World and its food forever shaped the history of Spain and Europe. In the case of Spain, the potato becomes the base of the *tortilla española* and other well-known dishes such as *patatas bravas*. Corn was one of the first crops brought back to Spain with records showing cultivation as early as 1494 (Franconie 23 in Wild). Tobacco became an important staple. Peanuts and tropical fruits such as pineapple made their way into the Old World (Nunn and Qian 163 in Wild). Nunn and Qian explain that the influx of new foods from the New World not only had gastronomic consequences for Spain, but also for them, "the New World foods had an important effect on the evolution of local cuisines" (Wild, 167).

Back to allegorical history, the ancient Greek and Roman scholars applied a very specific rhetorical meaning to allegory. Originally, allegory meant a brief trope but Schlegel expanded the concept of a general tension in literary language. Such expansion in scope of meaning demonstrates how literary works always aspire to express that which cannot be expressed, even to the commentary of De Man that narratives can even betray their own system of values (allegory, *Princeton*).

Current trends allow for varying degrees of allegorical expression. The fictional autonomy of the text and how many different ambient factors point to another set of principles, actions or circumstances, are both important considerations in allegorical expression. Ambivalence in allegorical language is an artistic sign in composition that the text will allow for different interpretations. An allegorical interpretation helps preserve the author's intent and, in a sense, it canonizes it. Historically, allegorical strategy resulted in the exegesis of a text not as mythology but rather as sacred text. The relationship of allegory to sacred texts provided an authority, at the same time a vision of the future yet to be written, only in prophesy.

The *auto sacramental* should be defined as well, short, usually one-act, theatrical allegorical representations had such allegorical characters as the Pilgrim, Avarice, The Roman Catholic Church, Sins, the life of Christ or the Virgin Mary. They were represented either in the church or the public square to a largely illiterate public without much decoration or costuming. By the end of the Middle Ages, there were more and more apocalyptic forms, more related to death, more macabre than the ascetic, satiric or courtly love scenes to develop later where sex/food would certainly be implied.

With the inspiration of the Italian Renaissance from the late fifteenth century on and neoclassic period, those changes between fiction and fact became a rather formal design. Spaniards never just accepted anything exactly as rendered in another language, but rather Hispanicized everything from outside, returning to medieval elements. Around the seventeenth century, how one text related to another was revealed in the relationship of imaginative language to formal structure. Structural decorum reigned and the sixteenth-century Italian critics, under the influence of Aristotle's Poetics, insisted on the formalities of composition including unity and credibility. Spanish dramatists such as Lope de Vega in the first Golden Age century and continuing with Calderón de la Barca in the second, had begun to elaborate on the language and mythological themes, using various parade floats Mardi Gras style, to render more colorful, complicated scenes that moved through the public square. They would focus on a particular religious celebration, Lent, Corpus Christi or the Immaculate Conception. The allegory was reserved precisely to give credibility to the fantastic back then.

Afterwards, in the eighteenth and nineteenth centuries, critics such as Giambattista Vico maintained that an image could separate from its abstract concept, preferring symbols and myth over the allegory. By the time of Sigmund Freud and Carl Jung, myth critics and psychoanalysts employed their psychological and anthropological theories to explain the myths and symbols as deep structures. Walter Benjamin points out that the romantic symbol obscured the effect of time and impeded the unity of the ephemeral object with an eternal idea, a kind of dead allegory (allegory, *Princeton*).

The Christian Cosmovision had extended to include a variety of mythological stories. What roles do motivation and censorship in the name of the Inquisition play in creating an allegory? Whatever an author holds sacred is often left behind in his writing as traces on the page. That preconscious level was not exploited in the structuralists' literary criticism, although it provided a unique system in the form of a grid to judge literary works. The arbitrary nature of the sign, as postulated in Ferdinand de Saussure's *Course in General Linguistics,* was the basis for the modern structuralist movement. Since a structure is a system of differences, studied independently of what it or its parts might mean outside of the system, a structuralist appears to view words only in their differential relationship to other words on anthropological or linguistic terms.

Choosing to move beyond a particular critical reading, such as a structuralist one, to a rather eclectic set of theoretical underpinnings allows an allegory to emerge. The use of allegory results in a rather formal ideology or discourse that is ritualized with symbolic values. We can follow Plato's description of poetry as an imitation of an imitation, twice removed from the truth, to Saussure's writings couched in Western metaphysics, which presumed *logos* as Webster's philosophical definition of the 'rational principle that governs and develops the universe', based on the Greek translation of *logo* as word. The transcendental signifier revealed the power of *a priori* knowledge and *parole* was prioritized over *langue*, leaving writing in a displaced second place.

The philosopher, Jacques Derrida, showed that speech was subject to the same logic as writing, extending Saussure's arbitrary nature of the sign to speech which must be inscribed as the signifier of the signified absent to both systems. He then proceeded to deconstruct that tradition of logocentric metaphysics (always assigning origin of truth to *logos*, the spoken word, voice of reason or word of God) by means of a new science called "grammatology," foregrounding writing in preference to speech for tracing the displacement of signifiers. Derrida chose to deconstruct the value of voice over the mute signs of writing, reversing the binary historical and cultural oppositions common to phono centrism. In that way such concepts as voice/writing, sound/silence, being/nonbeing, reality/image, thing/sign, truth/lie, presence/absence, signified/signifier were reversed.

Derrida imagined a science before it even became one, presenting grammatology as a radical challenge to structuralism. Jacques Derrida also found in the work of Claude Levi-Strauss the analogy of the differential sign in describing myths as bundles of relations or differences. The author's interest in advancing the argument of writing over speech could be revealed through his reading of Levi-Strauss. In *Structure, Sign and Play in the Discourse of the Human Sciences,* Derrida focused on the peculiar idea of structure as a totalization for any system, presuming to give closure and coherence, which he said could not work with the element of play in the signifier.

Supplement, as used by Levi-Strauss, possessed a double meaning, to supply the missing, as well as supplying another something. In that manner, there was always something more to be understood. Derrida described this process as a floating one, emphasizing the double direction of the process taking it back to Saussure. "The strange structure of the *supplement* appears . . . by delayed reaction, a possibility produces that to which it is said to be added on" (Harland 130). Such philosophers as Frederick Nietzsche and Martin Heidegger also reviewed that ontological dilemma.

Perhaps Derrida's strongest argument for his claim that writing precedes speech rested upon his rejection of the German philosopher Edmund Husserl's phenomenological theory of language as presented by Richard Harland in *Superstructuralism.* Husserl's human language posited an absolute distinction between human and natural signs. That German philosopher felt true language had to be willfully intended by an utterer because relation to non-verbal phenomena making it incidental to linguistic signs could also form association. That necessity that words mean only because someone means them to mean something naturally pushed Husserl's theory of language toward speech. (For example: what I meant was . . . what I was trying to say was . . .). Husserl was the promoter of pure phenomenology or a science of the essence of meaning.

Derrida totally reversed Husserl's argument by seeing written language as self-sufficient: "The structure, peculiar to language alone, allows it to function entirely by itself when its intention is cut off from intuition" (Harland 127). Again, in *De grammatologie,* Derrida insisted that writing was language at its most self-sufficient because it was language at its most spatial. It did not exist briefly and transparently as sound waves but rather as solid, enduring marks on a page. There was no need for those marks to be propped up by their maker's presence. Actually, that person was always absent, maybe dead.

Writing releases thought from consciousness, functioning as an *aide-memoire.* Derrida said "writing, a mnemotechnic means, supplanting good . . . spontaneous memory, signifies forgetfulness . . . its violence befalls the soul as unconsciousness" (Harland 128).

The bottom line of Derrida's model was language-superseded speech. Phonetic languages fit the model, but in Chinese and Egyptian that have hieroglyphic and ideogram scripts, the written sign does not need the spoken sign to signify. Historically, the development of those scripts preceded phonetic scripts. Derrida denied the logical assumption that the truest form is the original one. So, even though speech precedes language in human development, there is no rational justification to assume rediscovering primitive communication will explain language. With this radical separation of historical and conceptual priority according to Spinoza, Derrida said the fact of writing followed from the fact of speech, but the idea of speech depended upon the idea of writing. Writing became the logically fundamental condition to which language aimed.

Derrida reversed Husserl's mental meaning behind verbal meaning as a means of controlling the verbal message. Instead, the writer only discovered the meaning in the act of writing. He said, "before me, the signifier on its own says more than I believe that I meant to say and in relation to it, my meaning-to-say is submissive rather than active" (Harland 132). The writer just became another reader, which is exactly where this reader-researcher is leading with these details.

Derrida refused any conscious meaning in the sense of movement from marks on the page to mental concepts. When we could find only absence and emptiness for the elusive signified, Derrida told us that the signified was merely an illusion that we invented not to deal with the materialism of language. The signifiers are always signifying, pointing away from themselves to other signifiers, constantly in motion in a state of dissemination. That concept was different from *univocity*, which is 'the state of single meanings maintained by the signified in the reader's mind.'

Dissemination goes on in perpetuity as unfulfilled meaning in the absence of all signifieds. Language supplanted human control, revealing its own creativity to which writers and readers alike must succumb. There was no social or individual responsibility. In that endlessly unbalanced state, words no longer pushed against each other at the same time, they pushed successively, like falling dominoes of causal units.

The Saussurean *langue* that bounced from positive to negative now flowed from pole to pole in electrical terms. With that new model, Derrida brought a new dimension of study to structuralism, the dimension of time, which was excluded from the structuralist model. This helps explains to students how to approach different literary works from a variety of critical processes. With *differance*, Derrida provided two meanings: difference as distinction, inequality or discernibility and the interposition of delay, the interval of a spacing and temporalizing, which allowed for the presently denied to be put off until later. Thus, the conception of time deferred meaning only for the present and in time, the deferred meaning flowed over into it. An uttered word existed by its deferring of unuttered words. From Plato, in particular, to the Greek language in general, *parole* to *langue* was generated in that theory of language.

Another area of deconstruction of structuralism was opposing traditional philosophical dualism of mind/matter, soul/body, spirit/natural world. Derrida saw a tremendous inequality in those oppositions. "In a classical philosophical opposition, we are not dealing with the peaceful coexistence of a vis-a-vis, but rather with a violent hierarchy. One of the two terms governs the other . . . or has the upper hand" (Richard Harland 142). Rising up against this mind-soul-spirit concept was the unconscious mind in the form of writing, which Derrida called arch-writing, a theory Harland contended he derived from Sigmund Freud, especially in his essay "Note on the Mystic Writing Pad" (143).

He used Freud's mechanical model for perception and memory in the neurological system of the brain, where a force in the perceptual circuits opened up a pathway or trace of lowered electro-chemical resistance. That trace then remained as the physical form of an unconscious memory, a rut along which future forces could flow more easily and follow. Derrida connected that theory to the writing inscribed upon the waxed base of the "mystic writing pad," with the channel hollowed out by the stylus.

The important part was that Derrida combined the sign with causal force that had the effect of deconstructing the phenomenological concept of an absolute present moment, the idea of things themselves. The legibility of writing came not from the stylus pressing down, but the darkness of the base that showed up. "Writing . . . supplements perception before perception even appears to itself" (Harland 144). That was a valid advance to the philosophical idea of psychic vision as a movie theater, a non-stop picture show inside the head. Derrida's theory is particularly apt for an explanation of the creative process that is allegory. As the preceding outline of allegory's history revealed, it has been described as a trope, a metaphor, or discourse.

Derrida saw consciousness as an illusion that humans invented fearing a purely materialist conception of the brain. Mind was a signified that we ascribe to the brain, divine spirit as a signified, we connect to the natural world, etc., etc. All of those impressions were in

Derridean terms mere versions of logos, just a type of wishful thinking that his theory of writing as a theory of materialism deconstructed. That type of materialism provided for a path akin to meditation, a comparison made by Harland, as an expanding, unfolding general meaningfulness. Beyond the historical literary definition of allegory as trope, metaphor, or discourse, then is this meditation or open reading.

In that way, linguistic claims of truth underwent a transformation, resulting in an opening up of literary language. By connecting its creative play with strategies of power, with real historical forces, writers could undercut authority, destabilize institutions, and realign social values and hierarchies by demystifying with revolutionary aims. That was the real paradox of literature already commented on by Sören Kierkegaard in *God Becoming Man in Christian Theology*, William von Schlegel, who linked it closer to poetry and irony in the human experience, and Wordsworth in "Composed Upon Westminster Bridge" (Princeton Encyclopedia 8). We could compare these strategic power plays with the way contemporary fine dining today rescues lost provincial and peasant foods and elevates them to a higher status with deconstructed versions of provincial stews such as the Spanish *fabada or cocido*.[9] Just look online to see the number of recommendations of the best restaurant to enjoy "authentic" regional recipes of each of these. Also, equally applicable are the literary and cultural images and symbols in novels, films, and poetry, as well as commercial ads and tv programs. Food metaphors are used more than sports metaphors in food ads, clichés and idioms to express emotions, feelings, desires, beliefs, social and economic standing, the social importance of celebrations, business transactions and relationships.

With new online capacities popping up every day, students are provided with visual insights from online entries, *Wikipedia*, and search engines that provide external links such as animated mini-series and audiobooks by simply clicking classic Spanish works such as *Lazarillo de Tormes*. But, there are many works about the significance of the *pícaro* or rogue in Spanish literature that they will not find there and especially about *Lazarillo de Tormes* as the precursor or prototype of the picaresque genre in sixteenth-century Spanish literature. There is also ample criticism documenting the picaresque works as a significant stage in the evolution of the modern Spanish novel. Historically, this sixteenth-century classic reveals a satirical account of the Toledo *Cortes*, the Spanish parliament in 1538 during the reign of Charles V. In the twentieth century, Harry Sieber provided a semiotic reading of *Lazarillo* documenting the rhetoric and power of hunger through semiology.

Discussing this broad structural and semiotic criticism after the historical account, pushing forward, as in any survey course, provides a summary of pertinent critical works to guide them. That history is necessary to understand why "Lazarillo is both the story of the '*fortunas y adversidades*' (good fortune and adversity) experienced in becoming a dishonorable *pregonero* (town crier) and the story of a *pregonero* who becomes an honorable author. The totally oral status of Lázaro as town crier of Toledo is converted into his "persona" as writer" (Siebert ix).

The Archbishop of Toledo, invited by Charles V to obtain not only support of the clergy, but also the Commoners, presided over the Cortes proceedings in 1538. This was the last time that year that the three estates, the Nobility, the Clergy, and the Commoners, met to raise the necessary funds to build up the king's depleted treasury. The proposal, known as the *sisa*, was to impose a general tax on food. When the Nobility cast the final vote and walked out, they left behind an act that effectively abolished parliamentary procedure. The following *Cortes* merely sanctioned every call to refill the king's coffers.

The historical meaning becomes a political allegory and is important in understanding the semiotic reading. Also, students in literature of Spain classes are usually required to read only the first three of the seven chapters, those included in the Del Río anthology that includes too many historical parallels to ignore. Critics have noted since as early as 1915 with Bonilla San Martín and afterwards by Lázaro Carrreter that the hunger theme is what supports the first three *tratados* and that the author simply needed more episodes to transition to the other main themes.

Lazarillo serves three different masters in the first three chapters: the blind man, that would be the Commoners, in chapter i, the priest who represents the Clergy in chapter ii, and the squire as the Nobility in chapter iii. Lazarillo runs away from his first role model, the second master throws him out and he is abandoned by the third. Students can find in *Wikipedia* how *lazarillo* became an accepted term as a guide to a blind person and a quote regarding the blind man and the priest:

> The self-indulgent cleric concentrates on feeding himself, and when he does decide to give the 'crumbs from his table' to Lazarillo, he says, 'toma, come, triunfa, para tí es el mundo' "take, eat, triumph—the world is yours," a clear parody of a key communion statement." Finally, the squire leaves his honor in disgrace since he cannot provide food for himself, much less for his servant (Andrade).

Rodolfo Cortina documents that the word *sisa* was used by Lazarillo's author figuratively not to mean tax, but theft. This was the first documentation of that usage in Spanish. Sieber follows with acknowledgement that hunger is not merely a theme of this work but actually provides the narrative structure for the first three chapters. Historically, this would be the effects of the tax (*sisa*) on all food products so that Charles V could continue the constant warfare necessary to stay in power. His people were hungry.

At this point, a little background on the picaresque genre in general is necessary. These roguish adventures, usually rather formulaic, are typically the real, or supposed to be the real, biography of a humble anti-hero, a low life who satirizes the life of the different masters. This under-view rather than overview of society follows the formula and Lázaro provides a faithful picture of his picaresque surroundings, as well as a satire of those social conditions reflected in earlier idealistic medieval books of chivalry or the pastoral novels with sweet masquerading shepherds. In the Marxist view, he is poor little proletarian in a protest novel. The penetrating realism and parody of life in general were in direct contrast to the predominantly Neo-Platonist literature of the epoch such as Garcilaso de la Vega's flowery sonnets or the beautiful writings of the mystics, such as Saint John of the Cross or Santa Teresa de Jesús. It was also a reflection of Spain's expensive ventures in the New World (the founding of New Spain, Mexico, 1535 and the viceroyalty in Peru, 1543).

The chivalrous attributes of the knight errant were negated by every picaresque action as Cervantes did in *Don Quixote*. The knight was usually a nobleman by birth, brave of heart, generous in deed, dutiful, chaste in love, with honor as his watchword. The *pícaro*, on the other hand, was of low birth, of which he was mockingly proud, and a coward at heart. His only profession appeared to be living by his wits. Honor did not enter into his spiritual pattern and if chaste love ever stirred his heart, he was not aware of it. He displayed no will power other than a desire to satisfy his hunger and other immediate needs. Despite all of the above, he was intelligent, observant and certainly had a sense of humor.

Lazarillo roamed about, changing masters in quest of a livelihood, allowing the anonymous author to evaluate the society within his range of vision, graphically painting a picture of existing conditions, including the political issues of overtaxed food, leaving a hungry populace. Although not overly didactic in nature, Lazarillo's story is an interesting social satire. This social satire has been debated, interpreted and discussed in terms of dating, authorship, perspective and point-of-view in all manner of critical discourse for centuries. There had also been many studies of the social, legal and theological context of honor without dealing directly with the issue of language. Harry Sieber's work was the first semiotic analysis in the twentieth century. In his prologue, Sieber is explicit regarding his examination of the wider social implications of the language of honor because the text itself functions as a sign of honor (viii).

The conversion of the text to a sign of honor is in the Ciceronian notion of the power of persuasive speech to effect action. Thus, a whole series of social problems become apparent through language alone, including the language of honor. Beginning with this notion of a language of honor, the author made clear he was dealing with structuralism and semiotics, leaving aside most of the other important past contributions except the notion of Lazarillo as an "epic of hunger" in the sense that honor did not enter into the spiritual pattern of this parody of the knight errant who displayed none of the quijotesque will power to not eat even in the presence of sumptuous banquets if it did not suit his chivalrous manner. The *pícaro* satisfied his hunger and other immediate needs even if theft was involved. In spite of all of the above, he was, as the faithful squire, Sancho Panza of the *Quijote*, intelligent, observant and certainly had a sense of humor.

Using semiology to deal with the relationship of the political allegory within the literary text itself, Sieber discusses the way language is articulated and doesn't deal necessarily with other important topics: the master–servant relationships, the function of folklore, thematic structure, social satire, style and the myriad of other issues involved with this work. For that reason, here are other past opinions on the cohesion of the hunger epic narrative structure of the first three *tratados*. As early as 1915, Bonilla San Martín noted from the fourth *tratado* that the narrative becomes rushed and there is a certain waning disinterest that happens when the hunger leitmotif begins to falter (30). Lázaro Carreter followed the same idea, notices this same gradation as the hunger theme that serves as the vertebrae of the first three chapters is worn out, there is a kind of fatigue or creative impotence that seems to take hold of the author. But, he still needs to find equilibrium, he suggests that was the reason for adding the other episodes. Thus, with a respectable transition he could take Lazarillo to the dishonorable marriage; therefore, Carreter concludes that the other three *tratados* were simply of arquitectonic necessity (4). Francisco Ayala also noted the structural change when he said the action culminates in the third treatise_and sees the fourth and sixth as very brief, with a nervous style and little narrative expansion (5). The last tratados are also very short and really do not seem to add any other special cohesive element to this classic political allegory of hunger.

The important issue here is Lazarillo, the protagonist, in his everyday fight against hunger. Since the style is autobiographical and subjective, there are anecdotes and even more objective descriptions of reality only colored by his naïve introspection. Harry Sieber describes a kind of linear linguistic development with his definition of the relationship between Lazarillo and his masters as linguistic rather than psychological and it is the language of metaphorical and real hunger. This is more than just satire of the clergy to a rather absorbing investigation of sacramental discourse as visible language within Lazarillo's own linguistic games of trying to get back at his masters for his ever-present hunger. Lazarillo's increasing susceptibility to his own language are:

> his gaining access to the priest's chest of bread; his invention and experience as a mouse (the product of his own discourse); and his becoming the serpent (the product of the discourse of others). The key that admits him to the chest of bread is clearly the most important element, for it also opens and closes his fiction. (Sieber 18)

The treatment of sacramental discourse is well-documented in the text. Sieber refers to the structural relationship implicit in the act of Holy Communion (26), which he observes to be the same as the linguistic mediation between Lazarillo and the priest. Lazarillo's figurative description of the bread is revealing:

> he worships the bread, not daring, however, to receive it . . . he then kisses it . . . and even later, he speaks of the persecuted bread, and he treats the chest as if it were the body of the crucified Christ after he inflicts a gaping hole in its rib cage. The pierced side of the chest, which yields Lazarillo's bread of life, bespeaks an act of breaking and entering his "*paraíso panal*" breadly paradise. (21)

In the third *tratado*, Lázaro returns to the beggar's discourse of the first *tratado* but now he does not have a blind master. He must deal with a new language of honor on the part of his new master, the squire. While the psychological interplay is intriguing, the protagonist will once again show the verbal power of hunger by providing beggar's bread for the pretentious squire. This treatise has more dialogue than any of the others, which provides more direct linguistic interchange. Sieber properly notes the "nonreciprocal semantic power apparent in the choice of pronouns with which Lazarillo and the squire address each other" (39). Students can relate this sixteenth century usage with the *vos* form that has replaced *tú* as the form of address for equals or those who perform services. A linguistic equality based on their shared poverty is denoted by the *tuteo* used by Lazarillo in his silent asides to his master. While the squire speaks to Lazarillo as master to servant, Lazarillo responds with various modes of address, beginning with the relatively neutral *señor*, soon introducing the respectful but more socio-linguistically significant *vuestra merced* (your grace) and ending with a much lower, almost denigrating *vos*" (39).

The relationships between speech and production, honor and economy, honor and Toldedo's linguistic system are based on the town's economy. This community places no value on the squire's old code from the Valladolid manorial system. In other words, his honorable language cannot provide for their mutual hunger. Seiber's historical justification of "a power semantic based, not on wealth, but by birth" . . . not functioning in "a speech community whose language is simply an extension of the economy" . . . is well-footnoted with comments on the sixteenth-century nobility in Valladolid and the distribution of the merchant class in Toledo (31). "These mutually-dependent relationships between speech and production, honor and economy, commercial and manorial systems" (44) provide the apparent struggle between servant and master. There are progressive stages in the servant's perception of the usefulness of language to satiate his hunger, coming full circle from a few metaphors to even the power of silence to communicate. This semiotic explanation serves to interpret the text, along with more traditional, historical, social, theological, psychological and other forms of literary criticism. This relationship between food representation in the form of a political allegory results in a text of resistance in the face of historical oppression.

Globalization has been changing our outlook and access to Hispanic food culture here in the United States for some time now. In bringing together others' course descriptions using Hispanic food culture in the higher-education classroom, adding a few suggestions and analyzing an old iconic Golden Age work as a political allegory, this work has shown the student interest and instructor insight in building new courses and reimagining old literary works for higher education.

Notes

1   Fry, Michael: www.comics.com
2   www.actfl.org/sites/default/files/publications/ACTFLPerformance_Descriptors.pdf
3   A simple search will also produce a multitude of Latinx bilingual children's books on food as culture and heritage like the one below: teachinglatinamericathroughliterature.wordpress.com/2016/11/03/10-

latinx-childrens-books-on-food-as-culture-and-heritage/
4   https://www.amherst.edu/academiclife/departments/spanish/courses
5   See Esteban, José. *La cocina en Galdós y otras noticias literario-gastro-nómicas*, Gázquez Ortiz, Antonio. *La cocina en tiempos del Arcipreste de Hita and A la mesa con Don Quijote y Sancho* by Pedro Plasencia.
6   https://www.iberianature.com/spainblog/2019/12/rabbit-roman-coin-of-hispania/

Bibliography

"Allegory." *The New Princeton Encyclopedia of Poetry and Poetics*. 1993.

Allende, Isabel. *Aphrodite : The Love of Food & the Food of Love*. Flamingo, 1999.

Almodóvar Martín, Miguel Angel. *El hambre en España*. 2003.

Anderson, Benedict. *Imagined Communities*. New York: Verso, 2006.

Andrade, Marcel Charles. *Lazarillo De Tormes: Adapted for Intermediate Students*. Lincolnwood, III: National Textbook Co, 1987.

Ashley, Bob et al. "Food and Cultural Studies." *Studies in Consumption and Market*. New York: Routledge, 2004.

"Autosacramentales."curiosidadesdelenguayliteratura.blogspot.com/2011/02/autossacramentales. html visual depictions of those described in this writing.

Ayala, Francisco. *El Lazarillo reexaminado*. Ed. Taurus, S.A.: Madrid, 1971.

Barthes, Roland. "Towards a Psychosociology of Contemporary Food Consumption." *Food and Culture: A Reader*. Eds. Carole Counihan and Penny Van Esterik. London: Routledge, 2007, 28–35.

Bataillon, Marcel. *Novedad y fecundidad del Lazarillo de Tormes*. Anaya, S.A.: Barcelona, 1968.

Burgos, Carmen de. *La cocina moderna*. Valencia: Prometeo, 1918.

Carreter, Fernando Lázaro. *Lazarillo de Tormes en la picaresca*. Ed. Ariel: Barcelona, 1972.

Cortina Gómez, Rodolfo. "On Dating the Lazarillo." Philadelphia: *Hispanic Review*, Vol. 45, Issue 1 (Winter 1977), 61–66.

Counihan, Carol and Penny Van Esterik. "Time, Sugar, and Sweetness." *Food and Culture: A Reader*. London: Routledge, 2007, 91–103.

De Man, Paul. "The Rhetoric of Blindness: Jacques Derrida's Reading of Rousseau." *Blindness and Insight: Essays in the Rhetoric of Contemporary Criticism*. Minneapolis: University of Minnesota Press, 1983, second edition), 102–41.

Del Río, Angel y Amelia. *La vida de Lazarillo de Tormes*. Ed. H. J. Chaytor. Manchester, UK: Manchester University Press, 1922.

Derrida, Jacques. *Of Grammatology*. Baltimore & London: Johns Hopkins University Press, 1997.

——. "Structure, Sign and Play in the Discourse of the Human Sciences," John Hopkins University. 21 October 1966,

Douglas, Mary. "Deciphering a Meal," *Food and Culture: A Reader*. Eds. Carole Counihan and   Penny Van Esterik. London: Routledge, 2007, 44–53.

Esteban, José. *La cocina en Galdós y otras noticias literario-gastronómicas.* Madrid: Ediciones El Museo Universal, 1992.

Esquivel, Laura. *Como agua para chocolate.* Barcelona: Bibliotex, S.L., 2001.

Fletcher, Angus. *Allegory: The Theory of a Symbolic Mode.* Cornell: Cornell University Press, 1964.

Garth, Hanna. *Food in Cuba.* Stanford, California: Stanford University Press, 2020.

Gázquez Ortiz, Antonio. *La cocina en tiempos del Arcipreste de Hita.* Madrid: Alianza Editorial, 2002.

Goody, Jack. *Cooking, Cuisine, and Class: A Study in Comparative Sociology.* Cambridge, UK: Cambridge University Press, 1982.

Gutiérrez Flores, Daniela. "ACS 28622 SPAN 26822 Women and Food in Latin America." Chicago, Ill.: *University of Chicago 2021–2022 Catalog.* collegecatalog.uchicago.edu/thecollege/latinamericanstudies/ Accessed online May 1, 2021.

Harris, Roy. *Interpreters of Saussure.* Edinburgh: University of Edinburgh Press, 2001, 171–188.

Heywood, Sam. *Foods of Latin America Project.* Center for Latin American Studies at University of Arizona, las.arizona.edu/foods-latin-america-project-based-learninexperience
accessed May 1, 2021.
las.arizona.edu/sites/las.arizona.edu/files/Middle%20and%20
Elementary %20Lesson%20Full-converted.pdf

Levi-Strauss, Claude. "The Culinary Triangle." *Food and Culture: A Reader.* Eds. Carole Counihan and Penny Van Esterik. London: Routledge, 2007, 36–43.

La vida de Lazarillo de Tormes. Prefacio de Gregorio Marañón, Espasa Calpe: Buenos Aires, 1948.

Mead, Margaret. "The Problem of Changing Food Habits." *Food and Culture: A Reader.* Eds Carole Counihan and Penny Van Esterik. London: Routledge, 2007, 17–27.

Mennel, Stephen, Anne Murcett and Anneke H. Van Otterloo. *The Sociology of Food: Eating, Diet and Culture.* London: Sage, 1992.

——. *All Manners of Food: Eating and Taste in England and France from the Middle Ages to the Present.* Urbana, IL: U of Illinois Press, 1996.

Mintz Sidney. *Sweetness and Power: The Place of Sugar in Modern History* (1986).

Mintz, Stanley. "Eating Communities: The Mixed Appeals of Sodality." *Eating Culture: The Poetics and Politics of Food.* Eds. Tobias Doring, Markus Heide and Susanne Muhleisen. Druck: *Memminger Medienlentrum,* London, Routledge, 2004, 19–34.

Muhleisen, Susanne. "Globalized Tongues: The Cultural Semantics of Food Names." *Eating Culture: The Poetics and Politics of Food.* Eds. Tobias Doring, Markus Heide and Susanne Muhleisen. Druck: *Memminger Medienlentrum,* 2003, 71–88.

Plasencia, Pedro. *Cocina madrileña.* Madrid: Editorial Everest, 1995.

Pérez, Dionisio. *Guía del buen comer español: inventario y loa de la cocina clásica de España y sus regiones.* Madrid: Sucesores de Rivandeneyia, 1929.

Pardo Bazán, Emilia. *La cocina española antigua.* Madrid: Sociedad anónima renacimiento, 1913.

——. *La cocina española moderna.* Madrid: Sociedad Anónima Renacimiento, 1917.

"Porcus, puerco, cerdo." *El cerdo en la gastronomía española.* Madrid: Alianza Editorial, 2000.

Portnoy, Sarah. *The Culture of Food in Hispanic Los Angeles.* Urbana-Champaign, Ill.: University of Illinois Urbana-Champaign Dept of Spanish and Portuguese, 2018. www./spanport.illinois.edu/node/206 Accessed May 1, 2021. www.lataco.com/how-to- teach-students-spanish-using-tacos-and-pupusas-meet-professor-sarah-portnoy/ "rabbit," www.iberianature.com/spainblog/2019/12/rabbit-roman-coin-of-hispania/ Accessed May 1, 2021.

Saussure, Ferdinand de. "Saussure's Third Course of Lectures in General Linguistics 1910–1911)." *Notebooks of Emile Constantin.* (Language and Communication series, vol. 12). French text edited by Eisuke Komatsu & trans. by Roy Harris. Oxford: Pergamon Press, 1993.

Sharp, Michelle M. "Family Responsibilites. A Recipe for the Modern Spanish Nation: Carmen de Burgos' and Emilia Pardo Bazán's Cookbook Discourses." *S/He Sex & Gender in Hispanic Cultures.* Ed. Debra D. Andrist. Sussex Academic Press, 2017, 5–22.

Sieber, Harry. *Language and Society in La vida de Lazarillo de Tormes.* Johns Hopkins Univ. Press: Baltimore. 1978.

Sieber, Harry. Language and Society in *La vida de Lazarillo de Tormes."* *Modern Language Review* 74 (1979): 580–98 *faculty-staff.ou.edu/L/A-Robert.R.Lauer-1/picaresca.html*

Valbuena y Prat. *La novela picaresca.* Aguilar: Madrid, 1968.

Valdivieso, José de. "El peregrino del cielo." *Autos sacramentales eucarísticos.* Madrid: Ed. Cervantes, 1952, 91–92.

Wild, Matthew J., "Eating Spain: National Cuisine Since 1900" (2015). *Theses and Dissertations—Hispanic Studies.* 24. Accessed May 1, 2021.

3

Vitamin F: First Wave Feminist-Fueled Home Economics— A Dialogue of Trends in North America and Spain

MICHELLE M. SHARP

The presumption that the tasks of domesticity are inextricably linked to the female sex was a sociological development in western Europe `and North America that can be traced to the eighteenth and nineteenth centuries. With the rise of the middle class and successive waves of migration from rural to urban populations, adult women, especially those of the middle and upper classes, served their families as the angel of the hearth. Assuming that a biological capacity for motherhood defined the ultimate aspiration of a woman, this social assignment prioritized the rearing of children and the maintenance of the domestic space above any professional wage-earning employment outside of the home. The less fiscally productive a woman was, the more respectable her family. There was strong social pressure to adhere to this domestic role. Mary Nash explains that in the case of Spain,

> The discourse of domesticity legitimated a negative attitude toward women's right to employment in the labor market, even among the working classes. Another significant long-term consequence was the redefinition of housework as non-work and services, thus leading to its invisibility, lack of monetary value and ultimately, its low social status. (28)

Women were relegated to a passive and reactionary role with a limited horizon. Asexual and yet defined by their sex, women in much of western Europe and the United States lacked the legal protections and universal suffrage that white men enjoyed. This restriction of women to the domestic space became a cultural norm, a seemingly intrinsic value that was to be seen as natural. "It can be argued that the theoretical glass ceiling of the Spanish women's movement was the inability to challenge motherhood as the nucleus of female identity" (Nash 40). Women who rejected their socially constructed "natural" role would have been committing a taboo act.

A challenge of the social reform movement of moderate feminism was how to advocate for the equal legal standing and public rights of women while elevating the respect of the domestic role that many women fulfilled and some embraced. Radical feminism that rejected motherhood and family life was off-putting to many people, including women who wished to be recognized for their efforts on the domestic front. Home economics, which approached the domestic sphere through a scientific lens, offered a compromise of sorts. While some feminists were disgusted by the notion that housework and motherhood could be recast as a career, home economics was an enlightening possibility for others. As Laura Shapiro explains:

> The women promoting it wanted to peel back the sentiment wrapped around domestic life, dismiss its old-fashioned trappings, and free the American home to take its rightful place in the modern world. Under the rubric of home economics, or so its founders dreamed, all women would study the science involved in cooking, cleaning and childcare; and those who wished to study further could earn an academic degree representing their intellectual fitness for the job of wife and mother. (109)

This was a woman's profession that could exist within a man's world. It elevated the drudgery of repetitive and uncompensated work to something technical that required training. Therefore, completing these tasks merited respect for its successful mastery. Home economics managed "to remove domesticity from the realm of the emotions and place it among the sciences, to make it an activity for the brain rather than the heart" (113). When trained professionals completed the tasks included under the broad umbrella of home economics, the whole nation would benefit (112). This benefit lent itself both to individual women and to a nation confronting the rapid modernization of the first half of the twentieth century. Home economics offered a pathway forward that promoted a common good through its educational intent.

Spanish first-wave feminist Carmen de Burgos (1867–1932) (Figure 3.1) believed that motherhood could be compatible with outside interests rather than the one existing at the exclusion of the other.

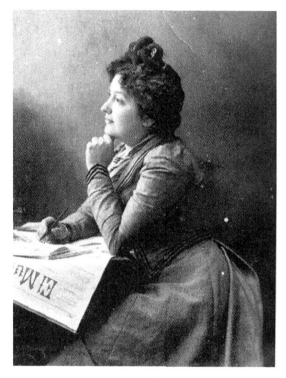

3.1 Carmen de Burgos.

A social reformer and defender of women's and children's rights, Burgos denied being a proponent of feminism even after publishing a treatise in favor of legalizing divorce in Spain in 1904. It wasn't until 1921 that she publicly identified as a feminist. It was essential for her to be able to reconcile her celebration of motherhood and family life with legal rights, protections, and non-domestic public roles for women. Feminism, for some, was unlike other political movements that sought to achieve power in its own right. For reformers like Burgos, "[Feminism] sought a redress of grievances, but not to take power; instead they wished to share power, and to change their societies for the better by exercising what political theorist Kathleen Jones has since termed 'compassionate authority'" (Offen 13). In time, Burgos saw that feminism could work to address the imbalance of power between the sexes in Spain. Burgos was a respected leader among Spanish liberals:

> Burgos can be considered one of the most distinguished proponents
> of Spanish feminism in the lead-up to the Second Republic . . . [A]t

the beginning of her career Burgos was a moderate feminist, becoming increasingly radical by the 1920s. Secondly, in line with international first wave feminism, she strongly believed in the urgency of legal reform, manifested most notably in her life-long campaigns for divorce and the vote. (Louis 3–4)

Feminism could be in harmony with her Krausist view of Spanish society by promoting grassroots educational efforts in order to elevate the entire nation's population, starting with the most disenfranchised. In this way Burgos could promote the autonomy of women while advocating for a strong family base as the cornerstone of the nation. Without this strong foundation of a harmonious family unit rooted in mutual respect and dignity for all its members, the Spanish nation would not thrive.

Carmen de Burgos's engagement with social reform was largely through her writing career. She was a prolific author who published 75 short novels, nine novels, 27 practical manuals, three cookbooks and a number of translations, including Helen Keller's biography and Paul Julius Moebius's *The Mental Inferiority of Women*. She also served as a war correspondent in Morocco and published regular newspaper columns in the *Diario Universal* and the *Heraldo de Madrid*. Burgos is noteworthy for a variety of reasons in Spanish literature and politics including the fact that she was among the first women to earn a living from her writing and public speaking.

Burgos wrote extensively about food, the care of children and the maintenance of the home in her newspaper articles and the traditionally feminine texts of domestic manuals and beauty guides. Domestic manuals and beauty guides are considered to be feminine texts because their content predominantly considers the female experience of the world.[1] These cookbooks and domestic manuals reinforce and enhance the feminist educational efforts of her treatises on divorce, universal suffrage and women's rights. While titles such as *Arte de ser elegante/The Art of Being Elegant* (1918) and *El arte de ser amada/ The Art of Being Loved* (1918) may seem otherwise, Burgos maintained a consistent focus of female empowerment regardless of the format or forum of her writing. Her domestically themed texts are not throw-away aberrations from her corpus of essays and novels written out of financial necessity. Instead, they were an opportunity to reach a broader audience that she could educate about their rights and appropriate expectations. Her multiple levels of writing were intentional and deliberate:

The diversity of editorial projects suggests that her writing engaged women at different levels of education, literacy and economic means. The market for these inexpensive texts [domestic manuals] allowed her ideas to reach reader-consumers who might not have encountered them by attending her feminist speeches or by seeking out her overtly political writing. (Ingram 182)

It is important to note that Burgos published these domestic texts throughout her entire literary career, regardless of her financial position.

Seemingly innocuous feminine texts such as cookbooks and domestic manuals may be discounted by contemporary scholars in search of "true" or "pure" feminist thought. In doing so, they risk missing out on the richness of the daily messages that women received regarding social protocol and norms. Janet Theophano proposes that "There is much to be learned from reading a cookbook besides how to prepare food—discovering the stories told in the spaces between the recipes or within the recipes themselves" (6). Additionally, she states that, "It was in domestic literature such as cookery books that women could develop both their concepts of the feminine ideal and their opinions on social and political issues ranging from women's education to temperance and religion" (6). These domestic manuals provided women with a space to share, to think, to question, and, most importantly, to express themselves within the domestic space in which they were conventionally restricted. Women could use these non-threatening feminine texts to build community. Restructuring the care and execution of their domestic spaces could give all women a starting point towards greater autonomy and self-worth. They could be the master of their own domain.[2]

At the same time, twenty-first century scholars must bear in mind that Burgos's publication of her own cookbooks *La cocina moderna/The Modern Kitchen* (1906), *¿Quiere Ud. comer bien?/Do You Wish to Eat Well?* (1916), and *Nueva cocina práctica/The New Practical Kitchen* (1925) was a gender subversive act. Between 1880 and 1920 the best-known cooking manuals in Spain were all written and published by professional men.[3] With the publication of her own cookbooks, Burgos challenged male authority. The covers themselves of Burgos's cookbooks are a noteworthy element of this question of gender authority. While the texts' introductions, as will be discussed shortly, clearly address middle- and aspiring-middle-class women in urban environments, the covers themselves are much more open to interpretation. *¿Quiere Ud. comer bien?* has two different covers. In Figure 3.2, the cover displays an opulent dish ready for a feast.

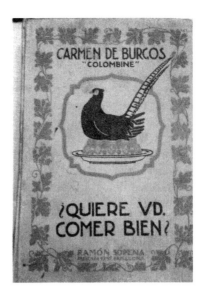

3.2 *¿Quiere Ud. comer bien?*

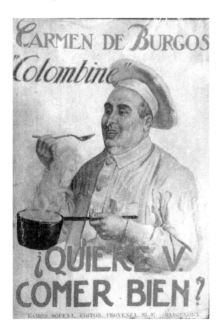

3.3 *¿Quiere V comer bien?*

In Figure 3.3, there is a corpulent male French-style chef tasting a dish in process. Neither of these covers, aside from the prominent display of Burgos's name as the author, emphasize the feminine nature of the text. In fact, given the question that serves as the title for the cookbook and the distinguished covers, it's hard to imagine anyone responding 'no.' It's as gender neutral as can be.

For the cover of the 1925 *Nueva cocina práctica* (Figure 3.4), however, the cover features a well-heeled table with two elegant women in the spotlight. One of them appears to be preparing a dish for service. They are dressed as elegantly as everyone else at the table, eliminating any question of them being household staff. In this cover, published after Burgos has become vocally active in Spanish feminist organizations, two poised women control the table. Their delectable dish, the arrangement of the table, and the ability to execute this event together are surely thanks to the advice and guidance of the cookbook whose cover they grace. Burgos sent her readers a message with these covers. Her cookbooks will allow them to flawlessly execute complicated dishes, rival a professional male chef, and partake in elegant evenings. She will provide them with the necessary tools to let them be in control, to be an active agent rather than a reactionary participant in their households.

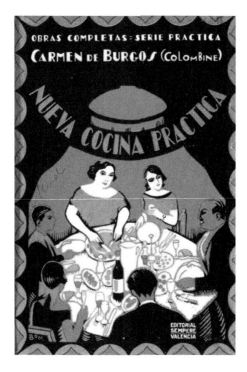

3.4 *Nueva cocina práctica.*

Her cookbooks were directed to home cooks and their staffs. She used her cooking manuals as an opportunity to teach women about the domestic laboratories of their homes (Burgos, ¿*Quiere Ud?* 5). The presence of her manual in a home affords her the opportunity to teach her reader about broader food trends, skills necessary to manage a household, and how to organize daily family meals as a special occasion. In looking at how women practice food acquisition, preparation, and presentation within their homes, there is a confluence of food and gender studies: "One of the most basic assumptions of scholarship in both food studies and women's studies is that the daily life of ordinary people is not only worthy of study but necessary to any understanding of past and present worlds" (Avakian and Haber 16). These prescriptive texts allow for an analysis of the advice circulating throughout the early twentieth century as women encountered a ceaseless influx of new technologies. They may be criticized as a "history of social ideas" that may "[emphasize] gender norms rather than the way individual people might have resisted or complied with those norms" (Neuhaus 3). At the same time, there is great potential of what these popular texts, referring to texts published for a general, middle-class audience, can teach us "because they enable us to reconstruct the norms, visual images, and received truths that encased and thus could not help but influence daily lives" (Neuhaus 3–4). Burgos's focus in all of her writing was individual empowerment through education. The combination of elements in her cookbooks and domestic manuals were strategically arranged so as to break the cycle of enforced ignorance that dominated Spanish women's instruction.

Burgos's writing confronted the angel of the hearth discourse, that idealized feminine role in the western world beginning in the Victorian era persisting into the twentieth century. This notion of feminine domesticity stipulates that a woman best serves her community as a wife and mother. The proverbial and literal heart of the family must do her best to ensure that the domestic space is a family haven from the demands and discomfort of the outside world. The woman's entire realm consists of the domestic space; her glass ceiling is the roof of the family's house.

Burgos did not deny the importance of the domestic sphere. Remember that, for Burgos, the family is the cornerstone of the Spanish nation. In order to dismantle the angel of the hearth as the supreme ideal, she had to undermine the simplicity of the archetype. By emphasizing female education and instruction for domestic management, she negated the concept that there is anything innate about caring for a home or a family. One needs training in order to complete the range of tasks required to maintain a modern home and hygienically care for its inhabitants. Burgos counteracted the low social status of domestic occupation, "By insisting on the importance of good household management, cookbook authors asserted the importance of the 'women's sphere' to the productivity and stability of the market economy" (Neuhaus 16). While still not a wage-earning role itself, the production of the external capitalist system depended upon the efficiency of the woman at home. Through a portrayal of the domestic tasks as essential, Burgos sought to increase respect for the repetitive work completed behind the scenes in the name of home and family care. Writing about the importance of the wife and mother in prescriptive texts recognized the value of the demanding work done on behalf of the household in an explicit way.

Turning now to specific textual examples, *La cocina moderna* includes history lessons and international recipes—a bold move given the geographical and cultural isolation of Spain at Burgos's time. Titled "Importancia del arte culinario/The Importance of the Culinary Arts," the introduction to this cookbook includes detailed accounts of royal families' involvement in the invention and careful preparation of dishes such as Madame Dubarry's "los filetes de truchas" (filets of trout) and Madame de Pompadour's "los filets de volaille" (filets of chicken) (11). She also notes how much care regal figures took in the menu-planning for, and daily feeding of, their spouses. By high-lighting the culinary and domestic achievements of Catherine de Médicis, Queens Alexandra and Victoria of England, and Empress Maria, widow of Tsar Alexander III, among others, Burgos elevates the daily act of food preparation to something regal, making it a weighty matter (10–13). This is a savvy move that elevates a non-work invisible labor into something worthy of royal attention. In this way, "Female political figures demonstrate that food preparation is a meaningful social practice, nor merely domestic labor that belongs to women of inferior status. Paradoxically, this discourse both normalizes the idea of women laboring in the kitchen at the same time that it converts cooking into a social practice that shapes politics" (Ingram 188). This paradox is consistent with the balancing act of moderate feminism where a woman proficient in household maintenance may also seek external endeavors and personal enrichment. Burgos was one of the original proponents of the claim that women could have it all—both a fulfilling private and the public life.

This melding of politics and private life lends itself to an explanation of how these regal figures are able to execute multiple roles with such dexterity. In *La cocina moderna*/The Modern Kitchen, Burgos notes that "todas las hijas de la reina de Dinamarca/all the daughters of the queen of Denmark" and "todas las princesas hijas de Eduardo

VII/all of Edward VII's daughters" (12) had a formal education that prepared them to complete their domestic tasks with refinement and skill. Schools focused on female education with a unique curricula had existed since the nineteenth century. However, early iterations of segregated female curricula "focused specifically on household chores to the detriment of building skills in reading or writing" (Scanlon 17). Domestic hygiene and needlework along with skills of entertainment like reciting poetry or playing piano were considered essential for a career as an upper-class wife and mother. Burgos sought a distinctive educational model for all women, regardless of social class, that more closely aligned with home economics as previously discussed. Home economics allowed for a public role, one that expanded housekeeping from the home to social and even municipal contexts. Burgos sought the common good in her endorsement of a more rigorous training program for women that included science, accounting and management skills. "Burgos's proposal to make cooking part of education reform would create a domain for a professionalized workforce of women . . . Like the US-American home economists, Spanish women would be prepared to address cooking and nutrition as part of social policy . . . In this context, cooking becomes a social practice with relevance to national health" (Ingram 190).

Burgos is explicit in her declaration that there is a science to cooking. The introduction to *¿Quiere Ud. comer bien?/Do You Want to Eat Well?* begins with a colorful description of the household kitchen, "La cocina es el laboratorio doméstico donde se preparan los alimentos, y debe reunir en lo posible todas las condiciones de comodidad, de salubridad y de economía deseables/The kitchen is the domestic laboratory where foodstuffs are prepared and all desired modes of convenience, good health, and economy possible should be brought together in it" (5). This reference to the kitchen as a laboratory separates it immediately from any romantic notion of domestic bliss. There is no rosy glow from the hearth nor freshly baked treats cooling on the stove. A laboratory is a place of work, a professional and sterile environment in which its director conducts investigations. It is to be a domain that merits respect because only a competent individual will effectively manage a laboratory. There must be a hierarchy. Its director manages the inventory, procedures, and labor of all involved in the space. Burgos's wife and mother is a household manager who directs this space.

Burgos makes no assumptions as to the knowledge that her potential readers have in managing their domestic laboratory. For example, in the chapter titled "Elecciones de las carnes/Selecting meats," she provides descriptions of each butchered portion of beef, veal, mutton and pork so that a cook knows what's appropriate for a roast, a stew, and so forth (27). When the cookbook moves into recipes, Burgos's instructions are full of guidance and support. To introduce the classic dish of "cocido español/Spanish stew," Burgos explains, "Por primitivo que sea el cocido y fácil en apariencia, requiere gran cuidado para hacerlo bien; no consiste en meterlo todo en la olla y dejar que se guise; hay un arte delicado que observar, y hasta el fuego ha de estar graduado/In spite of the rustic nature and easy appearance of the stew, it requires great care to make it well; it does not work to simply put it all in the pot and let it cook; there is a delicate art that must be observed and even the heat of the fire needs to be adjusted)" (62). Beyond food preparation, Burgos also includes recipes for medicinal products, as is traditional of cookbooks of the eighteenth and nineteenth centuries, when these texts were thought of as repositories of all necessary domestic knowledge. Burgos includes extensive information regarding the nutritional value and digestive time of a number of foods, subjects that would be covered in a home economics course.

Burgos recognized that the existence alone of guidebooks such as her own feminine texts and articles was insufficient to prepare women for the demands of the task before them. She was an outspoken advocate for domestic-training schools, even more so after visiting several of them on her state-sponsored tour of western European educational systems. She cites examples of their success with the upper class and nobility across Europe—something that would definitely bolster the cache of this sort of education. These schools provided women with useful educations in accounting, hygiene, food science and other necessary skills for running a home. Burgos speaks with authority on this subject as she is identified on the title page of *La mujer en el hogar/The Woman at Home* as "Profesora de esta asignatura en la escuela superior de artes industriales de Madrid/Professor of this subject in the upper school of industrial arts in Madrid." This professional title does not appear on her works of fiction or essays, it is a unique identifier intended to bolster the status of the domestic manuals. These are professional texts written by a trained woman for women who will benefit from the knowledge gained through her expertise. She is proficient enough in her own domestic skills so as to be able to help others better themselves in their management of these tasks.

Burgos defines the ideal feminine education and its benefits in the introduction of *La mujer en el hogar/The Woman in the Home*: "Así, de una educación sólida, a la vez práctica é intelectual, que no se detiene en un extremo para caer en la erudición falsa de la marisabidilla ni en el analfabetismo, se obtiene la verdadera influencia femenina/Therefore, from a strong education, at the same time practical and intellectual, which does not stray to one extreme to lapse into the false knowledge of the know-it-all nor in illiteracy, one obtains true feminine influence" (18). The better a woman's preparation through formal education, the more effective she can be in managing a moral and proper household. This is a far cry from the mantra of ignorance being the surest way to maintain a woman's purity and innocence. A woman must be trained as a moral guide for her family; this is something of utmost importance since the Victorian reform of marriage saw it as a couple united in love with the woman's role as the teacher of the next generation (Coontz 178). Burgos asserted that these schools and its graduates would enhance Spanish society, making it stronger, helping it to modernize. This training also elevated the importance of the tasks women undertook in the home. Within the domestic sphere, there is still a question of power at stake. Food and its processing are a prism that reflects the values of a culture. The treatment of the people who make and prepare the food that feeds the nation tells a story. Without adequate nutrition and a healthy home life, a nation cannot meet the challenges of the changing world that surrounds it.

Guidebooks alone could not provide women with equal access to the scientific discoveries nor the comprehension of them needed to participate as modern citizens of the twentieth century. The early twentieth century was revolutionary for food science both in terms of production and understanding the properties of the foods consumed. For example, Dr. Elmer V. McCollum, a biochemist, developed an experiment to evaluate the nutritional value of fats in 1912. He discovered that rats fed a diet rich in butterfat thrived while those fed a diet rich in olive oil did not. This led to the identification of "Vitamin A," a discovery that changed the concept of the nutritional value of foods (Ziegelman and Coe 44).[4] A desire to understand these food values generated research into vitamins, calories, minerals, and the human digestive system at a rapid pace during the First World War and the ensuing European food shortages. The Great Depression then made food allocation a concern for the United States Government, further accelerating nutritional science research. What diet was appropriate for a soldier, a child, or a nursing mother? Could people avoid rickets even when food security was a challenge? How would people respond to the new technologies of food production and preparation at the level of the farm, the factory, and the home in addition to the population shift from rural to urban?

The answer to these questions brings us back to home economics: a movement that intended to make every home a modern and efficient one. This movement proposed that, "Being a wife and mother, according to home economics, wasn't a job managed by love, it was a job managed by serious rational work" (Shapiro 113). This was to be the end of the angel of the hearth discourse. This also counteracted notions of women's limitations due to hysteria, a uniquely female condition that supposedly diminished her capacity to contend with the demands of the outside world. Burgos used this scientific subject matter language throughout the domestic manuals to ennoble the repetitive tasks that filled women's days. It also allowed her to suggest the possibility of work outside of the home once a woman mastered the domestic sphere. There was no reason why a woman could not have a variety of interests: Burgos demonstrated this in her own writing. Why wouldn't she publish both essays examining the legalization of divorce and domestic manuals for women, full-length novels and beauty guides? Burgos sought to debunk the myth that one cannot be both beautiful and intelligent, interested in the home and engaged in the public sphere. She herself, as stated previously, was a professional in the field of domestic science who managed her own home, albeit with the help of her sister, and maintained a public presence through her writing and speaking engagements.

There is a noteworthy parallel for this particular educational reform movement among European nations and the United States in the first third of the twentieth century. Burgos cited in her foundational 1927 essay titled *La mujer moderna y sus derechos/On Modern Women and Their Rights* examples of women's equality throughout western countries and the positive impact that these reforms had on the nations themselves. The fourth chapter of this essay details women's contributions to the arts, business, medicine, and law. After highlighting exceptional examples of women who have enjoyed success in the public sphere, Burgos focuses more generally on the need for universal education for all women. She stresses that the perceived positive attribute of ignorance is a pursuit of folly that weakens the nation:

La mujer que sólo sea buena para perpetuar la especie con su vigor físico, no esté dotada de vigor intelectual, no podrá ser jamás 'esa guía que el hombre necesita en el duro batallar de la vida'. No será ni siquiera su compañera digna. Precisamente la falta de cultura de la mujer perjudica más a los hombres . . . Hay que fomentar la cultura, la afición a la lectura, para lo que es el factor más importante: la mujer/The woman who is only good for perpetuating the species thanks to her physical vigor, but is not endowed with intellectual vigor, will never be 'that guide that men need in the hard battle of life.' She will not even be a decent partner. It is precisely because of this lack of education that women are more detrimental to men . . . We

must promote education and love of reading for the sake of the most
important factor: women. (127)

Burgos places the question of female education and autonomy as a
matter of national strength. Without adequate application of the
tremendous resource that is the female portion of Spanish society, or
any society for that matter, a nation risks falling behind, losing out on
the advancements of the twentieth century, because it is clinging to an
antiquated notion. Men should further the advancement of women if
only to benefit themselves. Her arguments may not fit into a neat
definition of feminism, but Burgos's urgency for the need for universal
female education in the form of home economics is palpable.

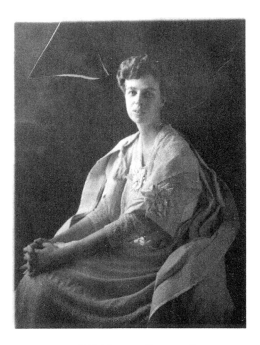

3.5 Eleanor Roosevelt.

Across the ocean, Burgos had a powerful ally in the promotion of
female empowerment through home economics in Eleanor Roosevelt
(1884–1962) (Figure 3.5). While there is no existing correspondence
between them, the parallels in their advocacy is striking and merits
further consideration in order to better comprehend the breadth and
depth of the home economics movement. As the First Lady of the
United States, Roosevelt dedicated herself to the education and

empowerment of women. Through her 7500 "My Day" columns, 556 magazine articles, 27 books and 496 radio and television programs, she was a one-woman teach-in. In spite of her popular public persona, Eleanor Roosevelt was frequently criticized in the press during her tenure as First Lady for the quality and quantity of food at White House dinners. Word spread that if you received a White House invitation, you should always eat beforehand. Her critics failed to understand that the meals were the direct result of her embrace of the science of the home economics movement. They were an effort to connect with the realities of many Americans during the Depression and through the nation's economic recovery. Home economics inspired Roosevelt from the moment that she discovered it. No matter how packed her schedule, she always made time to attend the annual conference at Cornell University in New York, the heart and head of the home economics curricular movement. As Laura Shapiro states in *What She Ate:*

> Everything she [Roosevelt] heard about home economics made sense to Eleanor. The women promoting it wanted to peel back the sentiment wrapped around domestic life, dismiss its old-fashioned trappings, and free the American home to take its rightful place in the modern world. Under the rubric of home economics, or so its founders dreamed, all women would study the science involved in cooking, cleaning and childcare; and those who wished to study further could earn an academic degree representing their intellectual fitness for the job of wife and mother. (109)

For Roosevelt, being the First Lady was a teaching opportunity. She used the stage of the White House dining room table to show the power of the budget lunch and to inspire America's home cooks. Roosevelt knew that embracing its lessons in her own household was the best way to lend the movement her full support. (Ziegelman and Coe 199). Roosevelt lived the ethos of the home economics movement.

Making cooking scientific made it a tool of female empowerment. Actually applying rigorous science to the workings of the home-made sense to her. "Scientific cookery, a cuisine of female empowerment, spoke to the feminist in Eleanor" (Ziegelman and Coe 203). In her 1933 text, *It's Up to the Women*, defined by Ziegelman and Coe as "Part political manifesto, part homily and part homemaking manual" (203), Roosevelt devoted an entire chapter to the Cornell diet. In her chapter titled "Budgets," Roosevelt stated, "In considering the family food expense and in preparing menus, it would be well to go over Miss Flora Rose's menus or any menus prepared by a home economics college and see if it is possible to buy one's supplies more economically and have a nourishing and balanced diet at a lower cost" (41). Roosevelt discusses the extension courses offered by state colleges of agriculture as a resource for rural women. She seeks to convince her readers of the need for changes in dietary habits with warnings like, "Children can eat a great deal and still be undernourished and the adults in the family also may eat and not get the maximum amount of good out of their food, so the mother of a family should look upon her housekeeping and the planning of meals as a scientific occupation" (58). Roosevelt suggests that this training should extend to hygiene, caring for the sick and childbearing. She also insists that:

> Not only the girl but the young boy should be taught something which will fit him to be a husband and father . . . both of these young people should know something about the care of a baby if they are going to be given one to bring up, to educate and to start on its way through life. There are books to-day that teach all of this. They are worth reading but I would suggest that not only in colleges of home economics but in every school and college there be given some practical instruction along these lines to both men and women. (78)

Bear in mind that these are suggestions of the sitting First Lady of the United States to the women and men of her nation. She sought to be a reform activist as First Lady that was informed by home economics. In an article published in *Ladies' Home Journal* in May 1941, Roosevelt writes again of the role of home economics courses and how girls would benefit from a year of compulsory service as part of home defense:

> I should like to see set up, in the schools, highly efficient courses in home economics. The schools could be used as laboratories by providing free hot lunches for every child, or the girls could run school cafeterias by way of practice in properly feeding groups of people. This again would achieve a double end by improving the health of the children in the community, and by giving the girls the knowledge and experience which would help them to raise the standards of their own future homes. (25)

Like Burgos, Roosevelt proposes this training so as to strengthen the family unit, which in turn bolsters the nation.

A potential limitation of home economics was that "it was a woman's profession in a man's world. No lines were crossed, no fief-doms challenged, but the women gave heart and soul to work they cared about" (Shapiro 114). A key element to Shapiro's definition is that it was a movement that rallied women together. It taught them to organize and to work together when there was something that they found of mutual value. Due to its way of creating a new space within the patriarchal system, it found appeal among many moderate feminists. The rise of home economics and its emphasis on science was an important step forward within first-wave feminism. Considering home economics through the lens of gender and how it was used to empower women gives us greater knowledge of how this social and academic movement influence twentieth century lives: "Gender effects not just the factual content of historical knowledge—what is included and what gets left out—but also the philosophical assumptions underlying our interpretations of the nature and meaning of social processes" (Felski 1). While this gender empowerment was perhaps diluted by the time I took a cooking class through the home economics department as a high school course elective in the 1990s, the course still sought to teach its students life skills for how to care for themselves. By then, the course was no longer strictly for girls. All students, regardless of their gender, were expected to clean dishes, maintain an organized kitchen, and learn how to follow the recipe instructions carefully.

The development of the home economics movement marked an organization founded by women for women. This was grassroots empowerment. This was an extension of the community created by the act of women writing about cooking. Both Burgos in Spain and Roosevelt in the United States promoted this course of study within their own countries and throughout their global travels as a way of increasing the common good. The organization of this educational reform movement laid the groundwork for further feminist reforms. Writing about domestic subjects and learning the science of home economics gave women a voice to continue exploring their sphere. This consideration of the role of the home economics movement as a part of first-wave feminism encourages a reexamination of a largely gendered movement that sought to create a new empowered space for women.

Notes

1   For further discussion of the definition of feminine literature and the challenges that it faces see Sharp, Michelle M. "*La perfecta casada*: Carmen de Burgos's new feminine feminist perfection" in *Multiple Modernities: Carmen de Burgos, Author and Activist*. eds. Anja Louis and Michelle M. Sharp. New York: Routledge, 2017. 197–213. Print.

2   Isabella Beeton, the author of the original *Book of Household Management*, is a pivotal figure in the creation of one of the first ency-

clopedic reference books for domestic tasks that elevated the role of the woman who maintained the domestic space. In Beeton's words, the lady of the house, "[O]ught always to remember that she is the first and the last, the Alpha and the Omega, in the government of her establishment . . . She is, therefore, a person of far more importance in a community than she usually thinks she is" (239).

3   The most notable cookbooks in Spain were published by Ignacio Doménech who openly criticized Carmen de Burgos and Emilia Pardo Bazán for being cookbook authors.

4   It was named Vitamin A because it was the first vitamin identified. Subsequent discovery and identification of vitamins followed this same pattern. There is nothing inherently "A-list" about Vitamin A, not B-list about the variety of B vitamins (Ziegelman and Coe 44).

Bibliography

Avakian, Arlene Voski and Barbara Haber. *From Betty Crocker to Feminist Food Studies: Critical Perspectives on Women and Food*. Amherst: U of Massachusetts P, 2005.

Beeton, Isabella. *Book of Household Management*. London: S.O. Beeton, 1861.

Burgos, Carmen de. *La cocina moderna*. Valencia: Prometeo Sociedad Editorial, 1906.

——. *La mujer moderna y sus derechos*. 1927. Pilar Ballarín, ed. Madrid: Editorial Biblioteca Nueva, 2007.

——. *Nueva cocina práctica*. [*La cocina práctica*.] Valencia: Editorial Sempere, 1925.

——. *¿Quiere Ud. comer bien?*. Barcelona: Sopena, 1916.

Coontz, Stephanie. *Marriage, A History: From Obedience to Intimacy or How Love Conquered Marriage*. New York: Penguin Group, 2005.

Felski, Rita. *The Gender of Modernity*. Cambridge: Harvard UP, 1995.

Ingram, Rebecca. "Bringing the *escuela* to the *despensa*: Regenerationist Politics in Carmen de Burgos's cookbooks." *Multiple Modernities: Carmen de Burgos, Author and Activist*. Anja Louis and Michelle M. Sharp, eds. New York: Routledge, 2017, 180–196.

Louis, Anja. *Women and the Law: Carmen de Burgos, An Early Feminist*. Woodbridge: Tamesis, 2005.

Nash, Mary. "Un/Contested Identities: Motherhood, Sex Reform and the Modernization of Gender Identity in Early Twentieth Century Spain." *Constructing Spanish Womanhood: Female Identity in Modern Spain*. Victoria Lorée Enders & Pamela Beth Radcliff, eds. Albany: SUNY P, 1999, 25–49.

National Park Service. "Eleanor Roosevelt National Historic Site" https://www.nps.gov/nr/travel/presidents/eleanor_roosevelt_valkill.html

Neuhaus, Jessamyn. *Manly Meals and Mom's Home Cooking: Cookbooks and Gender in Modern America*. Baltimore: Johns Hopkins UP, 2003.

Offen, Karen. *European Feminisms, 1700–1950: A Political History.* Stanford, CA: Stanford UP, 2000.

Roosevelt, Eleanor. "Defense and Girls." *Ladies' Home Journal* May 1941; 58, 5; ProQuest 25.

——. *It's Up to The Women.* ed. Jill Lepore. New York: Nation Books, 2017.

Scanlon, Geraldine M. *La polémica feminista en la España contemporánea (1868–1974).* Trans. Rafael Mazarrasa. Madrid: Akal, 1986.

Shapiro, Laura. *What She Ate: Six Remarkable Women and The Food That Tells Their Stories.* New York: Viking, 2017.

Theophano, Janet. *Eat My Words: Reading Women's Lives Through the Cookbooks They Wrote.* New York: Palgrave. 2002.

Ziegelman, Jane and Andrew Coe. *A Square Meal: A Culinary History of the Great Depression.* New York: HarperCollins, 2016.

4

Family Responsibilities: A Recipe for the Modern Spanish Nation— Carmen de Burgos's and Emilia Pardo Bazán's Cookbook Discourses

Michelle M. Sharp

This chapter considers the often-overlooked culinary contributions of two celebrated Spanish first-wave feminists. While known for their popular fictional texts, Emilia Pardo Bazán and Carmen de Burgos each wrote cookbooks: Pardo Bazán's *La cocina española antigua* [*Historical Spanish Cooking*] (1913) and *La cocina española moderna* [*Modern Spanish Cooking*] (1917), as a part of her published series the *Biblioteca de la mujer* [*The Woman's Library*], and Burgos's *¿Quiere Ud. comer bien?* [*Do You Want to Eat Well?*] (1916), *La cocina moderna* [*The Modern Kitchen*] (1918) and *La cocina práctica* [*The Practical Kitchen*] (1920). These rich texts have been largely overlooked in the study of these authors since, as encyclopedic non-narrative texts, they lack the prestige attributed to the narratives or essays that dominate the canon. By devaluing these practical texts, we risk missing insight into Spanish women's daily lives. Scholars also lose access to how these authors tried to influence their readers' self-definition, both in terms of the application of practical feminism and efforts to define and modernize the Spanish nation with a role for women as a crucial part. Even though they created their cookbooks in different fashions, the end-result is a benchmark of the authentic situation of middle-class Spanish women in terms of their social limitations, social expectations, and the general education or preparation that they received in order to execute the tasks demanded of them.

Exploring why these authors devoted themselves to writing texts on domestic matters allows contemporary readers and scholars to appreciate the astounding depth and breadth of their multifaceted writing profiles. Taking into account the socio-cultural context of the time, we are able to recognize that seemingly mundane texts now considered to be feminine and traditional were not so easily defined at the time. These cookbooks sought to liberate their readers, largely newly literate women of the middle class, from the *ángel del hogar* [angel of the hearth] discourse that intended to confine them to the domestic realm. These cookbooks were bold educational tools written by women in a field dominated by male authors. While women were in charge of the daily meals of the family, they were excluded from professional writing about the topic. The simple act of publishing these texts challenged that norm.

Before delving into the texts themselves, one must answer the question of what they contribute to a contemporary discussion of the rise of the feminist movement and to our goal of better understanding daily life, especially the experience for women, in the first decades of twentieth-century Spain. In Arlene Voski Avakian and Barbara Haber's ground-breaking text, which sought to merge food and gender studies, they present how food historian Anne L. Bower "reads cookbooks as fictions because they have settings, characters, and plot—all the necessary components of literature. Like most of women's art . . . recipes and cookbooks are a distinct genre that has not been recognized by a patriarchal literary establishment" (18). Feminine literature, that is, anything that deals predominantly with the female experience of and in the world, is often undervalued both at its moment of publication and also by critics and scholars who later overlook the texts for not being "real" literature.

From this disadvantaged position, cookbooks must prove their worth. They are prescriptive rather than descriptive texts, which mean that they provide readers with guidance on how to carry out their tasks according to a certain ideology. As Carol Gold explains, "Cookbooks relate what the authors expect from their readers—what they ought to be eating and how they ought to eat, if not necessarily what they do eat" (12). As documents of social history, cookbooks have the power to reveal the concerns and priorities of those who wrote them. This chapter will examine how Carmen de Burgos's cookbooks were educational tools that furthered her feminist notion of reform for women of urban Spain. She designed her cookbooks to be manuals of instruction that detailed the physical design of the household and the treatment of its people. Emilia Pardo Bazán also wrote her cookbooks with the middle-class woman in mind, but her instruction had less to do with the management of an urban household and everything to do with a definition of what it meant to eat and cook like a Spaniard. While Burgos included a range of international recipes to encourage her readers to think beyond their national borders, Pardo Bazán sought to establish the preeminence of Spanish cuisine as part of a nation-building project. Yet, of course, Pardo Bazán could not know if her readers rejected French-cooking trends nor could Burgos ensure that the lady of the house demanded respect and fair treatment from her husband. The strength of any form of prescriptive literature, especially cookbooks, is that they serve as flags: "Cookbooks, while they certainly reflect changes in society, also themselves constitute these changes . . . As society changes, as new middle classes evolve, cookbooks capture the changes and, in so doing, help the changes along" (Gold, *Danish* 13). Burgos's and Pardo Bazán's focal points in their texts provide an orientation to the priorities of Spanish first-wave feminists and early twentieth-century social reformers.

The notion of education through cookbooks and cookbooks as a reflection of educational levels reveals much about the development of a society, particularly in relation to the training of its women. The Spanish publishing industry entered a new phase of production in the early twentieth century thanks to technological advances that made low-cost publishing possible. Also key to the success of printing at this time was a sharp increase in literacy levels, especially among urban populations.[1] We know that both Burgos's and Pardo Bazán's cookbooks were directed towards middle-class women, not professional chefs. In *La cocina española moderna*, Pardo Bazán goes so far as to state in the prologue that, "Esta obra, sin embargo, no será muy útil á las personas que pueden pagar cocinero, porque no es, ni por semejas, tratado de alta cocina, y conviene más á los que, limitándose á una mesa hasta casera, aspiran sin embargo á que cada plato presente aspecto agradable y coquetón, y á poder tener convidados sin avergonzarse del prosaísmo de una minuta de <<sota, caballo, y rey>>" / "This text, however, will not be very useful to the people who can pay for a cook because it is not, nor does it resemble, a work of haute cuisine, and will better agree with those who, even if limited to a rudimentary table, still desire that each meal be pleasant and agreeable, and to be able to have guests without being embarrassed by the quick meal of the same old dish of meat, vegetables and sauce" (II).[2] If this is to be Pardo Bazán's true audience, this indicates a certain level of both literacy and numeracy among her target population so that they can successfully read and manipulate the recipes (Gold, *Danish* 13). The same applies for Burgos when she dedicated *¿Quiere Ud. comer bien?* as "Obra indispensable para cocineras y para las señoras que deseen intervenir en la cocina y en la dirección de la casa" / "An indispensable text for cooks and for those women who wish to take part in the kitchen and in the management of their homes" (title page).

The advent of the modern cookbook and that of the existence of the urban middle class are tightly linked. It is easy to underestimate the impact of the flurry of societal structural changes along with the variety of technological innovations on people's daily rhythms. As populations shifted from dominantly rural to urban, there was a great need for education to guide women through this radical transition: "Cookbooks . . . offered recipes designed to appeal to women just beginning to establish themselves firmly as middle-class. Such women sought advice and information to help delineate the newly forming boundaries of middle-class life, which demanded more elaborate meals to reflect rising class status" (Neuhaus 14). While Jessamyn Neuhaus's research focus is the cultural shift in the United States, her point holds for Spain, albeit several decades later than the early nineteenth-century sweep of the example that she references here. Cookbooks, by nature of being prescriptive, instructed women on the nuances of this new way of life. This also marks a shift in women's resources as the printed word supplants oral sources of information.

Leading the charge in the establishment of the modern cookbook was Isabella Beeton, the author of the original *Book of Household Management*. This text, first published in England in the 1860s, is described by Kathryn Hughes in *The Short Life and Long Times of Mrs. Beeton* as "not simply a reference book, [but] it is a manual of instruction" (196). As was popular in Victorian literature, it is encyclopedic in nature, designed to instruct the new middle-class woman in everything that she needs to manage her household. Her principal thrust of "convincing her readers to overcome their prejudices and accept that household management is a socially and economically crucial activity, as skilled and deserving of respect as any job carried out by men" (Hughes 6) sets her apart in her charge to elevate women's new roles. This is a direct challenge to the low capital value of women's domestic work, at times even labeled as non-work (Beetham 20). While essential for the household, since it did not participate in the external economy of production, it was devalued, "thus leading to its invisibility, lack of monetary value and ultimately, its low social status" (Nash 28).

Beeton's charge to women largely supports the tenets of the angel of the hearth discourse. She does so, however, while insisting upon a woman's importance both for herself and for society at large. The woman's role was of great strategic significance, "The Commander of an Army" (Hughes 238) and she encouraged her readers with the exhortation that: "She ought always to remember that she is the first and the last, the Alpha and the Omega, in the government of her establishment . . . She is, therefore, a person of far more importance in a community than she usually thinks she is" (239).[3] Burgos's and Pardo Bazán's cookbooks follow the model of an encyclopedic text with a pedagogical focus, seeking to charge their readers with a sense of mission that elevates the supposedly simple preparation of meals to part of a greater social movement. The key to deciphering the prescriptive code of a cookbook is to take note of the cohesive message of the recipes, the overarching guidance, and the audience of the book.

Cookbooks, as considered by scholars including Edvige Giunta, Carol Gold, María Paz Moreno, Jessamyn Neuhaus, Louise DeSalvo, and Janet Theophano, have been established as rich modes of understanding women's lives and livelihoods. Their consensus is that if we look beyond the recipes and into the author, the style, and take into account the historical and social context of the text, there is much to be learned. Janet Theophano, a professor of foodways in the United States,[4] asserts that "There is much to be learned from reading a cookbook besides how to prepare food—discovering the stories told in the spaces between the recipes or within the recipes themselves" (6). Cookbooks written by women are not merely listed collections of domestic knowledge. Rather, they serve as vehicles for women to express their voices, assert their individuality and build community. Initially, these domestic texts would have been produced in the home and only shared among family members or close friends. However, with the rise of the publishing industry and some increase in both female writers and readers, these texts enjoyed wider distribution and, by extension, had the potential to reinforce current social rules or to establish new ones (Floyd and Forster 4).

Food and its preparation are an opportunity for self-expression and individuality, something not found within the majority of the standard domestic tasks assigned to women in the domestic economy: "Unlike many other domestic chores, cooking offers opportunity for creative expression, for experimentation, and public and private appreciation" (Neuhaus 2). There can be a pleasure to cooking that may be reflected in cookbooks. Within a patriarchal culture such as the Italian American community considered by DeSalvo and Giunta, "providing food is the only kind of power women are permitted to employ" (8). Given what we know about the social structure of early twentieth-century Spain, this likely holds true for Burgos's and Pardo Bazán's readers as well. Furthermore, cooking provides an opportunity for women to distinguish themselves in their establishment of signature dishes, family preferences, and the variety of her skills. Developing a personal repertoire and sharing dishes within one's community contributes to both individual and collective identities: "People articulate and recognize their distinctiveness through the medium of food" (Counihan 7). Above all, the distribution of and the information within cookbooks offer insights into women's daily lives in a way that few other texts can. As Theophano explains, "Cookbooks are celebrations of identity. Connections to people, places, and the past are embedded in the recipes women kept and exchanged, transformed and adapted to their changing world" (8). Thus a cookbook shows the suggested parameters of a woman's role within her home and her greater community. It also gives a contemporary reader a sense of the challenges that the original readers navigated as they managed their homes and sought to shape their individual identities.

Given their richness in defining culture, the question remains of why these domestic texts have not been readily studied by literary scholars, even in the current academic environment that encourages a wider breadth of avenues of discovery. In part, their pertinence to daily life works against them. These texts are dismissed for being too accessible, too present. Women who may not have read Burgos's or Pardo Bazán's fiction or scholarly essays may have had their cookbooks on their shelves. When Burgos's works were censored under the Franco dictatorship, her cookbooks and domestic manuals were not pulled from circulation. Even at that juncture, they were simply overlooked: what progressive danger could there be in a cookbook?

Cookbooks may not tell us what people actually ate, but they can tell us about household size, ingredient availability and sample menus based on proportions and other instruction (Gold, *Danish* 12). Cookbooks provide a bridge from the high literature of the canon to the repetition of the ordinary. This is fundamental to a complete comprehension of any culture for, "The daily life of ordinary people is not only worthy of study but necessary to any understanding of past and present worlds" (Avakian 16). Hazel Gold has addressed why in Hispanist studies scholars have largely overlooked these domestic texts: first, there is the marginalization from the canon of popular genres that display obvious feminine character, including magazines by and for women, conduct manuals and domestic manuals—meaning anything that deals primarily with the home and/or the family. Second, there is the tendency to privilege narrative texts over those texts like cookbooks that have an encyclopedic structure; this is a reflection of what is considered to be a part of the literary canon and what is not. Third, in the specific case of Emilia Pardo Bazán, there is the difficulty of reconciling the image of her as a tireless defender of women's rights while participating in a supposed angel of the hearth discourse as she edits cookbook editions (313).

This line of thinking, where we ignore or generally discredit works that don't support the progressive image that we wish our first-wave feminists to have, is counterproductive. By ignoring these texts, we risk missing out on an encapsulation of how practical feminism was (or was not) being presented to everyday women in Spain. In the case of Carmen de Burgos, her cookbooks are consistent with her feminist notion of reform. By writing a cookbook Burgos shows that a woman can have a variety of interests; why shouldn't she publish both edited texts examining divorce and domestic manuals for women, full-length novels and beauty guides? Burgos's notion of feminism sought to incorporate domestic family life with the possibility of outside interests and even professional aspirations. All of her published texts contribute to her overarching mission of desiring to educate women and to by breaking the code of ignorance that had long been the status quo of women of the middle and upper social classes in Spain. She wants her readers to understand the meaning behind what they do on a daily basis. Indeed, she first wants women to question the world around them with the hope that this questioning will lead them in pursuit of the reasons. Pardo Bazán also has an educational focus, though hers places greater emphasis on the strengths of Spain's culinary traditions. As cited above, her cookbooks were published as part of the *Biblioteca de la mujer* series, which had initially been devoted to educating Spanish women about European trends in feminism and other progressive political movements. While she presented the publication of her cookbooks as evidence of the failure of feminism in Spain, she persisted in offering social reforms. Her insistence on the existence of a Spanish cuisine is a strong message about the need for a national culinary identity based on the strengths of Spain's culinary tradition.

Additionally, publishing their own cookbooks constitutes an act of gender subversion on the part of Pardo Bazán and Burgos. Between 1880 and 1920 the best-known cooking manuals in Spain were all written and published by professional chefs such as Ignacio Doménech and Teodoro Baradají. With the publication of their own cookbooks, Burgos and Pardo Bazán challenged the status quo that only men are permitted to speak with authority about the act of cooking. Women should only speak to other women about the domestic space. The publishing of these texts sought to dismantle the *ángel del hogar* [angel of the hearth] discourse that activists like Burgos and Pardo Bazán rallied against at the beginning of the twentieth century. To clarify, the concept of the *ángel del hogar* refers to an idealized domesticity where the woman best serves her community as a wife and a mother. She is the proverbial and literal heart of her family and is to do her best to ensure that the domestic space is a refuge and haven for her family from the demands and discomfort of the outside world. The women's entire realm consists of the domestic space; this is to be enough for her. This was a new role for women that spread throughout Western Europe in the nineteenth century, facilitated in large part by the rise of the middle class and the sharp increase in urban populations.

The greater a woman's leisure and lack of profit-making activities were, the greater the social status of her family. Within these parameters, women are effectively eliminated from the economy of production (Labanyi 34–39, Nash 27–28). This notion of the angel of the hearth is encompassed within a gender discourse that came to define social expectations of male and female roles in late nineteenth-century Spain. Mary Nash explains that for Spain, as well as the rest of Western Europe and North America, "This model of good mothering and housewifery—the product of male thought—generated the notion that women's ambitions had to be exclusively limited to home and family. Motherhood figured as the maximum horizon for women's self-fulfillment and social role. Women's cultural identity was shaped through marriage and motherhood to the exclusion of any other social or professional undertakings" (27). Burgos and Pardo Bazán question this status quo in the many textual formats available to them, which allows them to participate in a feminist dialogue about the status quo. Simply put, "Feminism is the name given to a comprehensive critical response to the deliberate and systematic subordination of women as a group by men within a given cultural setting" (Offen 20). Since the preparation of food for the family and the care and decoration of the domestic realm have been considered women's work throughout the nineteenth and twentieth centuries, it seems unlikely to stake a claim for women's independence within this realm. Yet this is precisely what Pardo Bazán and Burgos strive to do with their culinary texts. It is a complex balance of power between women and food, for it can result in being both an empowering and a disempowering aspect of women's lives depending on the approach (Forster 147).

It may seem a bold claim that a cookbook could dismantle a domestic discourse, yet both Burgos's and Pardo Bazán's cookbooks seek to do so. Through their presentation of strong opinions, detailed technical information, a bit of science, and an awareness of broader trends throughout the Iberian Peninsula and beyond its borders, both writers challenge the status quo and seek to stir the pot, as it were, well beyond the instructions in their recipes.

As already stated, Pardo Bazán's cookbooks are part of her *Biblioteca de la mujer*. This is an eleven-volume series that began in 1892 with the purpose of introducing Spanish women to ideas about feminism that were circulating throughout the rest of Europe. In the prologue to *La cocina española antigua* Pardo Bazán presents reasons why she chose to write a cookbook. She laments that there is little interest in feminism in Spain and so she decided to use her press to pursue other topics that may be useful to women. She states, "Puesto que la opinión sigue relegando a la mujer a las faenas caseras, me propuse enriquecer la Sección de la Economía Doméstica con varias obras que pueden ser útiles, contribuyendo a que la casa esté bien arreglada y regida" / "Since public opinion continues to push women into domestic chores, I proposed that I might enrich the School of Home Economics with various works that can be useful, contributing to a well-established and well-governed home" (ii). She is also motivated to write this cookbook as an effort to preserve dishes that she has enjoyed since childhood and are traditions within her family. She acknowledges the fact that some readers may be surprised to find her writing a cookbook since her studies are usually "más habituales en el otro sexo" / "more typical of the opposite sex" (ii), but she defends her interest in Spanish cooking since "La cocina, además, es, en mi entender, uno de los documentos etnográficos importantes" / "Cooking, furthermore, is, in my understanding, among the important ethnographic documents" (iii). The dishes of Spain have a history along with its government, its literature, its art, and its very people.

It is no accident that Pardo Bazán used this first of her two cookbooks to explore the history of Spanish cooking. This allows her to establish "the centrality of cuisine as a national discourse" (Ingram "Popular Tradition" 264). Rebecca Ingram has poignantly noted the frequency with which Pardo Bazán employs the possessive "nuestra" [our] both in reference to the culinary traditions and the specific national and regional dishes of Spain and its people (265). The shared experience of these foodstuffs, their preparation, as well as their flavors, evokes Benedict Anderson's notion of a shared national community (Anderson 1991). Pardo Bazán legitimizes both her own writing of a cookbook and the preparation efforts of her readers with her choice of inclusive vocabulary: "In these ways, she asserts the centrality of cooking to the national imagination and the canonical importance of her own volume" (Ingram 265). A challenge to the establishment of a shared identity is the ephemeral nature of any given meal. Collecting and writing the recipes into existence creates a permanence that each prepared dish cannot achieve. By writing down and organizing these 583 recipes into nine different sections, those of her family traditions and those of the many regions of Spain, Pardo Bazán defines the foundation of the Spanish diet. This cookbook does not contain recipes for other household items such as soaps or elixirs, as was common at the time. Instead, Pardo Bazán sets this text apart from other cookbooks, especially those authored by women, as a tool for understanding Spain's history: "Hay platos de nuestra cocina nacional que no son menos curiosos ni menos históricos que una medalla, un arma o un sepulcro" / "There are dishes of our national cuisine that are no less worthy of attention nor less historical than a medal, a weapon or a tomb" (iii). Knowing its dishes is a valid and important way of knowing Spain. Pardo Bazán' text provides access to that knowledge.

Pardo Bazán thus clearly views her cookbook as much more than a collection of recipes destined to satisfy the nutritional needs of one's family. She seeks to teach her intended audience, who for this text are women of the upper and middle classes, about their national cuisine. While she praises the virtues of the cooking "pueblo" [common folk], her target audience is of the higher social strata. "The *pueblo* is only relevant to the liberal national project when it is idealized and when its practices are converted to texts. In her discussion of the words that are used to describe foods in Spain . . . she signals that *cocina* itself is a philological project in addition to a folkloric one. Consequently, a different group of people will have the key role in practising the cooking that is significant to the nation . . . emerging or established middle-class women" (Ingram 269). Pardo Bazán extols the virtues of Spanish cuisine and cooking methods as a way of solidifying and promoting a national identity. She returns to this argument several times in the prologues of both of her cookbooks as well as in the included recipes. Pardo Bazán's call to aspiring cooks is one of patriotic pride: "La cocina española puede alabarse de sus sabores fuertes y claros, sin ambigüedad de salsas y de aderezos; de su pintoresca variedad según las regiones; de su perfecta adaptación al clima y a las necesidades del hombre" / "Spanish cooking can boast of its strong and simple flavors, without the ambiguity of sauces and dressings; of its picturesque variety among each of its regions; of its perfect modification to the climate and to the needs of each person" (*La cocina española antigua* v). For Pardo Bazán, Spanish cooking unifies the disparate people of the Iberian Peninsula through its simplicity and accommodating nature. She tells her readers that they should feel free to dabble in foreign cooking methods, but that they should always do so with a Spanish flair. Pardo Bazán is delightfully direct in her instructions, whether for individual dishes or her readers' general mindset as they undertake meal preparation. What is prepared and eaten should not be accidental: "La base de nuestra mesa tiene siempre que ser nacional. La mayoría de los platos extranjeros pueden hacerse a nuestro modo; no diré que metidos en la faena de adaptarlos no hayamos estropeado alguno; en cambio, a otros (y citaré para ejemplo las croquetas), los hemos mejorado en tercio y quinto" / "The fundamental basis of our table must always be national. The majority of foreign dishes can be made in our own style; I don't claim that when placed in the task of adapting them that we won't sometimes have missteps; however, for others (and I cite as an example croquettes), we have improved them in spades" (*La cocina moderna española* i). Pardo Bazán's assertion of Spanish culinary superiority continues throughout the presentation of the recipes themselves. For example, in her recipe of "Sopa a la marinera" [Sailor's Soup] she states "Y es mejor y más lógico que la *bouillabaisse* francesa, porque en ésta no se pone pescado dos veces y se desustancia todo el que se puso" / "And it is better and makes more sense than French bouillabaisse because in this recipe one doesn't add fish twice and turn everything that you've added into mush" (*La cocina española antigua* 30).

Pardo Bazán's style of writing is chatty with frequent asides, stories of how she procured certain recipes, endorsements such as "manjar superior" [superior delicacy], and criticisms (most notably of *langosta a la catalana* [Catalan style lobster] by the renowned chef Ignacio Doménech, an open critic of both Pardo Bazán and Burgos in the press). It feels as if she's looking over her readers' shoulder as they undertake her cooking challenges. The most noteworthy aspect of her writing style is that she feels free to express her opinions, offer improvements, and chastise practices that she feels are inappropriate. For example, at the end of the recipe for *Pájaros fritos de Madrid* [Fried birds of Madrid] she states, "La caza de estos pajaritos debiera estar prohibida. Son tan bonitos y tan útiles, que da pena verlos llegar ensartados y muertos. La agricultura pierde mucho con la persecución de los pajaritos, que viven de insectos, larvas y gusanos" / "The hunting of these little birds ought to be forbidden. They are so pretty and useful that it pains one to see them arrive strung up and dead. Agriculture suffers with the persecution of these birds, which feed on insects, larvae, and worms" (223–4). For the sake of completeness, she elects to include this recipe as a part of the official record of traditional dishes of Spain, but she makes it clear that it is not appropriate to either make or consume it. For the long-term sustainability of food production, this dish is simply counterproductive as its production undermines the agricultural practices on which the Spanish people depend for their top-notch ingredients. Other dishes featured in the text for the sake of reviewing the canon of Spanish food history, but then promptly dismissed are: *Sopa de fideos* [Noodle soup], which is "vulgar y trivial" / "tasteless and trite" (29) or *Manteca de ajo* [Garlic butter], which "Tiene sus partidarios, y en España son innumerables. Los graves inconvenientes de este condimento no se reducen al mal olor que comunica al aliento, ni al carácter villanesco . . . Su acción irritante es indiscutible" / "It has its supporters and in Spain they are numerous. The serious disadvantages of this condiment cannot be reduced to the bad odor that it gives to the breath nor to its peasant-like personality . . . Its irritating effect is undeniable" (370). The pejorative dismissal of this condiment as being "peasant-like" dismisses the *pueblo* while it supports the earlier discussion of her target audience of the middle class for shaping the national cuisine of Spain.

Not all of Pardo Bazán's strong commentaries are negative. Throughout the recipes she makes suggestions for personal adaptations and advises her cooks to consider their preferences. For example, "Salsa de perejil—Hay quien le pone un diente de ajo, no es de rigor, a menos que guste" / "Parsley sauce—There are those who add a clove of garlic, it is not essential, unless one likes it" (360). Furthering her national pride of Spanish cuisine, she extols the contributions Spaniards have made to certain categories of dishes, such as the way the *tortilla* has enriched the reputation of egg dishes worldwide. To make clear which dishes in the historical collection have her approval for preparation and consumption, she indicates with an asterisk in the index all the recipes that have been tried, presumably by her. This mode of concluding the text reinforces Pardo Bazán's authority for this text. By highlighting certain recipes with an asterisk, it prioritizes them, attributing a positive value that affirms their part in the national cuisine canon that the other dishes lack.

Carmen de Burgos's cookbooks were also directed to the rising and current middle-class women of Spain. The title of her second cooking text, *¿Quiere Ud. comer bien?* intends for the reader to think about the desired results of time spent in the kitchen. Surely the answer to the question must be yes and so Burgos dedicates the text, as stated earlier, as an "Obra indispensable para cocineras y para las señoras que deseen intervenir en la cocina y en la dirección de la casa." She then outlines the wisdom contained in the volume as, "Contiene, explicado en forma clara y precisa, todo cuanto se refiere a la cocina y al servicio doméstico y una multitud de recetas para hacer toda clase de platos, desde los más sencillos hasta los más exquisitos y complicados" / "An indispensable text for cooks and for those women who wish to take part in the kitchen and in the management of their homes. It contains, explained in a clear and precise fashion, everything that has to do with the kitchen and with domestic service and a multitude of recipes to make all sorts of dishes, from the simplest to the most exquisite and complicated" (title page). The title page also announces the fact that there are numerous illustrations, both black and white and also a dozen "cromotipias" that are in color. These color pictures show elaborate table settings, identify cuts of meat, and illustrate the results of the most complicated recipes. Their presence lends a visual orientation to Burgos's text that enriches her educational efforts. There are no such pictures in Pardo Bazán's cookbooks.

Beginning with precisely the instructional guidance that a novice cook or housewife would need, the text leads with a discussion of the layout of the kitchen itself: "La cocina es el laboratorio doméstico donde se preparan los alimentos, y debe reunir en lo posible todas las condiciones de comodidad, de salubridad y de economía deseables" / "The kitchen is the domestic laboratory where foodstuffs are prepared and all desired modes of convenience, good health, and economy possible should be brought together in it" (5). Burgos's prologue sets the stage for a book that is designed to empower women in their undertaking of domestic matters. It casts the woman as the caretaker who can and will make the decisions as to what is best for her family. In this light, Burgos also includes recipes for medicinal products, as is traditional of cookbooks of the eighteenth and nineteenth centuries, when these texts were thought of as repositories of all necessary domestic knowledge. Burgos also details modes of preparing specific dishes for children, the elderly, and the infirm. Burgos includes extensive information regarding the nutritional value and digestive time required for a number of foods, subjects that would be covered in a home economics course. Burgos was an outspoken advocate for domestic-training schools, after having visited several of them on her state-sponsored tour of western European educational systems. These schools would provide women with useful educations in accounting, hygiene, food science, and other necessary skills for running a home. There is nothing inherently female about managing a household; women required training to be able to do so well.[5]

Burgos's emphasis on education and explanation was in line with her strong ties to Krausism. This philosophical movement was popular with Spanish liberal activists, and emphasized education, through improved literacy and direct instruction, as the key to modernizing Spain. It was a grassroots movement that sought to empower the individual. The woman—most commonly the mother—has great potential, for she was the primary guide to future citizens: "This social model meant that the mother was responsible for teaching future citizens to put group interest before their own, with the family seen as the blueprint for the social organism as a whole: The mother's private role is thus not so private after all" (Labanyi 60). In other words, a shaping of the culture of the new urban middle-class woman could be something that evolved rather than something fixed by the Victorian-inspired ideals of feminine domesticity.

Burgos's cookbook is designed for a woman with a hands-on role in her household and someone who is open to advice from experts; she is ready to learn. While the relegation of women to the kitchen may seem to be a detour from Burgos's usual feminist stance, her domestic discourse is tinged with subversive undertones, much like her melo-dramatic fictional works. She places women in a position of power as the managers of their own homes. Notably, she does so from a position of authority. On the title page of *La cocina moderna* she is identified as a[n] "profesora de esta asignatura en la escuela de artes e industrias de Madrid" / "instructor of this subject at the Madrid school of art and industry" (title page). She is not merely a woman writing about cooking, but rather she is a professional in the field, just like Ignacio Doménech or any respected male food writer.

In order to educate and empower her readers, she provides a broad cultural scope. In the introduction of *La cocina moderna*, Burgos details the history of feasting and banqueting in the western world as well as the innovators who created some well-known dishes, such as Louis the XVI and his prowess with the potato (11). She lists a number of regents who either cooked or were familiar with culinary matters, including Queens Alexandra and Victoria of England and the Empress of Germany (12). This is a way of elevating the task of cooking and empowering her readers. They must view this domestic task as one of high importance: "Her framing of the commonalities between her readers and powerful women opens a space for understanding women's cooking labor in their homes as relevant to the public sphere. In this way she deconstructs the binary between cooking as a private-sphere practice and its public-sphere socio-political impact" (Ingram "Bringing the *escuela* to the *despensa*" 189).

In contrast to Pardo Bazán's peninsular cuisine preferences, Burgos, with little fanfare, includes recipes from all over the world in all of her cooking manuals. A few items, such as *salsa de menta* [mint sauce], receive a bit of additional context, namely that it is popular in London (¿*Quiere Ud. comer bien?* 91). Burgos includes recipes for *sopa a la francesa* [French soup], *sopa a la alemana* [German soup], and *sopa holandesa* [Dutch soup] just after recipes for *cocido español* [Spanish stew], *cocido catalán* [Catalan stew], *pote gallego* [Galician broth], and *olla de berza* [collard greens stew] with no further introduction (63–4, 76–7). She presents them as if they are part of a normal Spanish diet and, as such, require no additional orientation. Other international dishes of note include *salsa india de currié* [Indian curry sauce] (90), *foies gras* [foie gras] (153), *kouscoussou* [cous cous], presented as an Algerian and Turkish dish (107), and the noted Italian dish of raviolis (105). In total, she includes recipes from over 20 countries, including Poland, Turkey, Egypt, and Brazil, as well as featuring multiple regions of Spain[6]. These international recipes are published alongside traditional Spanish dishes: salted cod fish, *tortilla*, croquettes, and roasts, organized within general categories such as *Huevos* [Eggs], *Carne* [Meat], or *Pescado* [Fish] so that it is possible for her readers to contextualize unknown dishes among traditional favorites. This inclusion of international recipes is part of Burgos's sweeping educational efforts to broaden the scope of information available to Spanish women. Providing access to unfamiliar modes of cooking gives women an opportunity to expand their horizons. It is impossible to know the frequency with which Burgos's readers incorporated these dishes into their family menu plans. The key is not whether they were consumed, but rather that they provided access to trends beyond Spain's borders.

Burgos's and Pardo Bazán's publishing of cookbooks was a subversive act that is consistent with their overall reputations as feminist writers. Burgos's encouragement that her readers direct their households while expanding their families' palates and Pardo Bazán's nationalist view of cuisine and direct commentaries provide a vision of their proposed pathways to change. Their respective cookbooks introduce innovations that seek to empower women as a part of the post-1898 efforts to modernize Spain. Evaluating this experience allows for their inclusion within feminist criticism for, as Patricia Meyer Spacks states, "I take feminist criticism to include any mode that approaches a text with primary concern for the nature of the female experience in it—the fictional experience of characters, the deducible or imaginable experience of an author, the experience implicit in language and structure" (14). Reading these texts through the lens of gender offers insight regarding the female experience. Through this lens of reading, one can begin to comprehend the weight of Burgos's and Pardo Bazán's task. They are working to (re)shape their nation through their prescriptive advice as to what should be on the Spanish plate. These texts pertained to people's daily lives and repeated behaviors, something that could allow for them to have a tremendous amount of influence: "Writing about food was often just as engaged with the wider national project as were other more canonical forms of cultural production" (Anderson *Cooking Up the Nation* (5)). By embedding their subversive visions in "low" literature they sought to reach new audiences, and to pull Spanish society towards the modern era.

Notes

1   See Michelle Sharp, "Carmen de Burgos: Teaching Women of the Modern Age" in *Kiosk Literature of Silver Age Spain: Modernity and Mass Culture* eds. Jeffrey Zamostny and Susan Larson. Chicago: Intellect, 2017. for a discussion of the effect of these innovations in publishing on kiosk novelettes, in which Burgos first published the majority of her fictional works.

2   All translations are my own.

3   For a more in-depth consideration of Isabella Beeton's contributions to the development of the modern cookbook consult Michelle M. Sharp's chapter "La perfecta casada: Carmen de Burgos's New Feminine Feminist Perfection" in *Multiple Modernities: Carmen de Burgos, Author and Activist* (2017).

4   Foodways is defined by Collins English Dictionary as "the customs and traditions relating to food and its preparation. https://www.collinsdictionary.com/us/dictionary/english/foodways

5   For an analysis of Carmen de Burgos's domestic manuals as they pertain to her over-arching feminist notion of reform consult Michelle M. Sharp's chapter "La perfecta casada: Carmen de Burgos's New Feminine Feminist Perfection" in *Multiple Modernities: Carmen de Burgos, Author and Activist* (2017).

6   See Burgos's *Misión social de la mujer* (1911), *La protección y la higiene de los niños* (1904), and *La mujer moderna y sus derechos* (1927) for her explanations about the benefits of and need for domestic education schools.

7   SAs an example, in *¿Quiere Ud. comer bien?* Burgos includes four different recipes for gazpacho: *gazpacho, gazpacho extremeño* [Extremaduran gazpacho], *gazpacho granadino* [Grenadian gazpacho], and *gazpacho jerezano* [Jerez-style gazpacho] in the section for *Ensaladas* [Salads] (237–8).

Bibliography

Anderson, Benedict. *Imagined Communities*. London: Verso, 1991. Print.

Anderson, Lara Bernadette. *Cooking up the Nation: Spanish Culinary Texts and Culinary Nationalization in the Late Nineteenth and Early Twentieth Century*. Suffolk and Rochester: Tamesis, 2013. Print.

Avakian, Arlene and Barbara Haber. *From Betty Crocker to Feminist Food*

Studies: Critical Perspectives on Women and Food. Amherst: U of Massachusetts P, 2005. Print.

Beetham, Margaret. "Of Recipe Books and Reading in the Nineteenth Century: Mrs. Beeton and her Cultural Consequences." *The Recipe Reader: Narratives, Contexts, Traditions* Eds. Janet Floyd and Laura Forster. Aldershot England: Ashgate, 2003. 15–30. Print.

Burgos, Carmen de. *La cocina moderna*. Valencia: Prometeo Sociedad Editorial, 1906. Print.

—-. *¿Quiere Ud. comer bien?*. Barcelona: Sopena, 1916. Print.

Counihan, Carole M. *The Anthropology of Food and Body: Gender, Meaning and Power*. New York: Routledge, 1999. Print.

DeSalvo, Louise and Edvide Giunta. *The Milk of Almonds: Italian American Women Writers on Food and Culture*. New York: The Feminist Press at CUNY, 2003. Print.

Floyd, Janet and Laurel Forster. "The Recipe and its Cultural Contexts." *The Recipe Reader: Narratives, Contexts, Traditions*. Janet Floyd and Laura Forster, eds. Aldershot, England: Ashgate, 2003, pp. 1–14. Print.

Forster, Laurel. "Liberating the Recipe: A Study of the Relationship between Food and Feminism in the early 1970s." *The Recipe Reader: Narratives, Contexts, Traditions*. Janet Floyd and Laura Forster, eds. Aldershot, England: Ashgate, 2003, pp. 147-168. Print.

Gold, Carol. *Danish Cookbooks: Domesticity and National Identity 1616–1901*. Seattle: U of Washington P, 2007. Print.

Gold, Hazel. "Del foro al fogón: narrativas culturales en el discurso culinario de Emilia Pardo Bazán." *La literatura de Emilia Pardo Bazán*. Eds. José Manuel González Herrán, Cristina Patino Eirín,A Coruña: Ermitas Penas Varela Fundación Caixa Galicia, 2009. 313–323. Print.

Hughes, Kathryn. *The Short Life and Long Times of Mrs. Beeton: The First Domestic Goddess*. New York: Knopf, 2006. Print.

Ingram, Rebecca. "Bringing the *escuela* to the *despensa*." *Multiple Modernities: Carmen de Burgos, Author and Activist*. Anja Louis and Michelle M. Sharp, eds. New York: Taylor and Francis, 2017. Print.

—-. "Popular Tradition and Bourgeois Elegance in Emilia Pardo Bazán's *Cocina española*." *Bulletin of Hispanic Studies*. 91.3, 2014, pp. 261–274. Print.

Labanyi, Jo. *Gender and Modernization in the Spanish Realist Novel*. Oxford: Oxford UP, 2000. Print.

Moreno, María Paz. *De la página al plato: El libro de cocina en España*. Gijón: Trea, 2011. Print.

Nash, Mary. "Un/Contested Identities: Motherhood, Sex Reform and Modernization of Gender Identity in Early Twentieth-Century Spain." *Constructing Spanish Womanhood: Female Identity in Modern Spain*. Eds. Victoria Lorée Endres and Pamela Beth Radcliff. Albany: SUNY P, 1999. 25-49. Print.

Neuhaus, Jessamyn. *Manly Meals and Mom's Home Cooking: Cookbooks and Gender in Modern America*. Baltimore: Johns Hopkins UP, 2003. Print.

Offen, Karen. *European Feminisms 1700–1950: A Political History*. Palo Alto, CA: Stanford UP, 2000. Print.

Pardo Bazán, Emilia. *La cocina española antigua*. Biblioteca de la mujer. Madrid: Ediciones Poniente, 1913. Print.

—. *La cocina española moderna*. Blblioteca de la mujer. Madrid: Sociedad Anónomia Renacimiento, 1917. Print.

Spacks, Patricia Meyer. *The Female Imagination*. New York: Knopf, 1975. Print.

Theophano, Janet. *Eat My Words: Reading Women's Lives through the Cookbooks They Wrote*. New York: Palgrave, 2002. Print.

5

Linking & Selling Sustenance & Space: Wine Labels in Spain

KIMBERLY HABEGGER

The wine-producing areas of northern Spain are becoming increasingly celebrated, not only for their wine but for the innovative architecture of the wineries designed and built during the last two decades. These structures are designed by the world's most renowned architects and incorporate aesthetics and technology in inspired and efficient ways.

The image of the winery is a common feature portrayed on the labels of wine bottles throughout the wine-producing world. Consider the model of the labels from Bordeaux that most often feature the *Chateâu* rendered in a detailed, representational sketch in black and white. Complementing the effort to promote wine and wine-tourism through the construction of iconic *bodegas* in Spain, the bottle labels offer the vineyards an additional opportunity to reference the architecture and to emphasize the wineries' prestige as the labels showcase structures of some critical acclaim. In additional instances, the label reflects different facets of the wine tourist experience other than the remarkable architecture, as we shall see.

As the architecture of the *bodegas* is contemporary, so are a number of the visual representations depicted on the labels. Not limited to the constraints of figurative representation, the label images evoke the architecture in more stylized, suggestive and symbolic ways. The traditional depiction of the façade is often abandoned in favor of alternative perspectives: aerial perspectives of the building and the grounds, the elaboration of an architectural detail or the adaptation of early architectural sketches. And the techniques used on the label are not limited to ink on a square paper label, as the label itself may take a shape that is suggestive of the architecture. This study will analyze the buildings and the labels they inspired in order to describe how the printed images evoke and interpret the original architectural structure. The wineries will be from the acclaimed wine-producing regions of Rioja and Ribera del Duero.

Bodegas Portia. Norman Foster. (Foster + Partners) for the Faustino Group. Gumiel de Izán.

Just to the north of Aranda de Duero in the Ribera del Duero wine area lies Norman Foster's Bodegas Portia, built in 2007. The unique trefoil plan of the bodega reflects the three principal processes of wine creation: fermentation in steel vats; ageing in oak barrels; and storage and refinement in the bottle. For the architect, the project provided "an opportunity to look afresh at the building type, using the natural topography of the site to aid in the winemaking process and create the optimum working conditions, while reducing the building's energy demands and its visual impact on the landscape" (Foster's 1). The three wings are controlled by an operations hub at the core and the barrels and bottle wings are partly embedded in the ground to produce cellar conditions. In contrast, the fermentation wing is exposed allowing carbon dioxide to be released. A road rises to the roof of the building allowing tractors to directly deposit harvested grapes straight into the hopper. Gravity aids in the movement of the grapes within the building maximizing efficiency and minimizing damage to the grapes (2).

Nieves Caballero of the daily, *El Norte de Castilla,* notes that the trefoil design has been described in different ways: by the bodega as a three-pointed star and as a flower with three petals with a center— as Foster himself proposed. Nevertheless, Foster also describes the impact of the design in more dynamic terms: "the building has a strong, masculine and muscular form" (Fuerte). The concrete building is clad in shingles of Corten steel and the deep overhang of the roof canopy provides shade. The partial embedding of the structure, the photovoltaic cells of the roof and the thermal mass of the concrete combine to control interior temperatures. At the center of the bodega, a raised public galley extends into glazed mezzanine areas that project deep into each wing allowing visitors to enjoy elevated views of the three processes. Public areas are lined with deep-stained old wine barrel slats to evoke the tradition of winemaking in Ribera del Duero (Foster's 3–4). As the building's form references the winemaking process, so do the materials of the structure to include fermentation with the steel, barrel ageing with the oak and the bottle ageing with the glass (Caballero Fuerte in Habegger *Architecture*)

Consider the label designed for the Triennia vintage made by the Grupo Faustino at Bodegas Portia. Both the name of the special vintage (a limited production of 3000 bottles of 100% tempranillo aged in French oak for 18 months) and the graphic image reproduced on the bottle refer to the trefoil design of Foster's structure.

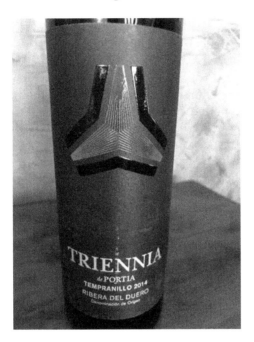

In the label's design, there is no attempt at representational imagery; instead an aerial view of the *bodega* is reduced to the basic shape of a triangle. The red interior of this triangle appears to reference the wine and the slight inward curves to the sides of the triangle approximate the curves of the walls of Portia as seen in the plan. The stylization of the architectural image harmonizes with the clean lines and the emphasis on efficiency and function of the architectural structure. This graphic image is easily decipherable by those familiar with the physical traits of the winery, yet stylized to the point that the uninitiated would not recognize the image/building association.

Marqués de Riscal. Ciudad del Vino, Frank O. Gehry. Elciego, La Rioja.

As noted by the local daily, *Diario La Rioja*, when visitors approach the hotel and vineyard from the town of Cenicero, the hotel has the appearance of what has been described as a medieval castle; arriving from the opposite direction of Laguardia, the site amazes visitors as it suddenly appears after having been obscured by the narrow winding roads of the village (Un Gehry 1).

Frank Gehry's hotel and the church tower frame the town of Elciego and, as the project architect Edwin Chan notes about the hotel, "it was important to have an identity of its own but it must also have a conversation with the surrounding historic properties" (Bold 3). This conversation meant playing off the steeple of Elciego's church; the curved titanium roof is intended to create symmetry with the steep roofline of the church. The hotel, inaugurated in October of 2006, coexists with both the town and the historic structures of the *bodega*. *The Wall Street Journal* notes that the angular sandstone foundation of the hotel blends with those of the century-old surrounding buildings of the winery and the landscaped garden beds that connect the different structures (Bold 2). Admirers consider the juxtaposition of new and old a success that recognizes its environment and they praise the originality and drama of the hotel; detractors question the appropriateness of the hotel competing with the traditional focal point of this and most other Spanish villages, the church. The prevailing opinion is a positive one, as portrayed in the cover photo of a 2008 edition of *Wine Spectator* that contains photos and an article on the wines, food and architecture of Rioja. The photograph features the dramatic interplay of the two buildings: the brightly illuminated church and hotel stand out against the soft natural light of the town in a harmonious yet vivid composition (DeSimone).

In addition to the building's relationship with its surroundings, the symbolic qualities of the structure are prominent. According to the architect, the building imitates an animal in movement over the fields in a festive, exciting expression, as wine itself (Un Gehry 1). The iconic curved titanium roof is said to mimic wine flowing from a bottle and the rose, silver and gold colors of the titanium sheets reference the classic wine bottle produced at this facility: rose for the wine, gold for the wire *malla* or mesh wrapped around the bottle and silver for the capsule. This understanding of the building allows the viewer to consider the hotel "architecture," according to Nelson Goodman's constructs. As per Goodman, a building that also has reference may be considered architecture. The Marqués de Riscal Hotel achieves reference through denotation: its suggestion of flowing wine satisfies the condition that this "building plus reference" is indeed architecture (Winters 84–85).

Although the exterior of the hotel is often photographed, well-publicized and critically evaluated, the interior has received less attention. Playing off Gehry's success with the Bilbao Guggenheim, this project is the most recognized of the winery structures in Spain today. Perhaps the denoted reference to flowing wine that so effortlessly leads the viewer to the connotative reference of wine consumption as a joyful and celebratory experience constitutes the essence of the acclaim (Habegger *Architecture*).

The prestigious Bodegas Marqués de Riscal has incorporated Gehry's architectural showcase to their label design in an innovative manner. One of Gehry's conceptual drawings of the hotel has been reproduced on a very select vintage: Vino Frank Gehry 2001. The exclusivity of the wine is connected directly to the stature of the hotel: the grapes are grown on vines that are a minimum of 40 years old, only 5000 bottles were blended, and the wine was aged for 22 months in barrels of new American oak. In 2001, the winery also produced vintages considered excellent throughout Rioja, thus augmenting the prestige of this vintage. Gehry's personal connection to the project is reflected on this bottle's label: he reportedly was convinced to accept the rather small-scale commission after he was offered a vintage from 1929, the year of his birth.

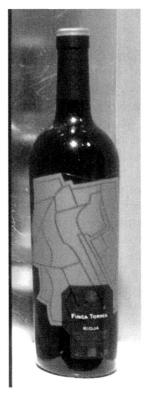

The unrestrained curves of the drawing insinuate the three-dimensional form of the final structure. The dark background of the label merges with the color of the wine itself thus creating the illusion of the wine flowing through the hotel image. Three colors of ink are applied to the drawing: white, gold and a rose-color which clearly connects to the colors of the titanium waves of the hotel and the colors' reference to the traditional values that coexist with innovation at the Marqués de Riscal (Marqués de Riscal).

Another vintage produced by the Marqués de Riscal, the Finca Torrea label design features what initially appears to be an abstract linear sketch. Yet, with further analysis, one discovers that it is actually an enlarged map of an area of the vineyard known as Finca Torre. Label designer Design Bridge explains how, for the Finca range, they blended Spain's ancient *terruño* with Google Earth images of the vineyards (Design Bridge). The winery's website summarizes the significance of the design: "the Finca de Torrea label "inspirándose en la línea del diseño marcada por el arquitecto Frank O. Gehry con el Hotel Marqués de Riscal/is inspired by the line of the design noted by the architect Frank O. Gehry with the Hotel Marqués de Riscal" (Marqués de Riscal) shows the connection between the Vino Frank Gehry and Finca Torrea labels.

Bodegas Ysios. Santiago Calatrava. Laguardia, La Rioja.

Bodegas Ysios by Santiago Calatrava is also located in the Rioja Alavesa, only a few kilometers from Elciego. A portmanteau formed from Isis and Osiris, the name pays homage to the Egyptian deities associated with wine. In his article on the architecture of wine publishing, Hugh Pearman acknowledges the importance of Bodegas Ysios as a destination in itself, the most successful "three-dimensional advertisement for its wine" (4). According to Pearman, "there is no question that [it is] the single most-published modern winery in the world, the one that no book or article on the subject could possibly afford to omit" (4). Although expressed while the Marqués de Riscal Hotel was still in under construction, Pearman's statement nevertheless indicates the importance of Ysios as an architectural destination today. The significance of Ysios is further illustrated by the fact that two books exploring the architecture of wineries feature Ysios on the cover (Richards, Webb). Books dedicated to the topic of the architecture of wineries not only in Spain but around the world, their authors selected Ysios to visually represent the content of their studies.

This building is the result of an investment by the giant firm Bebidas y Bodegas, the proprietor of 600 different labels. The 86,000 square-foot winery was constructed on the limited budget of $6 million. Its exterior materials include 85-foot laminated wood beams of Scandinavian fir, reflective aluminum sheeting for the roof, and horizontal strips of cedar on the south façade. The façade is accented by the addition of a reflecting pool with a mosaic border of ceramic tiles that runs the length of the building (Cohn Bodegas 242).

Certainly the most dramatic traits of the structure are its undulating north and south walls (in plan), the undulating roof line and the dramatic kick to the building's central curves so that the roof beams project an additional 33 feet into the air above the central entry (in elevation). This extra space is dedicated to an upper-level tasting room where guests can survey the view of the scenic village of Laguardia in the distance. The remainder of the interior is utilitarian in nature and consists of simple materials featuring the undulating walls and dramatic ceilings (242).

It is commonly noted that the *bodega* repeats the lines of the mountains that serve as its backdrop. The reflective nature of the aluminum and the colors of the wood complement the natural environment; the wood slats have been interpreted as homage to oak ageing barrels (Bold 2). David Cohn also notes that the building is in perfect alignment with the hilltop church of Laguardia (Cohn Bodegas 243), thus repeating the bodega/church relationship seen in Cenicero.

Comparisons with Gaudí's style are common: Pearman states that Ysios is as audacious as is the work of Gaudí (4) and the curvilinear mosaic reflecting pool seems to serve as a direct nod to Spain's most celebrated *modernista*. A writer for the *Wall Street Journal* compares the *bodega* to a modern cathedral (Bold 1). From this perspective, the dramatic exterior evokes the space that is the heart of many wineries: the cellar dedicated to the ageing of the most important vintages, also known as the cathedral. When viewed at some distance, the floating sculptural waves of Ysios manage to both harmonize with the natural environment and project a kind of transcendence (Habegger Architecture).

The label's representation of Calatrava's highly-acclaimed structure is a simple stylization of the overall façade of the winery. The most salient details are two curving lines running above and parallel to a horizontal line; a total of six waves suggest the distinctive curved roof line. In the center of the undulating lines, an arrowhead points upward, representing the gable of the grand, cathedral-like main entrance into the structure. Fine graphic details include small vertical lines within the arrowhead that appear to reference the glass window-

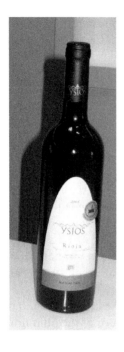
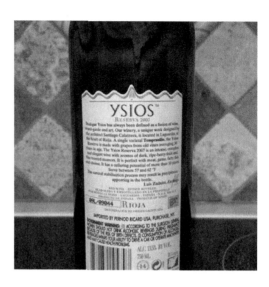

panes, allowing guests in the tasting room to survey the vineyards and the town of Laguardia. A more subtle detail still, a faint corner under the vertical lines suggests the upper-left-hand corner of the entrance. The horizontal line grounds the image, giving the viewer a sense of geographic orientation; other than this line, the image seems to represent only aspects of the architecture. However, the second undulating line could serve as a restrained representation of the striking rolling hills that serve as a backdrop to the architectural composition. The front label shape mimics that of the central arch of the "cathedral," while the label on the rear of the bottle places the representation of the entire structure on the upper edge of the label, which is cut out, following the wavy roof of the building.

Bodegas Viña Real (CVNE), vicinity of Laguardia, La Rioja.

On the top of the Cerro de a Mesa, just outside the town of Laguardia, one can easily view the Viña real de CVNE from the highway to Logroño and discern that the building is, in fact, a winery due to its unique, barrel-like form. Architect Phillipe Mazières originally hailed from Bordeaux (another connection to the French wine-growing region) and has worked on designed wineries in addition to Viña Real.

In 2006, the architect and his wife constructed and established a winery themselves, the Domaine de Collines, on the right bank of the Dordogne River.

The barrel section of the Viña Real facility (*nave de vinificación*) houses the vat fermentation area and the circular barrel-aging area immediately below; additional barrel-aging and bottle-aging occurs in two connected tunnels carved into the mountainside. The *nave de vinificación* is also connected to a bottling facility that links with a red-roofed warehousing structure. The reddish-brown color of the barrel structure, in contrast to the silvery steel of the other two edifices, reinforces the oak aging barrel reference. The winery's website declares that Viña Real "apuesta por la innovación y la experimentación/ committed to innovation and experimentation/" (Viña Real).

After passing through the main entrance featuring high ceilings that display offices that spiral upward from the nautilus-shaped reception desk, visitors proceed to the striking interior of the circular vinification area. The stainless-steel vats are placed in a large circle along the perimeter and the center consists of a Pantheon-like oculus supported by metal beams creating a lattice-like effect. Perfectly centered below the opening are eight slightly inclined pillars which serve as the base for the crane that transports the grapes into the top of the individual vats; the pillars also connect to and support the edges of the oculus. A more traditional detail is seen in the round wooden roof that features beams that radiate from the aperture to the periphery. The considerable volume and original architecture of this space impact visitors immediately upon entry.

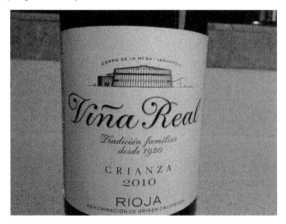

Gravity assists the transfer of the fermented grapes to the barrel aging area located directly below. Once more, the space is circular and the barrels are also positioned in a circular pattern. One barrel deep in the center of the space and four barrels deep around the circumference, the barrel placement allow expansive views of the aging area. The inclined cement pillars allude to those in the vat-fermentation area and their angle reminds visitors of the overall barrel-shape of the structure.

The labels of the different blends such as the acclaimed Imperial, vary. However, this example of a 2010 crianza does indeed feature the image of the iconic barrel silhouette of the bodega, a glimpse of the attached bottling and warehousing facilities and a profile view of the dramatic trellises. The clean, almost architectural style of rendering the winery contrasts with the labels we have seen for Portia, the Marqués de Riscal and Ysios, as these vineyards have opted for more stylized representations of their iconic architecture.

Bodegas Darien. Jesús Marino Pascual. Logroño, La Rioja.

While the winery is no longer in business, architect Jesús Marino Pascual built Bodegas Darien which is located several kilometers south of the urban center of Logroño. In contrast with the other architects of this study, Marino Pascual has designed a number of interesting wine projects in Spain (El Museo Dinastía Vivanco, el Centro de la Cultura del Rioja and Bodegas Antión). To some extent, the exterior of the structure resembles large, stacked rectangular boulders; the reference to the landscape is present while avoiding naturalistic representation. There is no single façade, "sino mil diferentes, dependiendo del punto geográfico desde el que se observe/rather a thousand different ones, depending on the geographic point from which it is observed" (Las bodegas Darien). The walkway guides visitors towards the entrance.

Similar to other new winery projects, the structure fulfills functions other than the processing, barrel aging and storage of bottled wine: a restaurant, workspaces, a tasting room, a convention hall and a museum are all located within the built volumes that allow natural light to flow through the interior and afford extraordinary views of the vineyards. The Museum of the History of Ceramics in Rioja features many wine vessels and containers traditionally used by *riojanos* to store and savor the fruits of the local harvests.

The incorporation of the architecture of Bodegas Darien into the design of the label is creatively achieved: the remarkable white volumes are referenced, not by designs printed on the labels, but by the design of the label itself. The label, in the shape of a trapezoid, gradually tapers inward from top to bottom (Bodegas Darien).

The background is black with white text and two wide white lines delineate the left and top edge of the trapezoidal label. A semi-circular indentation is cut into the top and extends from the middle to approximately 1.5 centimeters from the edge. The label itself is a representation of a detail of the structure—one of its striking architectural volumes. Black was chosen for the background of the label instead of the white of the exterior, yet the black blends with the background color of the glass as the white exterior of the building blends with the soil of the vineyards.

Bodegas Baigorri. Inaki Aspiau. Samaniego, La Rioja.

Recognized for its architecture in the San Francisco MOMA Museum exhibit, "How Wine Became Modern: Design and Wine From 1976 to Now," Bodegas Baigorri "es la arquitectura al servicio del vino/is architecture in the service of wine" (Martínez), according to Isabel Oliver, public relations director of the winery. Architect Inaki Aspiau teamed with winery owner Jesús Baigorri to design this "crystal box" at the foot of the Cantabrian Range in Samaniego. The most distinctive architectural trait of this structure is the ground floor called the "mirador" that allows unsurpassed 360-degree views of the surrounding countryside to include rolling fields of vine and spectacular mountains. The structure is embraced by reflecting pools that duplicate the glass structure and the magnificent environment. This detail not only adds an air of tranquility, it has a practical function as it can be used as a source of water in case of fire (Gosález 2). As do many of the new *bodegas*, Baigorri has been built to allow gravity to facilitate the grapes' movement from the harvest to aging barrels. Jesús Baigorri recognizes the role of the building's design: "la arquitectura es parte del proceso/architecture is part of the process" (Gosález 2). The design here clearly reflects Louis Sullivan's maxim of "form follows function." The seven floors below the 400-square meter *mirador* are terraced into the slope of the hill, each housing a different phase of the wine making process. The rear elevation of the structure recalls that of a Mayan pyramid.

Despite the initial peaceful impressions of the entire structure, there are many spaces in the winery to accommodate various activities in addition to wine production. Besides the *mirador*, the structure houses a restaurant, a shop, a multi-use room and a tasting room. These multiple spaces offer guests an opportunity to experience the wines of Baigorri in various pleasurable ways. Visitors to the winery follow the route of the grapes as they descend from the top of the structure to

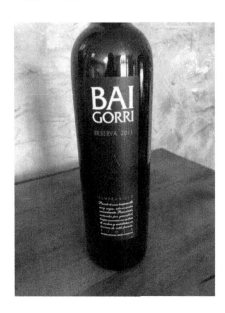

where the wine is fermented to the ageing cellars. This progression can be observed from both the interior and the exterior of the winery, thanks to a sidewalk that allows tourists to observe the different processes from the outdoors. Oliver of Baigorri observes that for tourists this "es un viaje graviatorio que merece mucho la pena en vendimia/is a trip in tracing the vintage that is very much worth the effort" (Martínez). The environment surrounding the winery is remarkably pastoral, even compared to that of other vineyards in the area and the *mirador* maximizes and integrates the beauty of nature into the structure. The minimalism of the Baigorri label may be said to reflect the simplicity of the edifice. The black rectangular label, free of excessive text, suggests the powerful rectangles of the *mirador,* the dominant flat roof and the surrounding reflecting pools. While the architecture is not directly referenced in the label, the strong lines of the rectangular   structure are insinuated in the simplicity, in the shape and by the color of the label itself.

Dinastía Vivanco

Much has been said of the importance of the Dinastía Vivanco in Briones in Rioja (Habegger, *Spain's Wine Museums* 5–8). The building is admirable for the creative architecture employed by architect Jesús Marino Pascual—but the truly significant aspect of this building is that it houses el Museo de la Cultura de Vino, a world-class wine museum that explores wine-making processes and the ways in which art has reflected the role of wine in different cultures. The extraordinary art collection includes works ranging from antiquity to still lifes by twentieth-century artistic geniuses such as Picasso.

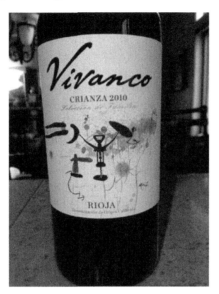

These two labels of their most-available wines (the *crianza* and the *reserva*) reference this art collection, that is to say, they allude to what is housed in the structure (apart from the wine itself) instead of the physical edifice. The *crianza* label appears to be inspired by the work of Joan Miró while the *reserva* label recalls the work of Juan Gris. While the compelling architecture of wineries in Spain is a major draw for tourists, in the case of Dinastía Vivanco, the exceptional Museo lures tourists to the winery, in additional to exceptional architecture, fabulous gardens and a highly-acclaimed restaurant.

Conclusions

Given the considerable effort and expenses incurred both by the *bodegas* and the local governments, it seems only natural that these extraordinary wineries are used to their maximum advantage. Originally conceived of as a manner to promote *enoturismo* and to raise the perceived value of local wines, this iconic architecture can also serve to promote the wines to those who have no direct knowledge of the structures. While Ysios and Portia feature stylized images of the entire building on the label, the Marqués de Riscal prints an early conceptual drawing on their special vintage and Darien constructs a label that suggests a detail of the building that blends into the surroundings. Dinastía Vivanco visually interprets the contents of the interior of their remarkable museum instead of focusing on the exterior architecture itself, while Viña Real presents a simple representation of the exterior. The connection between label and architecture in the Baigorri example relies on the commonalities of simplicity, boldness and the impact of the rectangular shape.

These unique labels are limited to only special vintages in the cases of Portia and Marqués de Riscal, while Ysios and Darien have employed them regularly. Nevertheless, it is interesting to note that a considerable number of other Spanish *bodegas* that have invested in iconic architecture, e.g., Aalto, Martín Berdugo, López de Heredia, have not, as yet, incorporated images of their recent architecture into the label design. Another spectacular winery, Protos, incorporates a drawing of the facility only on the bottle of their *crianza*.

In the cases studied here, the wine label itself has reinterpreted the building in a manner that parallels the creativity of the architecture of the *bodega*. Arguably, innovative architecture is best represented by such stylized images evoking the complexity of the multiple meanings of the architecture itself and the many nuances of wine consumption. The reinterpretation of iconic architecture by such open imagery enhances Humberto Eco's concept of what should be guiding architectural design today: "the architect should be designing for variable primary functions and open secondary functions" (200). In other words, architectural design should allow multiple physical functions that are open to fluctuating meanings. In the examples studied here, the more stylized labels, such as Portia's La Triennia, most successfully reflect the multiple primary and secondary functions of the architecture they represent.

Bibliography

Bodegas Baigorri. www.bodegasbaigorri.com
Bodegas Darien. https://musikundwein.ch/bodegas-darien/
Bodegas Dinastía Vivanco. www.dinastiavivanco.com
Bodegas Portia. www.bodegasportia.com
Bodegas Ysios. www.bodegasysios.com
"Bold Bodegas: Top Architects Change the Face of Spanish Wine." *The Wall Street Journal*. (Oct. 2008): 1–4. Web. 13 July 2011.
Caballero, Nieves. "Fuerte, masculino y musculoso." *El Norte de Castilla.* 29 Oct. 2010. Wed. Web. 10 Oct. 2011.

Cohn, David. "Bodegas Ysios." *Architectural Record.* 191. (May 2003): 242. Web.

Desimone, Mike & Jeff Jenssen. "Rioja: Wine, Food and Architecture Star in Spain's Premier Vineyard Region." *Wine Spectator.* 15 Dec. 2008, 77–84.

Eco, Humberto. "Function and Sign: The Semiotics of Architecture." *Rethinking Architecture: A Reader in Cultural Theory.* Ed. Neil Leach. New York: Routledge, 1997, 182–202.

"Foster's Faustino Winery Open in Spain." *Architecture Lab: Online Magazine.* 2 Nov. 2010. Web. 10 Oct. 2011.

Gosález, Patricia. "Seis sueños de arquitectura y vino." El *Viajero de El País.* 21 Oct. 2006. Web. 7 Nov. 2011.

Habegger, Kimberly. "Architecture Meets Viniculture: The Iconic Structures of Spain's Rioja and Ribera del Duero Regions." *The International Journal of Architectonic, Spatial, and Environmental Design.* Vol.6, no. 4, 2012–2013.

——. "Spain's Wine Museums: Where Age- Old Oenological Tradition Intersects with Contemporary Design and Modern Technology." *Crossroads: Time & Space/Tradition & Modernity in Hispanic Worlds.* Ed. Debra D. Andrist. Brighton: Sussex Academic Press, 2020, 3–18.

"How Wine Became Modern: Design and Wine from 1976 to Now." Exhibition. San Francisco Museum of Modern Art. Nov. 20, 2010–April 17, 2011. www.sfmoma.org/exhibition

"Las bodegas Darien aspiran a ser el referente en La Rioja del enoturimo y de los vinos de Calidad." *La Rioja.* 13 September 2007. Web. 27 May 2021.

Marqués de Riscal. ww.marquesderiscal.com.

Martínez, Inés. "Arquitectura al servicio del vino." *Larioja.com.* 31 Aug. 2016. Web. 2 June 2021.

Pearman, Hugh. "The Incredible New Architecture of Wine: A Publishing Phenomenon." *Gabion.* (May 2066):1–5. Web. 10 Oct. 2011.

Richards, Peter. *Wineries with Style.* London: Mitchell Beazley, 2004.

"Un Gehry al lado de casa." *Diario La Rioja.* 9 Sept. 2006. Web. 27 Sept. 2011.

Viña Real. www.cvne.com

Webb, Michael. *Adventurous Wine Architecture.* Mulgrave Victoria Australia: The Images Publishing Group, 2005.

Winters, Edward. *Aesthetics & Architecture.* London: Continuum International Publishing Group, 2007.

PART II

Sustenance & Physical Space/Objects

Introduction to Part II

A. THE MUSEUM: DRINK & ARCHITECTURE

A reprint from *Crossroads: Time & Space/Tradition & Modernity in Hispanic Worlds*, Habegger's "Spain's Wine Museums: Where Age-Old Oenological Tradition Intersects with Contemporary Design and Modern Technology," with photos, centers on the contemporary fashion of expanded wine museums and innovative architecture of Spanish wineries themselves. This reprint is included since it reiterates Habegger's preceding chapter from Part I on what the associated wine-bottle labels most frequently depict, i.e., some aspect of the physical architecture of the wineries which produced the wines.

B. THE KITCHEN: FOOD & PREPARATION & PRESENTATION

For some readers, who statistically will be either professionals in the fields related to the languages or cultures addressed in this collection on food and drink, my study on the kitchen and dining room, cooking and consuming, the preparation and presentation of food and/or drink, could be somewhat repetitive and/or cursory. However, my plan for the chapter was not to be comprehensive but to focus on a few, perhaps different and more specific, even lesser-known, aspects. The chapter begins with a Mexican American public kitchen "revival" history in San Antonio, Texas, plus a book and film which expand and include the indigenous roots before, after and beyond that "Chili Queens" phenomenon. In instances of ethnic kitchens, the demonstrated integration of food and identity therein, quite apart from being limited to any specific ethnic group per se, is illuminated further, and in other ethnicities, in chapters in Part V of this collection, in terms of works by a Lebanese/Mexican/U.S. writer, Rose Mary Salum, and in a novel by a Cuban, José Lezama Lima. The body of the chapter highlights but a few tools, utensils and other cook and/or serve ware and three linguistic aspects (naming of dishes) of the topic of preparation and presentation. Arguably, these are the lesser-generally-known specific cook and/or serve ware and drinkware items, including some "different" regional aspects of same—and the mention of some dish names with unique or surprising etymology, given the role of names in anticipatory contexts for the cook and the consumer of the meals, both in preparation and presentation of food and drink.

6

Spain's Wine Museums: Where Age-Old Oenological Tradition Intersects with Contemporary Design & Modern Technology

Kimberly Habegger

Since approximately the year 2000, innovative contemporary architecture has been incorporated into the creation and renovation of wineries in Spain. This tendency is part of a planned effort to differentiate Spain's wineries and their wines to a world market through a growing emphasis on wine tourism. Many distinguished architects of international acclaim have contributed to this redesign of the Spanish wine country to include Frank Gehry, Jesús Mario Pascual, Zaha Hadid, Richard Rogers, Santiago Calatrava, Rafael Moneo, and Norman Foster, among others.

A proliferation of wine museums has accompanied the appearance of design-oriented wineries. The website www.museosdelvino.es lists twenty-seven different wine museums in Spain at present. Some of these museums reflect the creative architecture of the new winery buildings while others place the contemporary museum interior into important pre-existing historical structures. While some museums are part of a private winery, others are sponsored by local governments to highlight wine culture and to educate visitors on the wines of their specific region. A theme common to the museums and the wineries is the juxtaposition of tradition and innovation in the wine industry in Spain today and the museum spaces explored in this monograph attempt to illustrate and explain this juxtaposition.

Wine museums are an important tool in the wine tourism promotion and said museums may contribute in different ways: through highlighting the history of wine in the region, through a portrayal of wine culture in general, or by allowing visitors the opportunity to explore the many facets of wine appreciation and tasting.

The *Cambridge Dictionary* defines a museum as "A building where objects of historical, scientific, or artistic interest are kept." To this definition, we should add the museum's critical function as not merely storing but displaying said objects for a particular audience. In Spain today, some wineries or *bodegas* serve as museums in addition to their primary wine-making function in their display of notable collections of art and historical artefacts as seen at Bodegas Otazu with their collection of contemporary sculpture and the former Bodegas Darien known for its collection of historic wine vessels, as examples. Due to their originality and captivating architectural design, other *bodegas* "feel like" or are experienced as contemporary museum spaces such as Bodegas Portia and Bodegas Protos in Ribera del Duero and Bodegas Marqués de Riscal and Bodegas Ysios in Rioja. Finally, some museums are structures dedicated to wine education and appreciation without the wine-making function or the purpose of promoting the wine of a specific vineyard.

The wine museum itself is of increasing importance around the world and its linkage to the wine industry and the wine tourism effort has been analyzed extensively, as we see in the cases of the Aragón Wine Museum and the Chilean Wine Museum (*Journal of Wine Research*, 2007, Vol 18, No. 2 pp. 121–123, more). In this study, we will address museums about wine, some of which are connected to specific wineries and others that are independent or publicly supported. The museums studied are found in three different wine areas in northern Spain and will include the Museo de la Cultura del Vino at the Bodegas Vivanco, the Museo del Vino in Valladolid, the Museo de la Cultura del Rioja, and the intimate wine museum at the Bodegas Fariña in the town of Toro in the Toro D.O. in western Spain.

The Museo de la Cultura del Vino is part of the Dinastía Vivanco winery located in Briones, Rioja, designed by architect Jesús Marino Pascual. Dedicated in 2004, Dinastía Vivanco offers wine tourists an incredible array of wine-related experiences. This obligatory stop on the Rioja wine trail provides the many expansive spaces required to accommodate these experiences as well: the facility includes ample parking, an excellent restaurant, a spacious gift store, a wine bar with *tapas*, beautifully planned gardens, a historical archive containing 5000 books on wine (accessible by appointment), and a world-class museum exploring wine culture around the world. Structurally, the museum and the winery are combined into one large structure consisting of multiple volumes. Architect Marino Pascual has created

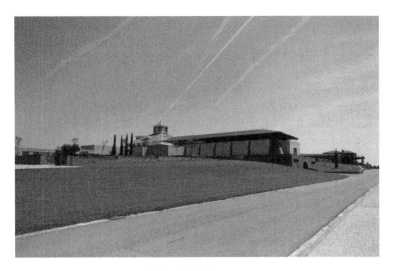

Dinastía Vivanco.

a number of other viniculture-oriented spaces in Spain: Bodega Antión and Bodega Darien are both located in Rioja, as is the Centro del la Cultura del Rioja in Logroño that we will discuss later. In addition, Bodegas Irius in Somontano is a spectacular example of Marino Pascual's work.

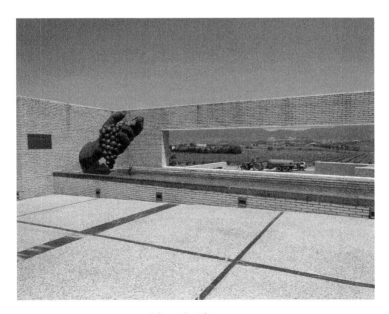

Dinastía Vivanco.

Approaching Dinastía Vivanco from some distance, the observer notes that the overall design consists of a number of inter-locking volumes reflecting some neoclassical influences through details such as a large rotunda placed towards the center of the complex and a square-shaped entry area, both crowned with lantern-like structures (the appendage over the entry actually functions as a chimney providing natural ventilation). In contrast with the neoclassical influences, a more contemporary sensibility is felt in the manner in which these volumes and others are varying dimensions connected with trellises and walkways of large, square cement pavers. Despite the contemporary feel, the grouping of these architectural volumes actually is characteristic of vernacular *bodega* structures and is reflective of the complexity of the wine-making process to be revealed through exploring this museum (Divisare).

The exterior materials, including oxidized copper, glass, and colored concrete (waves of purple on the perimeter wall and terracotta-toned areas of concrete on the building exterior) echo the colors of the landscape and the wine itself, all replicated by reflecting pools. In addition, the golden stone ashlar employed in the structure is indigenous to the Rioja Alta region thus further linking the *bodega* to its environment. The grounds surrounding the winery/museum display a garden of over 200 varietals (said to be one of the most significant private ampelographic collections in the world) and the well-manicured grounds and patios showcase statuary that pays homage to wine culture ranging from classical representations of Bacchus to a copious, stylized handful of grapes. This second sculpture is located to the side of a large open frame that features a superb view of the vineyards themselves with a vintage tractor visible in the distance. The entire vignette seems to honor the concepts of labor, nature, and abundance that constitute the process of creating wine.

Mostly underground, the interior of the winery, the museum space, and the social spaces are airy and contemporary leading the visitor on a multi-sensorial exploration of wine, wine making and wine appreciation. The collection of art and archaeology spanning from Antiquity to the present complement the educational experience of visitors as they proceed through the museum: historical implements used in the cultivation of grapes and the processing of wine, a collection of over 4000 corkscrews, and accessories and vessels for serving wine. The third floor houses the fine art and significant historical artefacts one would find in an archaeological museum such as an Egyptian frieze and original Picassos—all portraying some aspect of wine culture. In addition to the collections of objects, there are stops in the museum where guests learn about barrel making and the oaks used in their manufacture and how the use of glass and cork allow for the proper storage and aging of wine. Visitors also have access to experiential opportunities available through stations where the qualities of wine color and aroma are displayed, and guests are invited to test their abilities to distinguish the different nuances. Several videos placed throughout the museum dramatize aspects of the growing seasons and their corresponding vinicultural activities.

Owner Pedro Vivanco began safeguarding the family's traditional wine making equipment as the *bodega* modernized; these implements would serve as the starting point for the museum that is the result of 40 years of artefact accumulation (Robinson) now curated by son Santiago Vivanco. Pedro Vivanco has expressed the intention of the public display of the collection observing that the family feels compelled to "give back to wine what wine has given us" *(source)*. As an offering to Bacchus or as a gift to contemporary wine consumers that have contributed to the success of Bodegas Dinastía Vivanco, the collections of the winery reward both the gods and mortals alike.

So, in fact, this carefully curated collection was originally a family collection of tools of the trade of wine production and artistic works inspired by the final product of the family's labor, the wine itself. In his observations on the nature of collecting, critic Greg Noble reminds us that collected objects make our cultural world concrete, that objects are mnemonics for a complex world, and that our private acts of consumption are indeed profoundly social (235). The items in Dinastía Vivanco's Museo de la Cultura del Vino both reflect and are tangible fruits of the family's endeavors across several generations; yet their public display ensures that society is the beneficiary of the Vivanco's desire to "give back to wine what wine has given us." This cycle of labor resulting in wealth to be shared with those who contributed to the creation of this wealth is both an act of thanks and an investment in the future. Visitors should become consumers better informed about and more appreciate of wine culture who, in turn, should enthusiastically support the wine industry through the consumption of wine and the participation in wine tourism activities.

The Museo del Vino located in the town of Peñafiel was designed by architect Roberto Valle in 1999. The museum is a contemporary space that has been placed into the cellar of the Medieval Castle of Peñafiel located in the renowned Ribera del Duero wine producing area in the state of Valladolid in northern Spain. Visitors may purchase a tour of the Castle, a ticket for the museum, or both spaces can be experienced at a reduced price. The Castle is placed prominently on a hill that enabled domination of both the Duero and the Duratón rivers and this location allows for remarkable views both of the castle from

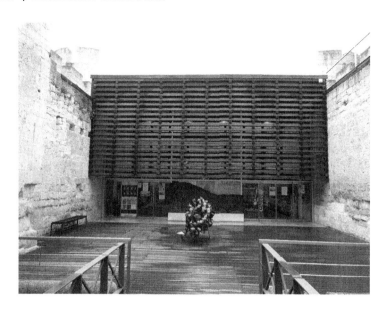

Museo de Valladolid.

a distance and from the castle as one surveys the town of Peñafiel and the neighboring vineyards and villages. The historic structure has its origins in the ninth entury although the present manifestation is attributed largely to Don Pedro Téllez Girónsu in the fifteenth century.

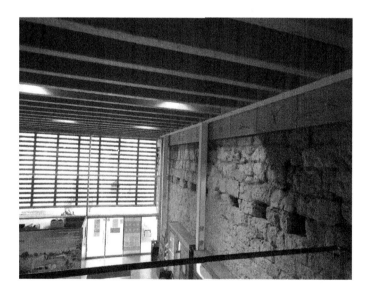

Museo de Valladolid.

In order to access the museum, one must descend to the lower level of the castle arriving at a landing where a contemporary work of sculpture constructed of metal ribbons suggesting grapes greets visitors. Moving through the museum interior, the juxtaposition of contemporary and historical architectural elements reminds guests of both the history and the innovation of wine in Spain today. The open floor plan allows easy passage through the exhibit space while also enhancing those historical architectural elements such as the stone walls and the original carved openings for the castle's structural beams. The museum contains sections dedicated to aspects of wine production and wine tasting (including professional tasting rooms)— at the same time many exhibits are clearly intended to illustrate the history and the characteristics of wine from the five DO's (denominación de origen) of Valladolid: Tierra de León, Ribera del Duero, Cigales, Toro, and Rueda and to the wines classified as Vinos de la Tierra de Castilla y León. One particularly unique display features garments and wine accessories used by the historic organizations of wine growers of the region over centuries while another showcases the bottles labels of many of the famous wineries of Valladolid including examples from the prestigious Vega Sicilia. Visitors can explore nine different sections such as "History," "Procedures," and those featuring types of wine presses, tools, bottles, and the specifics of wine tasting.

The museum space also includes smaller spaces that multiply the possibilities for visitor experiences such as the professional tasting room, the library, the shop and the auditorium. Interactive displays demonstrating wine traits and multiple audio-visual stations allow guests to process information through multiple avenues.

The Museo del Vino is clearly more than an area for display of historical artefacts and wine-related equipment, the province of Valladolid uses the museum to promote the wine not only of the acclaimed Ribera de Duero, but also of the other DO's mentioned previously. The Valladolid website expands on the mission with the following: "This unique museum space promotes the understanding, through the world of wine, of the province of Valladolid culturally and geographically as wine tourism has the ability to structure and connect all of the area's resources: landscape and nature, artistic patrimony, traditional arts, sport and leisure, festival and traditions, and of course, gastronomy" (www.provinciadevalladolid.com). The museum philosophy recognizes that viniculture influences and is molded by many different cultural aspects and therefore successfully demonstrates the interconnectivity between wine, history, and contemporary culture in Valladolid.

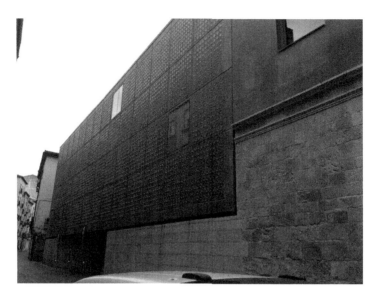

El Centro de la Cultura del Rioja.

The Centro de la Cultura del Rioja in Logroño was designed by Jesús Marino Pascual from 2008–2011. Situated in the historic center of Logroño, political capital of the state of Rioja, the museum occupies an entire block between Mercaderes, Ruavieja, and Marqués de San Nicolás streets. The original historical building was a sixteenth-

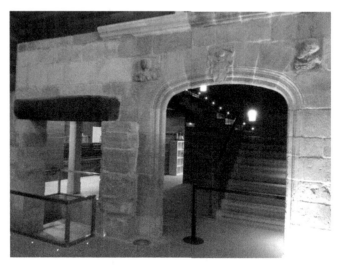

El Centro de la Cultura del Rioja.

century palace of the Yanguas family that has been a historical center of wine-making activities in the city. As in the case of Valladolid, this structure features the wines of the local area, and houses multiple wine-tasting purposes: wine store and bar, professional tasting rooms, temporary and permanent exhibits, all in significant historical buildings repurposed and reinterpreted by contemporary architecture.

The various spaces of the museum are situated amongst four levels of the building to include the cellar. The open area on the ground floor allows for only smaller L-shaped exhibit spaces on the two floors overhead. The expansiveness and abundant natural light augmented by contemporary fenestration render the entire floor quite appealing as other inviting spaces such as the shop and the wine bar greet visitor and promise the opportunity to savor local wines and culinary delicacies after the tour. The contrast between the historical architectural elements and those added by Marino Pascual are often delineated by the use of a wine-colored plaster application as seen in both interior and exterior views. A stairway original to the Renaissance palace has been carefully restored as it serves as the connection between the themes of the different floors. One display of particular interest is the original wine-aging cellar to the palace that was unearthed during the recent renovation work. Very distinct is the experience of a monumental metal sculpture of a bottle of wine that serves as the nucleus of the permanent exhibition space. Connecting the entire experience, a kind of computerized game queries visitors about their food and wine preferences at stations throughout the museum. The program makes a final wine recommendation and the end of the visit—conveniently as guests return to the ground floor's wine and epicurean shop.

Dedicated to the wine culture and gastronomy of Rioja, the Center hopes that visitors "can breathe history, tradition, innovation, design, and the wine of Rioja in a building of historical interest that combines exceptional architecture, artistic patrimony, history and innovation, design and tradition, wine and gastronomy" (website). It is interesting to note a small linguistic detail: the word "wine" does not appear in the museum's name although it is most definitely a wine museum. A visitor might expect some kind of general anthropological museum instead of one delving into numerous facets of wine cultivation, production, and appreciation. However, the part of the Museum's name: The Center for the Culture "del Rioja" references the celebrated wine of Rioja as opposed to the culture of Rioja in more generic terms.

Other less elaborate forms of wine museums also are found, among those is the Bodegas Fariña located in Toro, a wine producing DO in Castilla y León to the west of the more prominent Ribera del Duero. Toro (both a town and a DO) is a picturesque area with a growing

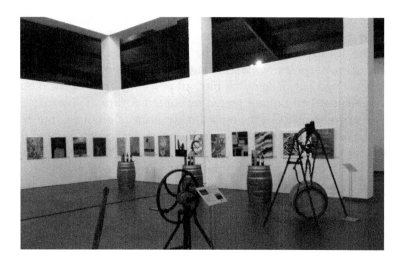

Bodegas Fariña.

wine industry that continues to receive increasing recognition for the quality of their its product. Founded in 1942, shortly after the grueling years of the Civil War, Bodegas Fariña is the oldest established winery in the area and consists of 300 hectors of wine featuring the varietal "tinta de Toro" a variation on the tempranillo grape. The winery

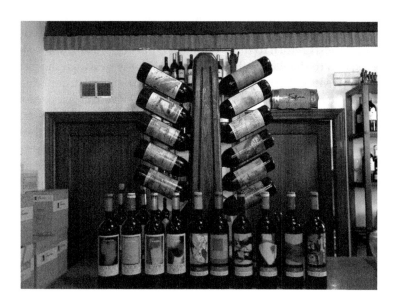

Bodegas Fariña.

offers tours, tastings, and an opportunity to visit their intimate wine museum. The museum space is located in a spacious agricultural structure modified to allow significant natural light and interesting construction details in the exposed roof frame. The objects in the museum include historical tools and wine presses formerly used in wine production and the most recent collection of paintings that are in competition to be selected as the image for the wine label of the current year's harvest. A large wine tasting bar complements the space and supplements an additional bar in the tasting room where purchases are made. The colorful bar in the tasting room displays the labels produced as a result of previous painting contests; the collection illustrates the variety, creativity, and quality of the artwork chosen since the inception of the competition. The museum offers a special treat for guests as they tour the winery grounds offering insights into the process of winemaking and the values and passions of the vintners.

Conclusions

Wine tourism can be analyzed from three distinct perspectives: (i) as a strategy though which destinations develop and wine-related attractions are marketed; (ii) as a form of consumer behavior that motivates wine lovers to travel to preferred destinations of wine production; (iii) as an opportunity for wineries and wine merchants to sell directly to consumers (Staging experiences). As seen in this essay, the four wine museums featured contribute to the promotion of wine tourism in unique and compelling ways. The availability of interactive experiences and the focus on engaging the five senses in wine education are key to the success of museums dedicated to the development of wine appreciation and to the understanding of wine producing cultures. The iconic architecture of three of the examples, the Museo de la Cultura del Vino, the Museo del Vino in Peñafiel and the Centro de la Cultura del Rioja, aligns with the critical acclaim of the design of numerous *bodegas* constructed in recent years and reflects a consistent theme of pairing the traditions of wine culture with technological and artistic innovations in contemporary Spain.

Bibliography

Bodegas Fariña. https://www.bodegasfarina.com

Buggelin, Gretchen. "Museum Space and the Experience of the Sacred." *Material Religion*. Vol. II, 30–51. Valparaiso University.

Cambridge Dictionary. https://dictionary.cambridge.org/us/

Coen, David. "Sacred and Profane." *Architectural Review*. 00038611X, March 2015, Vol. 237, no. 1417. Web.

Dinastía Vivanco. https://vivancoculturadevino.es Divisare. https://divisare.com website closed Dec. 15, 2018.

El Centro de la Cultura de la Rioja. www.centrodelaculturadelrioja.es/

Foucault, Michel. "Of other spaces: Utopias and Heterotopias." Trans. Jay Miskowiec. *Architecture/Mouvement/Continuité*. Oct. 1984. Web.

Habegger, Kimberly. "Architecture Meets Viniculture: The Iconic Structures of Spain's Rioja and Ribera del Duero Regions." *The International Journal of Architectonic Spatial, and Environmental Design*. Vol. 6, no. 4, 2012–2013.

Jackson, John Brinckerhoff. *A Sense of place, a Sense of Time*. New Haven and London: Yale University Press, 1994.

Llewellyn, Marc. "Inside the Extraordinary d'Arenberg Cube." *Good Food*. www.goodfood.com.au. June 16, 2017. Web.

Museos del Vino. www.museosdelvino.es

Noble, Greg. "Accumulating Being." *International Journal of Cultural Studies*. London: Sage Publications, 2004, 233–256. Web.

Provincia de Valladolid. www.provinciadevalladolid.com/enoturismygastronomia/ museoprovincialdelvino

Pikkemaat, Birgit, Mike Peters, Philip Boksberger & Manuela Secco (2009). "The Staging of Experiences in Wine Tourism." *Journal of Hospitality Marketing & Management*. 18: 2–3, 237–253. Web.

Robinson, Zev. "Making the Dinastia Vivanco Documentary." Feb. 16, 2011. http://zevrobinson.com/video/making-the-dinastia-vivanco-documentary. Web.

Shiner, Larry. "On Aesthetics and Function in Architecture: The Case of the "Spectacle." *Art Museum*." *The American Society for Aesthetics*. 2011, 31–41. Web.

Zamora, Jorge & Pablo Lacoste. "Tourism and Wine: A Marriage of Convenience or True Love?" *Journal of Wine Research*. 2007. Vol. 18. no. 2, 121–123. Web.

7

The Kitchen & Dining Room: Cooking & Consuming, Who, What, How in the Preparation & Presentation of Food & Drink

Debra D. Andrist

As particular phenomena of the time of the preparation of this collection of articles about food and drink, i.e., the first half of the 2021, the even more intense scrutiny of, and efforts towards, diversity movements & interest in attributing neglected indigenous and/or ethnic contributions to cultures, this collection and chapter begins by mentioning two, specifically Mexican American. One is embodied in on-line articles reviving the specific story of the Chili Queens of San Antonio, Texas; the other, a follow-up and much more general expansion by Texas-native chef & food writer, Adán Medrano. He has produced both a book, with recipes, and a film, *Truly Texas Mexican*. The Kitchen Sisters' blog details the basic history of the Queens themselves:

> Some kitchens are hidden by place, some by time—like the saga of the chili queens. For over 100 years, young women came at twilight to the Alamo and the plazas of San Antonio with makeshift tables and big pots of chili to cook over open fires. The plazas teemed with people—soldiers, tourists, cattlemen and the troubadours—who roamed the tables, filling the night with music. From San Antonio's earliest days as a Spanish military encampment, life in the town revolved around the plazas. They were the marketplace, the meeting place, the place of government and festivals—funerals, weddings and hangings. People came to argue politics with their neighbors, to listen to the sad songs of the troubadours, and eat the food of the legendary chili queens. The chili queens were romanticized in the press as being

exotic Spanish women with sable hair and fiery tempers. They became the stuff of tourist legend. No trip to the Southwest was complete without a visit to the chili queens. These women were often peoples' first introduction to 'that spicy, dangerous, Mexican food.' In the 1930s, Lydia Mendoza, the queen of Tejano music, began her legendary career singing in the plazas of downtown San Antonio with the chili queens. As San Antonio grew and modernized, the chili queens were periodically driven out of one plaza only to reopen their little stalls in another. In the 1930s, the health department finally lowered the boom. Health regulations and the war ended the chili queens' reign in the plaza of San Antonio.[1]

Medrano's film traces an overview of the whole topic, far before and beyond the queens themselves; according to Amazon.com:

> Over time and during conquest, *comida casera*, home cooking of Texas Mexican families sustained indigenous identity and memory. Cooking deer, cactus and tortillas, women led the cultural resistance against colonization. This road movie weaves through Texas cities, names the racism that erased Native American history. It celebrates a new type of encounter, one with a table where All are welcome.[2]

These integrations of food, drink and identity, quite apart from being limited to any specific ethnic group per se, are also illuminated in later chapters in Part V of this collection, in terms of works by a Lebanese/Mexican/U.S. writer, Rose Mary Salum, and in a novel by a Cuban, José Lezama Lima.

Beyond ethnicity and identity as related to food & drink, the preparation and presentation of food & drink may, or may not, *require* special tools, utensils, cooking or serving pieces. The preferences and choices of the cook/chef in the preparation and/or those of the consumer of the food/drink certainly inform what is used and how. Frankly, usually there are only slight physical variations of very many food-preparation tools, utensils and cookware, as well presentation, or serve ware, items, which are employed in cooking and serving across cultures, depending on needs and applications, i.e., what they look like or how they specifically function. For Mexican/Latinx/etc. examples, the *molinillo*/whisk/chocolate frother, a kind of hand-powered blender (Figure 7.1); or the *molcajete y tejolote*/mortar & pestle in Mexico or other Mesoamerican corn-based cuisines[3]—called *mortero y maja* (sometimes *batán* in countries in South America)/mortar & pestle in other Latin American areas, like the Chilean example (Figure 7.2); or the *metate*/grinder (of similar

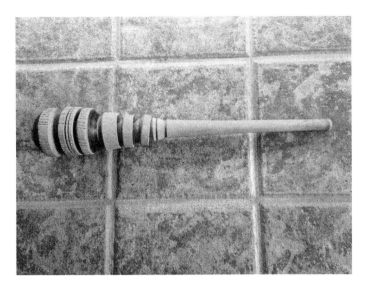

Figure 7.1

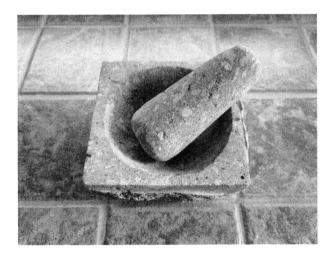

Figure 7.2

function to a mortar & pestle but with a flatter base and a rolling technique rather than crushing with a pestle of sorts); or the *tortilla* press; or the *comal*/griddle (Figure 7.3, modern electric combination of press and griddle). All fulfill the same basic function in the preparation of foodstuffs in other, sometimes vastly different, cultures in far-distant places. A pot is basically a bowl-like receptacle and probably neces-

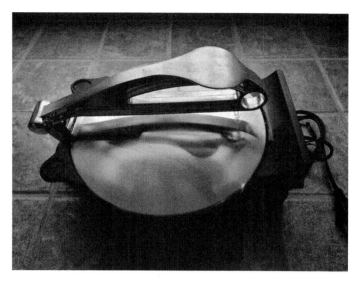

Figure 7.3

sarily heat-safe, a pan is a flatter item, nearly always heat-safe, however sizes and configurations may vary. Though seemingly different enough that the contrast is notable, chopsticks in the Eastern Worlds versus forks in the Western Worlds versus fingers in the Middle Eastern Worlds are all tools for manipulation of food in order to prepare or consume it. What is used for the equivalents of plates, bowls, cups, and so on, no matter the geometric shape, follows that general observation about function being the predominating factor.

Major differences lie in the materials from which the pieces are composed, frequently influenced by geographic features like kinds of stone or wood or clay, etc., readily available locally, beginning with natural, slightly modified pieces. More obviously, as production progressed, the types and colors of decorations which these pieces may exhibit/reflect geographic and/or ethnic influences. However, Hicks notes in her blog[4] about cookware worldwide from time immemorial that the evolving cooking techniques determined the basic types of ware used most.[5] The relatively similar cooking techniques and functions across geographies, i.e., heating, boiling, roasting, baking, grilling, etc. influenced cookware in a general manner rather than specifically. Local stones, wood, clay, etc., according to origin, by trial and error on the part of the cooks, became more or less popular according to their successful use. In any contexts, including Amerindian, Latin American and Iberian ones, far more individualities in terms of unique cookware and/or serve ware, although related to naturally occurring materials by geographic area or demographics, play important historical roles and the visual differences lie in specific configuration, color and decoration and, sometimes, technique, like coil or mold construction. Numerous sources agree that ceramic pieces, specifically (clay) pottery, were among the very first actively-human-crafted cook and/or serve ware worldwide, apart from the naturally occurring or adapted natural items. A note, this study focuses solely on cook and/or serve ware, not items, ceramic or otherwise, used for other purposes.

Human beings appear to have been making their own ceramics for at least 26,000 years, subjecting clay and silica to intense heat to fuse and form ceramic materials. The earliest found so far were in southern central Europe [keeping in mind the ubiquitous Eurocentric bias in history of everything] and were sculpted figures, not dishes. The earliest known pottery was made by mixing animal products with clay and baked in kilns at up to 800°C. While actual pottery fragments have been found up to 19,000 years old, it was not until about ten thousand years later that regular pottery became common.[6]

Of course, exact dates and places are controversial in any case. Remembering just how many different cultures of indigenous peoples of the Americas there were over the multiple thousands of years, many groups may well have been crafting all manner of sophisticated pottery items far, far earlier, certainly than at least the *arrival* of the Europeans in the Americas (see *Talavera* paragraph below). According to one source dedicated to pottery, though this study emphasizes what after the Treaty of *Tordesillas* became Hispanic America rather than Luso-Portuguese Brazil,[7]

In the Americas, evidence points to a surprising birth (or at least 'first') place: the Brazilian Rain Forest. Over 7,500 years ago, people of the Mina culture were making small bowl shapes resembling the later *tecomate* or cooking dish. Some of these first pots are plain, others are elaborately incised. Even at this early date, the Mina people knew to temper their clay with sand or ground shells to improve thermal shock. In fact, none of the excavations done so far have dug down to the earliest inhabited layers.[8]

But, referring back to what is attributed as the "first" American pottery, the Brazilian Mina peoples' *tecomate*, the Metropolitan Museum displays what curators refer to as an Olmec[9] *tecomate*. Olmec culture flourished on the east coast of today's Mexico from about the 12th to the 10th century BC.[10] In any case, this vessel type was nearly undoubtedly the earliest pottery cookware from the Americas, as the name refers to what

> is known as a *tecomate* ('gourd'), named after the gourds that inspired their original form. Some of the earliest ceramic vessels in Mesoamerica took the form of gourds captured in the more durable material of fired clay. *Tecomates* were important receptacles for community feasts, and many were subsequently placed in burials as important funerary offerings.[11]

Further, though the Inca Empire itself flourished later than either the Mina in Brazil or the Olmec in Mesoamerica, and in what is today western South America, evidence establishes that

> During the Inca Empire [c. 1400–1533 CE/AD] the production of pottery in the Andes was an art already developed in the region for thousands of years. The best example of pottery produced [even] before the days of the Inca Empire is found in the ceramic produced by the *Moche* or *Mochica* culture that thrived from 100 to 700 AD in the northern Peruvian coast. The Moche produced large amounts of pottery aided by the use of molds to create large quantities of specific shapes. Their color pallet was mostly limited to red, black and white. They used anthropomorphic figures and animal faces and bodies to shape their ceramic. They were the only pre-Inca culture to incorporate realistic facial expressions and emotions in their pottery work, a characteristic that the Inca pottery did not employ. One characteristic of Inca pottery is that it did not portray the human form, unlike other cultures that thrived before them, instead they used geometric patterns and shapes and heads of animals. The production and the use of pottery during the Inca Civilization had two purposes, utilitarian and ceremonial. [For the focus of this study, our interest is the] utilitarian pottery [which] was produced for everyday use and was usually thicker and less elaborate. The most common Inca vessel was the stirrup spout which is a bottle shaped vase intended for holding liquids with a long neck that forms the spout which usually serves as a handle . . . casted from a mold, whereas the stirrup spouts were handmade and welded into the vessel.[12]

Another example, not only still used daily in its country of origin, especially by rural peoples, but popular and currently selling on "gourmet" cookware internet sites worldwide (and even on Ebay), Colombia's *la Chamba* cook-&-serve ware has been found in archeological sites at least 700 years predating the arrival of the Spanish *conquistadores* in 1492. Made of a black clay containing mica in a traditional manner by the local villagers of La Chamba, on the banks of the Magdalena River in Central Colombia, the cook/serving ware is celebrated for both preparation and presentation of local dishes like *ajiaco*/chicken, potato & corn soup and/or nearly any other dutch-oven-type cooking since it heats and retains heat especially well due to the composition of the clay. Further, usage is unlimited as a rustic serve ware![13]

In terms of cook and/or serve ware, arguably the most-recognizable ceramic cook and/or serve items associated with Latin America, especially Mexico, outside Latin America today, apart from historic items in books and museums—and tourist pieces, may be *Talavera*[14] pieces (Figure 7.4).However, production techniques and decorations for this type of pottery were brought to the Americas by the Spanish conquerors in the 16th century, who got those from the Iberian Peninsula-invading Moors (711–1492 AD), but even so, not until about the 12th century AD.

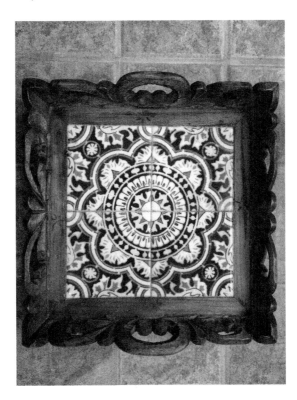

Figure 7.4

Moving to drinkware, in the opposite color from the black *La Chamba*, a naturally occurring white pigment from the Giacomo deposit near today's border between Peru and Chile, was mixed into resin by the Inca in Peru and used as decoration on *geros*, ceremonial wooden drinking cups, from about 1530, the time of the Spanish conquest of the country, to about 1570.[15] At that point, the Inca "switched to lead white, which the conquerors had brought from Europe," the most common source of white there versus the usual use of calcium carbonates, i.e., lime or chalk" (18). As archeologists examining the cups in museums discovered, the Inca usage of titantium dioxide preempted the so-called invention of titantium dioxide by a metallurgist named Auguste Rossi at a lab in Niagara Falls, New York in 1908, though Americans did not know this at the time. Rossi's "invention" was touted by some historians "as a chromatic revolution" (18) and what "color researcher, Matthijs de Keizer, calls the 'most significant contribution' to an explosion in 20th century pigment technology" (18), yet the Inca used it first several centuries before!

According to the website dedicated to overall information about another drink[16] specifically, *mate*,[17] plus the preparation and presentation of same, the bottle calabash gourd[18] or preferably *palo santo* wood[19] or horn brewing-and-drinking vessel, sometimes dyed or painted, decorated with *virola*/silver rim fittings, along with its accompanying *bombilla*/metal straw, usually silver, is one of the best-known Southern Cone (South American) drinkware items (Figure 7.5). Anecdotal history attributes the first usage of *mate* to the *Guaraní* Amerindians, who probably introduced it to other Amerindian groups and then to the Spanish *conquistadores*.

> The first to cultivate yerba mate trees were the Jesuit missionaries who had *yerba mate* farms in and around 1670. They were expelled from the Spanish territories in 1767 and this was a step back in the history of plantations of *yerba mate*. Yerba mate was again taken from the trees growing naturally in the forests. It remained so until more or less the early 20th century although in 1897 in the Paraguay district of Nueva Germania and the Argentinean district of Santa, Ana *yerba mate* was grown again in plantations.[20]

Still in wide usage in the South American countries of Argentina, Chile, Paraguay & Uruguay (also Brazil and some Middle Eastern countries like Syria and Lebanon) particularly, *mate* is called *terere* when served cold but this version is almost always served in a vessel made from horn or wood. Since the more common the gourd-made cups eventu-

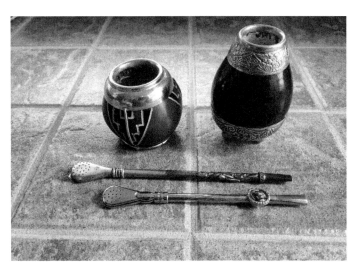

Figure 7.5

ally "sweat" from the associated moisture, some feature a tripod-like metal or leather support apparatus. These gourds are prized by

> Local people in Argentina [who] are unhappy to part with their gourds, even the old and broken ones. They repair the cracks using sheep intestines. They turn the wet intestines inside out and place the gourd inside. As the intestines dry out, they shrink and stiffen thus closing the crack of the gourd. The intestines add a decorative element to the gourd as they look like honeycomb. In some parts of Argentina, a cracked gourd is repaired by sewing with horsehair.[21]

For the most part, this study focuses on historic indigenous and Spanish food preparation and presentation, certainly recognizing the contributions and influences of other ethnic groups. As Diane Spivey, on the website, *Black Past*, emphasizes

> Africa has been a major contributor to the cuisine of North and South America although this contribution has long been overlooked, trivialized, or denied. The discourse contained in volumes on American cooking is usually consistent in its themes of celebrating what is considered the European influence . . . Africa's East and West Coast cultures made their indelible culinary marks through exploration, migration, and trade expeditions on the Olmecs and Mayans of Mexico, the Chavin of Peru, the Native American Mound Builders,

the Caribs of St. Vincent, and other indigenous cultures in the Americas, and these marks were made long before the so-called discovery of America by Christopher Columbus. Migration and trade between the Americas and Africa had made the exchange and trans-planting of foodstuffs between the three continents quite common. In other words, the African culinary influence on the Americas began long before the trans-Atlantic slave trade. The last stage of this culinary diaspora was the forced migration of Africans to the Americas through the slave trade, beginning in the 15th century, which brought numerous culinary artists and expert agriculturalists to the Atlantic coast stretching from Argentina to Nova Scotia. The continual influx and steady increase of Africans into the Caribbean and South America at the height of the human bondage trade ironically constantly reju-venated the African cultural input and fostered a culinary revolution under the influence of Africans that would permeate every aspect of cooking and cuisine in rural and urban areas of every country in the Americas.[22]

It is especially important to recognize the considerable African influ-ences on Latin American cook and/or serve ware post-importation of African slaves to the Americas. Whether pre- or post-Conquest and during the colonial years, African influence added other aspects to such cook and/or serve ware items, especially since one of the enforced labor tasks, particularly for slave women, was food and/or drink preparation for, and presentation to, their "owners," not to mention for their own usage. These items were frequently informed by the Africans' own ethnic preparation and presentation techniques and experiences. Since slaves were also used in production modes, their artistic talents and choices came to affect cook and/or serve ware in concept and appearance as it was produced.

But, moving to a more esoteric aspect of food and/or drink prepa-ration and/or presentation, naming dishes, whether for cooks' or consumers' benefit, highlighting ingredients and/or historical context, informs us of some unique provenances. The key concepts here are expectations and/or anticipations via the food or drink names. Though the Spanish language forcibly supplanted any Amerindian or African or other languages as the "official" *lengua franca* of the countries now known chiefly, whether truly accurate or not, as *hispanoamericanos*, the effect on naming of certain dishes and ingredients from those coun-tries and the indigenous languages therein went both ways in naming, of course. This supposition references back to the earlier chapter of this collection, positing that at least some culinary counter-conquest in terms of American-origin and/or European-import foodstuffs and ingredients also took place. However, due to socio-political issues post-Spanish conquest of Latin America and preceded by the numerous conquests of the Iberian Peninsula itself, I highlight only three uniquely named dishes, not ingredients from either culture, from the Spanish language rather than the myriad of those whose etymology is from the other cultures and languages in Latin America and/or Spain.

Rather obviously a Spanish import, particularly popular in Cuba, at least in name, the dish known as *moros y cristianos*/Moors & Christians, refers to the 700-year occupation of the Iberian Peninsula by Islamic peoples, particularly those from across the nine-mile strait from Northern Africa, specifically Morocco, and, most importantly, the successful *Reconquista* of same by the Roman Catholics. While this dish does not require any particularly unique tools, utensils or serving pieces, the arrangement of a pool of black beans surrounded by a ring of white rice is the traditional manner of presentation.

At least the Crusades-associated name of that dish refers to history and appears, on the surface at least, to be not as potentially offensive as what seems an even less-appealing reference in today's world—one of the terms in Spanish for a green bean, *judía verde*/green jewess, though that term is almost never used in Latin America at all for what will become the semi-obvious reason of its Arabic origin. Interestingly, the etymology of the name does not seem to support a popular but uninformed reaction. One layman's explanation reminds us that

> Green beans weren't brought to Europe until after the discovery of the Americas, so it's doubtful it was named that because of the Jews. The *DLE*[23] gives the etymology as "perhaps" from *judío*, but doesn't claim to be definitive. As pure speculation, recall some of the phonetic changes that occurred in various words Spanish: x (pronounced line English sh) went to j, interior o went to u, f went to an aspirated h went to silent or possibly to j, the d/l/r showed some variability . . . Thus a word like "hada" is, believe it or not, cognate with "fairy." So if *judía* didn't come from *judío*, it may have come from some earlier word like *xodío*, xurío, *forío*, etc. And, of course, there may have been another bean like plant called *judía* (for whichever reason that may be) that in turn gave its name to the American one.[24]

Much more scientific in terms of actual word etymology and in far more detail, another source underlines the incredibly involved evolution of sounds in pronunciation of Spanish through the various stages and additions of Arabic and Latin, vulgar (referring to the speech of the *pueblo*/town, i.e., the conquering Roman soldiers' vernacular, not referencing obscenity at all) and classical, as well as the botanical information which establishes the why of *chudiyas* in the first place:

(Arabic) *chudiyas* for judías . . . La palabra 'alubia' es de origen árabe. Ellos la llamaban al-lubilla. Hoy es la alubia y antes haba, frijol. En Asturias son 'fabes' y en el resto de España tambien 'judías,' esta última parece ser también de origen árabe *chudiya*. 'Haba' procede del latín *faba*, lo mismo que frijol, phaseolus. 'Habichuela' es de origen mozárabe, fabichela . . . Es una palabra Que viene del latín legumen y que también significa leguminosa. Es la planta que cria vaina. Judías, habas, garbanzos, lentejas, frijoles, altramuces, cacahuetes, guisantes, etc. pertenecen a la gran familia de las leguminosas . . . La judía, Phaselolus vulgaris, es la especie mejor conocida y más distribuída del género Phaseolus . . . Se piensa que se ha originado en la zona Oeste de Mejico-Guatemala, pero existen pruebas que sugieren su aclimatación en Centroamerica, a partir de especies ancestrales extendidas y polimórficas. Actualmente está muy extendida en distintas partes de los trópicos, subtrópicos y regiones templadas.[25]/(Arabic) chudiyas for beans . . . The word 'bean' is of Arabic origin. They called it *al-lubilla*. Today it is the bean and before bean, bean. In Asturias they are 'fabes' and in the rest of Spain they are also 'beans,' the latter seems to be also of *Chudiya* Arabic origin. 'Bean' comes from the Latin faba, as well as bean, phaselolus. 'Habichuela' is of Mozarabic origin, *fabichela* . . . It is a word that comes from the Latin *legumen* and also means legume. It is the plant that grows in pods. Beans, beans, chickpeas, lentils, beans, tart, peanuts, peas, etc. belong to the great family of legumes . . . The Bean, Phaselolus vulgaris, is the best known and most widely distributed species of the genus Phaseolus . . . It is thought to have originated in the western zone of Mexico-Guatemala, but there is evidence to suggest its acclimatization in Central America, from widespread and polymorphic ancestral species. It is currently widespread in different parts of the tropics, subtropics and temperate regions. (translation mine).

Tortilla is a foodstuff name which has frequently confused even Latin Americans aware of the history of corn-based cuisine and the indigenous flat-bread function of "their" *tortilla*, as well as Spaniards who make use of the American-origin potato in their own cuisine, basically a potato omelet, an appetizer and/or sandwich filling plus, "their" *tortilla* is usually qualified by the adjective, *española*. This is not to mention the confusion in other cultures and languages when this term is employed. Since the ingredients of both, traditionally cornmeal tortillas and white potatoes, are of American origin, many mistake the name as from indigenous roots. However, most etymology sources recognize that the term "dates from the 1690s, from American Spanish *tortilla*, from Spanish, 1a tart,1 literally 'a little cake,' diminutive of *torta* 'cake,' from Late Latin *torta* 'flat cake.'[26]

Thus, what might be considered a cursory overview scan of a very few iterations of the preparation and presentation of food and drink, especially focusing, not on food itself as does *Chapter 1* of this collection, but on Amerindian, Hispanic American and Spanish contributions, this brief study is so intended, not as a complete nor as a comprehensive look at the concepts of preparation and presentation of food and drink in those culinary traditions but as a highlight of a few, perhaps lesser-known, and varied aspects over a long history.

Notes

1 *The Chili Queens of San Antonio*—The Kitchen Sisters.

2 Watch 'Truly Texas Mexican' | Prime Video (amazon.com)

3 For those not familiar with said tools, in her blog, "Mexican Cooking Utensils," *Mexico in My Kitchen*, Mely Martínez describes what each looks like and how they are/were used. She emphasizes that "With the introduction of industrialization many years ago and many products ready to use in the markets, the *metate* is hardly used even in rural areas. Funny thing is that even in the early 1940's a *metate* was considered as an excellent gift for a newlywed woman." However, the *comal* and the *molcajete* are still commonly used in today's kitchen. She adds that "in Pre-Hispanic times [a chocolate drink was] a symbol of hospitality and wealth. Before the Spaniards arrived in America, the natives created the foam using two small gourd cups, pouring from the top of one another, repeating this process until the desired foam was formed. The *molinillo* we used today was created around the 1700's in colonial times." I add that the steel or iron *tortilla* press is also a relatively "new" tool since the traditional manner of preparing either corn or flour *tortillas* is to pat them out by hand or flatten them using what weights are conveniently at hand. And the contemporary electric press/griddle combination is an even newer, supposedly timesaving, appliance (but, in my personal experience, not as great in practice as it's advertised to be). See figures.

4 Evolution of cookware. Learn the history and innovation of cookware (booniehicks.com)

5 Evolution of cookware. Learn the history and innovation of cookware (booniehicks.com)

6 Ceramic—Wikipedia

7 "In 1494, a treaty named after the Spanish town in which it was stipulated was signed in Tordesillas."

The Treaty of Tordesillas maintained the north–south line [Pope] Alexander had drawn but moved it 920 miles (1,480 km) farther west. Supposedly, all Africa and Asia now "belonged" to Portugal; the New World to Spain. This westward shift of the line, however, brought much of the as-yet-undiscovered land later known as Brazil into Portuguese territory," Pope Alexander VI and Papal Bulls Divided Continents | Portraits From the Past (jw.org)

8 "Archive for Pre-Columbian Pottery," Pre-Columbian ceramics | This Day in Pottery History (wordpress.com)

9 Bowl (Tecomate) | Olmec | The Metropolitan Museum of Art (metmuseum.org)

10 Bowl (*Tecomate*) | Olmec | The Metropolitan Museum of Art (metmuseum.org)

11 Bowl (*Tecomate*) | Olmec | The Metropolitan Museum of Art (metmuseum.org)

12 Inca Pottery | Discover Peru (discover-peru.org)

13 *My Toque: Cooking Tools for the Home Chef.* About La Chamba Cookware & Authentic Black Clay Dinnerware—MyToque.

14 Talavera pottery—Wikipedia.

15 "The White Stuff: How the Inca Discovered a Prized Pigment," *Smithsonian*. Vol. 52, No. 03. June 2021, 18.

16 See Part III, Chapter 9 in this book to read about *pulque*, a fermented "wonder drug" drink from pre-Colombian Mesoamerica through the contemporary period.

17 Also regionally called *cimarrão* [Portuguese] or *cimarrón*, *mate* is a kind of tea made by soaking/steeping "the leaves of yerba mate plant (South American holly tree), *Ilex paraguariensis*," in water.

18 "Calabash is an annual climbing plant which grows up to 10 meters in height. It is one of the oldest farming plants in the tropic. It was known in Egypt some 3000 years BC and it was commonly utilized in South America well before Columbus discovered the continent." *Mate* gourds—*yerba mate* vessels made out of calabash (yerbamateinfo.com)

19 *Palo santo* wood gives a resin aroma to the *mate* but if used for hot *mate*, must be totally encased in metal. Three other woods are sometimes used but a *pampeano mate* requires a different brewing technique. *Wooden yerba mate cups (gourds): palo santo, algarrobo, lapacho, pampeano* (yerbamateinfo.com)

20 History of *yerba mate* (yerbamateinfo.com)

21 yerbamateinfo.com

22 TransAtlantic Food Migration: The African Culinary Influence on the Cuisine of the Americas • (blackpast.org)

23 Due to the large number of possible but related organizations and entities using this acronym, the exact source to which the writer refers is unclear.

24 etimología—Why are green beans called "green Jews"?—Spanish Language Stack Exchange.

25 judias verdes | Spanish to English | Idioms / Maxims / Sayings (proz.com)
26 *tortilla* | Origin and meaning of tortilla by Online Etymology Dictionary (etymonline.com)

Bibliography

Bowl (Tecomate) | *Olmec* | The Metropolitan Museum of Art (metmuseum.org)
The Chili Queens of San Antonio—The Kitchen Sisters.
Cole, Martin. *Native American Cooking Tools, Native American Cooking Tools* | *eHow* Yerba Mate Tea—information page (yerbamateinfo.com)
"Decrees that Divided Continents." *Pope Alexander VI and Papal Bulls Divided Continents* | *Portraits from the Past* (jw.org)
8 Foods That Highlight Latin America's African Roots (remezcla.com)
"etimología—Why are green beans called 'green Jews?" *Spanish Language Stack Exchange*
Hicks, Bonnie. "Evolution of cookware. Learn the history and innovation of cookware." Evolution of cookware. Learn the history and innovation of cookware (booniehicks.com)
The History of San Antonio's Chili Queens—San Antonio Magazine
Inca Pottery | Discover Peru (discover-peru.org)
judías verdes | Spanish to English | Idioms / Maxims / Sayings (proz.com)
Kenyon, Chelsie. "Methods Used in Authentic Mexican Cooking, the Spruce Eats." updated 8-14-2019. *Methods Used in Authentic Mexican Cooking (thespruceeats.com)*
Martínez, Mely. "Mexican Cooking Utensils." *Mexico in My Kitchen*. 2–23–2011/updated 4–15–2021. Traditional Mexican Cooking Utensils, Part I | Mexican Recipes (mexicoinmykitchen.com)
mate | Description, History, & Preparation | *Britannica*
Medrano, Adán. *New Documentary*, 'Truly Texas Mexican.' *Traces the Indigenous Food Heritage of the Borderlands*. Thttps://www.dallasnews.com/food/cooking/2020/09/04/
My Toque: Cooking Tools for the Home Chef. About La Chamba Cookware & Authentic Black Clay Dinnerware—MyToque.
Opie, Dr. Frederick Douglas. *Earthenware: A History of Table Traditions and Related Recipes*. Providence, RI: National Council for Education on the Ceramic Arts Keynote, Mar.
Pilcher, Jeffrey M. "American Latino Theme Study: Food." American Latino Theme Study: Food (U.S. National Park Service) (nps.gov)
Spivey, Diane. "Transatlantic Food Migration: The African Culinary Influence on the Cuisine of the Americas." Dec. 23, 2018. TransAtlantic Food Migration: The African Culinary Influence on the Cuisine of the Americas • (blackpast.org)
"Top 13 Latin American Food Blogs" | *Latin Discoveries.*
"*tortilla* | Origin and meaning of *tortilla*" by *Online Etymology Dictionary* (etymonline.com)

"Traditional Native American Cooking: Foods & Techniques." Traditional Native American Cooking: Foods & Techniques—*BrightHub Education*

TransAtlantic Food Migration: The African Culinary Influence on the Cuisine of the Americas (blackpast.org)

Watch 'Truly Texas Mexican' | Prime Video (amazon.com)

PART III

Sustenance for the Body & Soul:
Applications & Interpretations

Introduction to Sustenance for the Body & Soul: Applications & Interpretations

A. Food & Drink Applications for Medicine & Healing

The idea of food & drink conceived of, and/or used as, "medicines," perhaps even as being endowed with "magical" characteristics, dates from the very earliest documented human times. Humans not only took note of other animals' practices, what and how they did to ease or cure physical problems (just as domestic dogs are now known to eat grass for digestive upsets), but via trial and error, informed their choices. Indigenous peoples' successful usage of willow leaves and bark as analgesic, belladonna for cardiac applications, topical papaya for stings, topical honey to avoid infection, application of leeches, teas made from various leaves, among others, have stayed the course, preceding some "modern" medications still based on these particular plants and practices. The late 20th century revival of interest in, use of and publications about folk medicines, versus the modern age conception of the human body as a machine tended to by the physician-as-mechanic utilizing "artificial" tools, recognizes the applicability of, and progression in, those "natural" items which, in other cases, could/would be considered consumables solely for nutrition and/or sense-based enjoyment.

A specialist on Aztec topics, Jeanne Gillespie wrote the chapter "The Body Cured by Plants: Where Have all the (Chocolate and Popcorn) Flowers Gone?" for the first book in this series, *The Body: Subject & Subjected*. That chapter is reprinted in this volume since it focuses on food & drink in medical applications in that civilization. Her new chapter, "Healing Remedies and Patron Divinities: The Songs of *Pulque*," was written specifically for this volume about this Mesoamerican fermented beverage, *pulque*, historically a "wonder drug" in Mesoamerica, up through its contemporary "fashionable clubbing drink" use. For information about another drink, refer to Part II, Chapter 7, which highlights *mate*, a steeped South America plant beverage for centuries, mostly in the Southern Cone countries like Argentina, comparable to "morning coffee," and more, in continuing contemporary contexts.

My chapter 10 in this Part III is also a reprint but, in my opinion, bears yet another reprint since it explicates the actual science behind the magical realism depictions of food & drink in Laura Esquivel's *Como agua para chocolate/Like Water for Chocolate*.

A. Fᴇᴏᴏᴅ & Dʀɪɴᴋ Iɴᴛᴇʀᴘʀᴇᴛᴀᴛɪɴᴀᴠ ɪsʀᴄᴇʀᴇᴍᴏɴᴠ & Rᴇʟɪɢɪᴏɴ

A. FOOD & DRINK INTERPRETATIONS FOR CEREMONY & RELIGION

Given the heavy historical influence of Roman Catholic religious traditions in Hispanic worlds, i.e., Iberian and Post-Conquest Latin American, acknowledgement of the patron saint of cooks and the kitchen is appropriate at this point in this collection. St. Pasqual, or Paschal, of Baylón, born on the Feast of the Pentecost and named for that, was a 16ᵗʰ century Spanish Franciscan monk/mystic devoted to literally feeding the poor—and to the Eucharist. He is known in Church history for having defended the Eucharist against Calvinists.

The idea and function of Christian Communion as a rite of the Roman Catholic church (and other Christian denominations) worldwide has been expounded upon in literally thousands of religious and secular tomes. In this collection, John Francis Burke explains the ideas and functions of foods & drinks other than the "classic" bread & wine, ones associated specifically with Mexican American practices of Roman Catholicism. As Burke has emphasized in numerous others of his publications and presentations about *mestizaje*, the unique Latinx, specifically Mexican American, attitudes towards and practices of, spirituality and sacramentality, the *mixing of the divine and the human* which informs those practices, the amalgamation of religious and social realities, cannot be overestimated!

Ever so ubiquitous that the conspicuous absence of so-focused chapters in this collection must be at least acknowledged, the African religions' huge influences on cuisines and employment of food & drink, especially in the Caribbean, intended also for this Part III B, had to be deferred to the next volume in the series, *Rites, Rituals & Religions in Amerindian, Iberian & Latin American Worlds* for logistical reasons. In the meantime, a salient point is that the three major currents, *Santería, Palo Santo* and *Abacuá,* as well as *voudou,* are syncretized with Roman Catholicism, and that includes the employ of various foods & drink items in religious practice. For now, see Chapter 6, "Death/*Ikú* and the Spirits in Afro-Cuban Religions," in the seventh book in the series, *Death & Dying in Hispanic Worlds: The Nexus of Religions, Cultural Traditions and the Arts.* However, since that chapter focuses far more on death & dying practices than on food & drink aspects of these religions in Cuba, that chapter is not included as a reprint in this volume—but it includes considerable associated mention of food & drink in Afro-Hispanic religious practices.

8

The Body Cured by Plants: Where Have all the (Chocolate and Popcorn) Flower Gone? Recovering Healing Botanicals in Nahuatl Poetry

Jeanne L. Gillespie

How do science and art overlap in the process of documenting the Americas? What can an understanding of Mesoamerican strategies for storing knowledge add to our readings of documents compiled by European chroniclers? How did Mesoamerican and European knowledge storing systems preserve materials that could be useful or relevant in the 21st century?

We will approach these questions first from the perspective of the Spanish colonial administration, an organization that was very efficient and effective in documenting the vast territories they explored and claimed in the Americas. Spanish colonial expansion was an important strategy economically, politically, and socio-culturally. The processes employed in the documentation of new populations, lands and resources—the technologies of exploration and conquest, if you will—evolved from two distinct but related efforts in knowledge collection developed over the three centuries before the European colonization of the Americas. Upon arrival in the Americas, a third important sources for the technology of knowledge collection, that of Amerindian communities, also proved important to the documentation of exploration and settlement of the Americas. Both church and state recorders relied upon local informants to flesh out the details of their reports and to document and attempt to understand the intricacies of life in the Americas. In addition, knowledge storage techniques varied from community to community, so the vast amounts of materials collected in the *Archivo de Indias* reflects diverse approaches to the questions posited by the Spanish administration and the clergy.

In terms of secular models for data collection, the Spanish administration responsible for exploration and colonization built on the technologies for recording the details of regions and communities perfected during the administration of Castilian ruler, Alfonso X, "the Wise." In the thirteenth century, Alfonso X organized vast projects to collect and codify local heritage, to translate Arabic and Hebrew texts into Latin and Castilian, to record Spanish traditions including games and music, and to establish a legal code that would be a model for Europe and the Americas until the 19th century (and continues in Louisiana today!). Alfonso X's thorough exploration of the complexities of Iberian culture offered a precedent for collecting not only legal and scientific data, but popular culture and regional variation. In addition, Alfonso's legal treatise *Siete Partidas* (Seven Divisions) established a governing principle that included Christian, Jewish, and Moorish perspectives and commentary.

In the Iberian medieval era, the state and the church both had significant roles in the development of the ethnographic projects. While Alfonso X and his teams of scribes, translators, and data collectors were collecting materials from throughout the Peninsula, Franciscan missionaries were active in documenting life and practices in the Far East in attempt to Christianize the Mongol empire. Georges Baudot points out that half a century before of the publication of Marco Polo's fabulous travel narrative, Franciscan missionaries in service to Pope Innocent VI had documented a liberal and tolerant Mongol court and warned against an overly aggressive approach to conversion in Asia (376). Juan de Piano Carpini's *Historium Mongolorum* and Guillermo de Rubruk's *Itenerarium ad partes orientales* offered detailed, rigorous ethnographic documentation of Mongol society in hopes of securing a conversion to Christianity, and a favorable response to Franciscan missionization (376).

Although the Mongol world "fell" to Islam (at least in the eyes of the Christian administration), explorations to Africa and the West in the fifteenth century opened up new possibilities and new hopes for both imperial and religious prospects. In 1492, in the wake of the defeat of the Moors at Granada and the first voyage of Columbus, Antonio de Nebrija published the first grammar of Castilian Spanish. He also published the first Latin-Spanish/ Spanish-Latin dictionary. This new technology for the systematic collection of linguistic data would be vital to Spanish colonizing efforts and would provide a rich resource for ethnographic and linguistic study throughout the following 500 years.

In the early sixteenth century, eager and committed missionaries flocked to the Americas and began to collect linguistic data so that they could convert their subjects using indigenous languages and local cultural practices. These same priests worked to document "pagan" rituals so that their colleagues might recognize certain practices as counter to the missionary efforts. We have, from that time, grammars, vocabularies, dictionaries, *psalmodiae*, *doctrinae*, and other tools for catechizing in more than one hundred languages from Mexico and what is today the southern and southwestern United States. For example, a grammar and vocabulary in Timucua compiled by Franciscan missionary Francisco de Pareja is one of the few pieces of evidence that we have about languages from Spain's colonization of Florida. From Pareja's work and other documentation produced in Timucua, scholar Julian Granberry was able to construct a historical and linguistic narrative of this extinct language and to identify some cultural and ethnopoetic aspects of the people who spoke Timucua and their North and Central Florida communities (47–50). These Timucua texts have helped flesh out Amerindian life in the Florida colony.

Ethnopoetics was also a consideration of the documentary processes of Alfonso X and several of his heirs, who collected *cantigas*, *cancioneros* and *romanceros*, collections of songs in local voices that reflected local and regional themes and histories. These *cancioneros* and *romanceros* store a substantial repository of Castilian, Galician, Portuguese, and Catalan oral compositions as well as Arabic and Hebrew oral texts and poetry. This practice of collecting oral and performance texts also transferred to the Americas. At least two collections of documents that collected Nahuatl poetic texts also have survived from the colonial era. These are known as the *Cantares mexicanos* and the *Romances de los señores*. They are typical of "cancioneros/ romanceros" seen throughout Iberia in that they collect oral texts performed during the era, but they are also important because these texts are containers of Mesoamerican knowledge and part of the documentation of Mesoamerican historical, ethnographic, and ethnopoetic data as well.

The Franciscans Bernardino de Sahagún and Toribio de Benavente established substantial collections of ethnographic documentation in the Valley of Mexico beginning in the early 1530s. Another important Franciscan contributor in central Mexico was Alonso de Molina who complied his *Arte de la Lengua Nahuatl* in 1555. Miguel Ángel Esparza Torres explains that Molina's study of the language was heavily influenced by Nebrija and it has served as an extremely useful source for Nahuatl studies in the late 20th century (27–34).

These poetic texts themselves are treasure troves of many kinds of data, including ethnobotanical information related to local ritual and healing practices as well as texts that help us understand how the local communities adapted the teaching of the missionaries. Specifically, I would like to look at several texts that show ethnopoetic information from the Psalmodia crisitana by Sahagun and the Cantares mexicanos that can be linked to ethnobotanical data collected in the grammars, various medicinal texts and the *Relaciones geográficas*. To accomplish this, I would like to look at a selection of Amerindian texts that mention a specific flower, the *izquixochitl*, which is translated as "popcorn flower" in many English translations. It can also be translated as "roasted corn flower." This flower, generally identified as Bourreria huanita or B. Formosa, comes from a tree that is native to the Gulf Coast region and is often mentioned in conjunction with the cacao flower, *cacahuaxochitl*, from the same region.

In order to begin to unlock the possible meanings of this image, we must consult the Spanish sources as well as Amerindian sources and from here we will see what we can uncover. I would like to start with a psalm composed in the mid-sixteenth century for a celebration of St. Bernardino's day. This comes from Sahagun's *Psalmodia* and it gives us an idea of the lush and powerful images that the Americas offered.

MAY. St. Bernardinus's Day.
FIRST Psalm
Let us honor the cypress tree of quetzal
feathers, the silk cotton tree of trogon
feathers, which our lord God caused to
bud—St. Francis.

Everywhere in the world their covering,
their protection, shades all the
children of the Holy Church.
And in its shade, in its protection, we,
the people of New Spain, are here happy,
rejoicing greatly.

All the various heavenly flowers spread
[perfume] on it; all the various heavenly
precious stones grow as its fruit.
The heart flower, the godly popcorn
flower, the cacao flower, the Indian corn
flower, the cup flower, the red bone flower
there are all arched, fragrant; scattered

widely. They shine like the golden dew.
The emerald-green jade, the fine green
jade, the ruby, the pearl, the amethyst,
all the various precious stones lie massed
there, gathered together, gleaming there
—shining.
(Sahagún's *Psalmodia* fols. 89r-92r; Anderson's translation)

This offers an idyllic image. It is certainly easy to picture St. Francis of Assisi right in the middle of the scene. The treatment of the "godly popcorn flower" suggests a special category unique to this botanical. Upon examining a second collection of poetic texts, we begin to see how the popcorn flower is treated in other settings.

Beat your flower drum beautifully, singer.
Let there be popcorn flowers, cacao flowers.
Let them scatter let them sprinkle down
beside the drummer. Let us have joy.
There! The turquoise swan, the trogon, the
roseate swan is singing, warbling, happy with
these flowers. (Bierhorst, 190–191)

This is still a beautiful scene with the interesting addition of the drum and the song. It is also interesting that we are scattering flowers and having a joyous celebration, and again we have popcorn flowers and cacao flowers used together again. While I have taken these excerpts out of their context and that there are many more details and some problems with Bierhorst's translation that could be explored, but for now, I will continue to concentrate on examples using the popcorn flower. Here is another text from the *Cantares mexicanos*:

My song's begun within the House of Flowers, and at once I carry off my little princeling. I'll pleasure the little jewel. He dances,\his little babe, this little Ahuitzotl. / Cry no more my little princeling. These flowers and these bells of yours! You dance with these jewels. / I , a Mexican girl [female], am rocking the world! Off I go carrying my shield cradle, for there beyond where he lies, this treasure, this little war-flower babe of mine. . . My breasts [my created ones] are popcorn flowers. In bed with raven blooms [plumeria] we've been entwined [or we've been whorled with raven blooms]. (Bierhorst, 263–265)

Patricia Granziera helps us understand this reference a little better:

The Goddess Xochiquetzal (flower-feather), patron of artisans and sexual love, was associated with the popcorn flower *izquixochitl* (*Bourreira huanita* Hemsl.), a flower that, according to Francisco Hernández, was very much appreciated for its fragrant smell and curative properties. It was mixed with cacao to make *chocolatl*. The *izquixochitl* in [N]ahuatl means toasted maize flower (*Izquitl-xochitl*) because its seeds pop out like toasted corn. It has been considered a symbol of life, the metaphor of maize, and a basic plant in Mesoamerican alimentation. (187)

So, how does the *izquixochitl* imagery from the song connect the flower and the text to Xochiquetzal? What we see in this text is a baby boy "Ahuitzotl" in the House of Flowers. Ahuitzotl was an Aztec warrior and ruler who participated in the Flowery Wars, where adversaries set out on specific dates to engage in warfare to capture prisoners as sacrificial victims that would assure the proper rainfall and general cosmic well-being. Ross Hassig has written extensively about the practices of *Xochiyaoyotl* or Flowery Wars and Ahuitzotl's participation in this ritualized warfare (200–218).

The voice of the "Mexican girl" explains that she is pleasuring the infant ruler with her breasts . . . that are popcorn flowers. Actually, the Aztecs were obsessed with bodily fluids, and in this case, her pleasure is that of a nursemaid, suckling the warrior baby and rocking him in his shield cradle so he will grow up to be a powerful warrior. The popcorn flower here is a metaphor for her milk. There are few things sweeter than a nursing baby's breath and few more pleasured faces than those of a satiated baby. Mother's milk (or in this case, the nursemaid's milk) is linked to a flower that also produces similar effects.

Recent pharmacological research has identified hypnotic, anti-depressant, and anxiolytic properties in the *izquixochitl* (984–985). According to Indra Holzman and a team of Guatemalan and Brazilian researchers, "ethnobotanical surveys conducted in Guatemala have shown that the infusion of dried [*izquixochitl*] flowers is popularly used as a tranquilizer, to cure heart diseases and high blood pressure, as an analgesic, and as an antiseptic, mainly for skin complaints" (984). This flower was mixed into cacao to make a fortifying drink that the warriors would consume before battle, babies were offered this to strengthen them and lactating mothers also consumed this so their milk would be productive. In a sense, these little white flowers acted as a restorative with calming properties much like nature's mother's milk. The goddess Xochiquetzal is sometimes portrayed with these flowers in her headdress and she is the patron of midwives and doctors as well as artisans and sexuality (image source detailed in end of chapter note). In the Mesoamerican context, however, this is all designed to produce success in warfare, whether the battle of humans with their environment or actual organized warfare.

As we look deeper, and as Marie Sautron confirmed, "popcorn flower cacao flower" metaphorically represents the preparations for warfare (246–47). Further, each of these flowers comes from the Gulf Coast, adding an exotic touch to the conversation. Popcorn and cacao flower, like the chocolate they infused, were the ultimate luxury goods and had to be imported at great effort. If we look back at the second text in context with other similar songs, we find that the beating of the drum and the sprinkling of flowers also suggest the preparations for ritual before warfare or the celebration of a battle victory. The importance of these ingredients is reinforced with their mention and their representation in the images of the painted texts.

We begin to understand the links between the botanicals, the actions, and the actors in the metaphoric poetic practices characteristic of Nahuatl compositions. As we become more aware of how the botanical references reflect not only political, but pharmacological aspects, we see a dense, semiotically rich environment that the missionary priests may have not entirely understood. With the proper "homework" however, we can begin to tease out the deeper layers of meaning and understand better the Mesoamerican signifying practices being collected.

The *izquixochitl* is a tiny white flower that packs significant healing and olfactory attributes. The flower is used to adorn the headdress of one of the most important female divinities in the pantheon, and the flower itself is an additive to luxury consumption of cacao. In the pictorial and linguistic records of pre-Hispanic Mesoamerica, it receives significant attention. This flower was not chosen because of one characteristic, but because of the complex messages that it signifies: botanically, medicinally, geographically, culturally, aesthetically, and sensorially. The numerous layers of signification indicate an important role for this botanical. The *Cantares mexicanos* and other poetic colonial texts are rife with references to flowers and other plants, animals, and natural phenomena that indicate an extremely well-developed medical understanding of the natural resources of the region. Many of the other animals and plants that are referenced in Nahuatl "poetry" also have medicinal or other scientific properties. This is a call to reexamine Mesoamerican literary and pictorial arts with an eye for scientific and medicinal references. We have much to learn.

Note
Image source of Xochiquetzal with *izquixochitl* flowers in her headdress.
https://upload.wikimedia.org/wikipedia/commons/4/4b/Codex_Borgia
_page_60.jpg

Bibliography
Anderson, Arthur J. O. "The 'San Bernardino' of Sahagún's *Psalmodia.*" *Indiana.*9 (1984) 107–114. Online. http://www.iai.spkberlin.de/fileadmin/dokumentenbibliothek/Indiana/ Indiana_9/IND_09_Anderson.pdf
Baudot, Georges. "Amerindian Image and Utopian Project Motolinía and Millenarian Discourse." *Amerindian Images and the Legacy of Columbus.* Eds René Jara, Nicholas Spadaccini. Minneapolis, MN: U of Minnesota P, 1992. 375–400.
Bierhorst, John. *Cantares Mexicanos: Songs of the Aztecs.* Stanford, CA: Stanford University P, 1985.
Esparza Torres, Miguel Angel. "Nebrija y el modelo de los misioneros lingüistas del nahuatl." *Lingüística misionera III: Morphology and Syntax.* Eds. Otto Zwartjes, Gregory James, Emilio Ridruejo Alonso. Amsterdam: John Benjamins Publishing, 2007. 27–34.
Granberry, Julian. *A Grammar and Dictionary of the Timucua Language.* Tuscaloosa: U of Alabama. 1993.
Granziera, Patrizia. "Concept of the Garden in Pre-Hispanic Mexico." *Garden History* 29. 2 (Winter 2001): 185–213.
Hassig, Ross. *Aztec Warfare: Imperial Expansion and Political Control.* Norman: U of Oklahoma P, 1998.
Holzman, Indra. *et al.* "Psychopharmacological Profile of Hydroalcoholic Extract and P-Hydroxy-benzoic Acid Obtained from *Bourreria huanita* (Boraginaceae) in Mice." *Pharmacology & Pharmacy.*5 (2014): 983–995. Online. http://dx.doi.org/10.4236/pp.2014.511110
Sahagún, Bernardino de. *Psalmodia Christiana y sermonario de los sanctos del año, en lengua mexicana ordenada, en cantares o psalmos, para que canten los indios en los areytos que hazen en las iglesias.* México, 1583. Online. https://ia700807.us.archive.org/21/items/psalmodiachristi00 saha/ psalmodiachristi00saha.pdf
Sautron, Marie. "In izquixochitl in cacahuaxochitl: Presencia y significación de un binomio floral en el discurso poético Náhuatl prehispánico." *Estudios de Cultura Náhuatl* 38 (2007): 243–264.

9

Healing Remedies and Patron Divinities: The Songs of *Pulque*

Jeanne Gillespie

The maguey or agave (agave Americana) was and is a vital plant for ritual, medicinal and commercial uses. This study will concentrate on healing power and rituals surrounding the rich nectar it produces, *aguamiel*, and the production of the fermented product called *octli* or *pulque*. While this essay will only focus on this nectar and its fermented state, other parts of the plant were important medicinally, too. Mesoamericans extracted a preparation from the root that helped ease the symptoms of syphilis and tuberculosis. The juice from the leaves was used as a salve for skin lesions and deep wounds. The needles at the end of the leaves were used for sewing and for ritual purposes, as we shall see in a bit, and the fibers were woven into twine. Parts of this plant are collected, processed and distilled for the production of mezcal and tequila.

According to 16th century medical historian, Francisco Hernández, preparations to alleviate digestive and intestinal maladies, including stomach ulcers and dysentery, incorporated the sap from the roots. Remedies from the maguey plant helped dissolve and expel kidney stones and cleared out the kidneys and urinary tract. It was effective in the treatment for jaundice as well. Eighteenth century botanist and pharmacologist, Vicente Cervantes, confirmed that maguey preparations can be used as a "diuretic, sudorific, digestive agent, astringent, tonic, antiscorbutic . . . and diaphoretic as well as producing favorable results on venereal disease and tuberculosis" (*Atlas de las plantas de la medicina tradicional mexicana* "Agave"). It also possesses a fructans designated *agavin*, insulin compounds that "[d]ue to the high fructan and fructooligosaccharide (FOS) content . . . have been considered as an alternative source for prebiotic FOS syrups" that has "demonstrated beneficial health effects such as improving calcium absorption in postmenopausal women, iron absorption and colon cancer prevention" (Escalante et al. 11).

Other communities throughout Mesoamerica like the Otomi and the Huastecs enjoyed *pulque* consumption and were reputed to be heavy drinkers and valiant warriors. In fact, in 1946, one of the first studies of *pulque*'s nutritive value, determined that for the Otomi community studied, *pulque* was the second-most important food—only tortillas provided more nutrition—the vitamin C present in a serving of *pulque* consumed by the Otomi provided 48% of the daily dose, assuring that scurvy was nearly unknown in the region. The beverage also provided at least 25% percent of several B vitamins and 51% of the daily dose of iron. (Escalante et al.)

The discovery and production of this nutritional powerhouse is steeped in tradition and ritual. One origin story tells that the patron of maguey and nursing mothers, Mayahuel, discovered *pulque* walking through a maguey stand. According to the story, Mayahuel noticed a rabbit acting peculiar and upon further investigation discovered an agave plant with fermented *aguamiel* in its crown. She realized that the rabbit was intoxicated from the plant's juices.

Another legend tells of a romance in which the god of wind, Ehecatl-Quetzalcoatl seduced Mayahuel by whispering in her ear. She followed him from Tamoanchan (Paradise) to Earth where they formed a fused tree of two species. Ehecatl became the *quetzalhuéxotl* (*Salix lasiopelis*) and Mayahuel turned into a *xochicuáhuitl* (*Cordia megalantha*) and they intertwined. Mayahuel's grandmother, not pleased by this union, discovered the lovers and destroyed Mayahuel's trunk and branches. The devastated Ehecatl gathered the pieces of the shattered tree and buried them. From these grew the first agave plants.

Still a different account identifies Mayahuel's consort, Patécatl, as the creator responsible for developing the process to produce *pulque*. Patécatl has associations with Quetzalcoatl-Ehecatl, so this may not be the stretch it seems. In addition, sources identify Patécatl as the "father of medicine," further highlighting the importance of pulque and *aguamiel* in the Mesoamerican dietary and healing practices. Not only were the divinities that discovered and developed *pulque* remembered in oral narratives and pictorial texts, the process of cultivating agave, making, and using *pulque* also became part of the oral tradition. In this scene 68 from the *Codex Borgia*, Patécatl, seated on a throne, drinks *pulque* from the large foaming *pulque* jar in the center of the image while Mayahuel, as the embodiment of the maguey plant appears to dance (Figure 9.1). The ritual may be in commemoration of the eclipse illustrated above the *pulque* jar. It also appears that

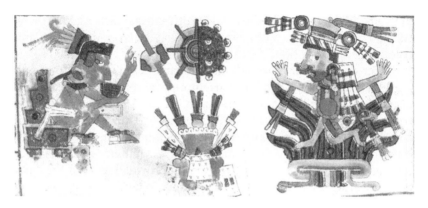

Figure 9.1 Patécatl drinks maguey during eclipse while Mayahuel
dances. *Codex Borgia* 68 FAMSI.

Pátecatl reaches for the digging stick that holds a crown removed from
the heart of the maguey plant.

Many indigenous pictorial manuscripts identify Mayahuel as the
embodiment or patron of maguey and *pulque*. In this role, she also
serves as patron of breast feeding. Some codices and indigenous documents depict her breastfeeding a child, a rabbit, or another creature.
The *Codex Laud* illustrates the connection between breast milk and
pulque. Mayahuel, seated on tortoise atop a snake, emerges from the
maguey plant. In her left hand and connected to her right breast,
Mayahuel holds a bone awl and maguey needle. In Mesoamerican
visual representations, penitents often employ bone awls and maguey
needles to perform auto-sacrificial perforation rituals to offer their
blood in exchange for divine favor. The use of these tools most
certainly indicates that she is practicing a sacrificial ritual, especially
because she holds bowl of ritual implements in other hand. Given the
posture, it is quite possible that she is offering breast milk for her sacrifice. Mothers' milk, like blood, is a precious, life giving fluid. We know
that midwives and healers used *pulque* as a healing tonic used to fortify
nursing mothers and to stimulate lactation. *Pulque* and breast milk
have similar color and consistency, linking them metaphorically. We
shall see later that there are other metaphorical links between mothers'
milk and *pulque*.

Returning to the image, a bowl of *pulque* similar to the one from
the scene with Patécatl and Mayahuel foams at right side of the
divinity, ready to be deployed in the ritual. In addition, an incense
burner and another bowl of sacrificial elements provide the tools to
support the offering. The digging stick that is used to transplant young

agave plants and to remove their crowns so that the plant can produce *aguamiel* stretches behind Mayahuel. The digging stick is a very important tool in the process of preparing the mature maguey to produce *aguamiel* as an invocation that narrates that process and invokes the divinities and tools involved in the process, as we shall see later (Figure 9.2).

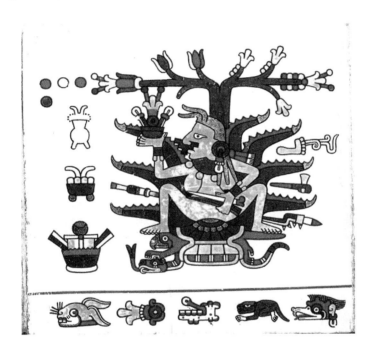

Figure 9.2 Mayahuel as maguey plant with sacrificial implements and *pulque. Codex Laud Folio* 9, FAMSI.

Pictorial and written narratives often combine to offer a better context for a particular aspect of life in Anahuac. One of the earliest texts collected by the missionary, Bernardo de Sahagún, the *Primeros memoriales*, records a hymn or *cuicatl*, in Nahuatl, as a gloss to an image of a woman embodying the maguey plant. The *cuicatl* "Ayopechtli" ("Seated on the tortoise shell") commemorates the act of giving birth and records the midwife's exhortation for the precious jewel baby to arise. This song celebrates the divinity who helps fortify a newborn baby.

Song of Ayopechtli [The Divine (?) One Seated on the Tortoise Bench]

There in the house where she [Ayopechtli] is seated on the tortoise bench, the expectant mother gave birth.

There in the house where she is seated on the tortoise bench, the expectant mother gave birth, there in her [Ayopechtli's] house the babies are born.

Begin your journey! Begin your journey, Newly Formed one! Begin your journey!

Begin your journey! Begin your journey, Precious Pearl! Begin your journey! (Seler 107–108; author's translation)

We see the mother giving birth and we hear the encouragement of the midwife calling the precious newborn to begin his/her journey. Although the text does not mention Mayahuel by name, Eduard Seler and others have attributed this text to her because she is almost always embodying the maguey plant and she is frequently represented seated on a tortoise shell as in the *Codex Laud* above. This is probably a fragment of a longer song. The midwife would have invoked the divinities responsible for childbirth as part of her exhortation, but we do not have this part of the narrative here, Seler notes that the place itself suggests a connection to the divine.

According to Seler:

Al parecer todo el canto es un himno de encantamiento, para hacer sencilla la labor de parto. En las primeras dos estrofas, por lo tanto, se da por cierto que en la casa de la fértil diosa se dan los nacimientos, esto es, son muchos y fáciles. Esto se supone que es un conjuro en relación con el nacimiento que es deseado en ese momento.

(Seler 109; It seems that the entire song is a hymn of enchantment to ease the labor of birth. In the first two stanzas, at least, it is given for certain that in the house of the fertile goddess births occur, that is, there are many and easy [births]. It seems that a conjure related to the birth is needed at the moment. Author's translation).

The pictorial texts and codices frequently not only portray Mayahuel as the embodiment of the maguey plant, but, also, they depict her nursing a human baby or an animal, further linking her to the care and nurturing through lactation. Sometimes she is depicted with many breasts, nursing many rabbits. As we shall see, while this event dates from pre-Hispanic times. birthing and christening rituals always included *pulque*, even well into the colonial era, despite attempts to squelch it.

While the previous examples were recorded in the mid-16th century, connections between Mayahuel, midwives, and *pulque* continued into the 17th century. A document compiled in 1629 by a priest named Hernando Ruíz de Alarcón dedicated to eradicating superstitions and witchcraft known as the *Tratado de supersticiones* confirms how important *pulque* and the midwife were in the birth and naming of a newborn, even more than 100 years after the Conquest. According to a native informant from the state of Hidalgo, at the time the child is born, the midwives tell the family that they must wait for their return until "[O]ne day before the children receive the Holy Baptism in order to remove the fire from them (212)." The midwives also order the family to prepare or provide *pulque*, tamales and a fowl and to invite the neighbors. The family is also instructed to have a fire burning. The midwives offer these gifts to the fire.

One midwife takes a bowl of water to the patio and places it in the center of the space. She returns to the fire and collects some fire in a pot. She then gathers the baby from the mother and brings the baby and the fire to the patio where she places the fire very close to the water and proceeds to bathe the newborn. As she bathes the child, the splashing extinguishes the fire and when it is out, the midwife asks what name the baby will be called. The midwife returns the baby to the mother and wraps the baby's head in a towel. She collects more fire in the pot which she uses trace a circle around the baby's head. She returns the fire to its origin and offers some of the *pulque* by pouring it in front of the fire. She then distributes the *pulque* to everyone present (212–213).

As we have seen, midwives used *pulque* at special events like a naming ceremony as well as to fortify mothers in labor and post-partum and to assure that newborn babies were hale and hearty. *Pulque* was used in many other rituals not related to the birth of a child. A 60-meter mural inside the pyramid of Cholula depicts an extensive celebration that seems to focus around the drinking of *pulque*. The *Codex Magliabechiano* illustrates a celebration with warriors and *ahuiani* [pleasure women] drinking *pulque*. A warrior wearing full battle regalia, including a nose ornament associated with *pulque*, drinks from a large foaming jar while another seated on a mat sips the beverage from a bowl. Women who were trained to attend the warrior class, the *ahuiani*, serve *pulque* and imbibe with the warriors. This celebration is probably to fortify warriors for battle. There would also be rituals in which *pulque* was consumed after the battle to cele-brate a victory and to help heal the soldiers. We have seen some of the ways that *aguamiel* and *pulque* have been used medicinally. We have also seen that medicinal and ritual use of this incredible plant are intertwined, as is the knowledge of the intoxicating power of the fermented product.

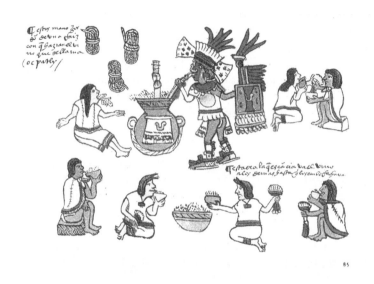

Figure 9.3 Warriors and *ahuiani* drinking *pulque*. *Codex Magliabechiano*. Page 171; Graz FAMSI.

For Mesoamericans, a careful balance had to be maintained because intoxication could lead to chaotic situations that could throw the elements of the cosmos out of balance. In general, people were not allowed to drink more than four bowls of the beverage at a time except for those over 70, who were allowed to drink until intoxicated. Here you see an example of elderly women becoming intoxicated from *pulque* as portrayed in the *Codex Mendoza*.

It is thought that the fortifications provided by *pulque* were healthy for the elderly and their intoxication would not disrupt other workings of Aztec society. In fact, in addition to drinking *pulque* to celebrate a birth, most rituals did include *pulque* as part of the festivities. While closely regulated, this consumption proved a healthy practice for the denizens of the Valley of Mexico.

Ruíz de Alarcón's *Tratado* also describes the steps and the invocations for planting young agave plants and preparing a mature agave to produce *aguamiel* to be fermented into *pulque*. While the priest calls the narrative a "conjure," it is really an oral tradition text that helps the *tlachiqueros* (extractors) in their work. This process is still very much the same as it entails significant steps that cannot be replicated

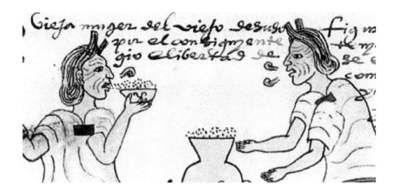

Figure 9.4 Elderly women drinking *pulque* and becoming talkative
Codex Mendoza folio 71r; Public Domain from Bodlian Libraries.

by machinery. *YouTube* has amazing videos of the collection and fermentation of *aguamiel* narrated by the *tlachiqueros* themselves.

The first step is to use the pruning stick/digging stick to remove the young maguey plant from the wild and place her in the proper row of the maguey field. The *Tratado* offers both instructions and words of comfort for her new resting place:

> Let it be soon! Come, priest, His [Ce atl]-tonal is One Water [i.e., the digging stick]. We will begin rooting out the Eight-flint-woman [i.e., the maguey— also translated "Noble Woman of Eight in a Row"], we will begin to set her upright. I am going in order to set her down. I am going in order to set her down in a place which is good, which is fine, where I have swept for her. There I will set her down; there she will be sitting. (Tratado 122)

Once the maguey plant, who is also perceived as his older sister, is properly placed, the *tlachiqero* petitions Tlaltecuhtli [the Earth Mother] to care for his charge, well:

> Be attentive to me, Tlaltecuhtli [i.e., the earth], indeed it is already in your hands that I place my older sister, [Noble Woman of Eight in a Row]. Carry her in your arms well. Embrace her well. It will not be a long time before I come to see her. Indeed, it only five instants before I will look upon her face, upon her headtop [i.e., before I come into her presence].

The translation of the name "Noble Woman of Eight in a Row" reflects a current discussion in the translation of the term "*tecpantli*" as "to count people twenty by twenty up to four hundred." We will examine these translations and what it may mean to the texts we are examining later in the discussion.

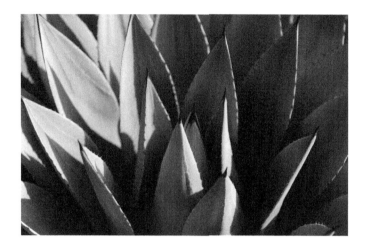

Figure 9.5 Agave bud: Freepik.com.

In this case, I interpret "headtop" as her crown and the five instants as the five years it normally takes for a maguey plant to mature. The headtop or heart will be perforated as soon as the bud forms on the flower stalk. The formation of the bud (Figure 9.5) signals the time to pierce the crown. Once again, the *tlachiquero* calls to his digging (now pruning) stick to assist him in the perforation and extraction of the heart:

> Come, priest, One Water [i.e., the pruning stick].
> Indeed, already the time has come.
> Indeed, you have become big, Noble Woman of Eight-in-a-Row
>   [i.e., the maguey].
> I will just insert the priest, One Water into your heart chamber.
> (Tratado 122)

This perforation of the maguey plant removes the crown or bud of the plant's flower stalk. The image of Mayahuel also illustrates the pruning stick behind her body. The image of Patécatl and Mayahuel (Figure 9.1) illustrates a maguey crown pierced by the pruning/ digging stick to the right of Patécatl's outstretched left hand. In this image, the marks where the leaves are cut from the heart so that it can be removed from the plant are also evident.

After a period of curing when the liquid does not flow or flows haltingly, the *tlachiquero* takes a set of copper scrapers/spoons and scrapes the walls of the basin so that the *aguamiel* will flow freely. As we have seen with the invocation to the digging/pruning stick "priest," an exhortation encourages the "Red Chichimecs" (the scrapers) to clean the maguey plant's walls to assure a good flow. If the digging stick is the priest, the red chichimecs are the warriors that perform the violent work of scraping the faces of the maguey to make her "cry." As they do their work, the maguey weeps and sheds her tears and even sweats the *aguamiel* from her "clean face." Tears and sweat are additional body fluids that Mesoamericans knew were vital to life.

> Let it be soon! Come, Red Chichimec [i.e., the spoon].
> Let it be now.
> Clean Noble Woman of Eight-in-a-Row
> in her heart chamber where you will live,
> where you will clean off her face.
> Indeed, already it is now that you will make Noble Woman
>   of Eight-in-a-Row shed tears,
> you will make her weep, you will make her sad,
> you will make her sweat; you will make her flow at the eyes
>   [i.e., exude *aguamiel*]". (Tratado 123)

Once the *aguamiel* begins to flow, the *tlachiqueros* must collect it twice a day for optimum harvest. The *tlachiqueros* carry the *aguamiel* back to their workshop in animal bladders, barrels or jars, and add it to previous collections. They also add a small amount of *pulque* to activate the fermentation process. In about a week, the *pulque* will be ready to consume. Not surprisingly, there are entities who oversee the consumption of *pulque*. These are the children of Mayahuel and Patécatl, the *Cenzon totochtin* (Four hundred rabbits). From the origin stories, we know that rabbits have a propensity for drinking. The *Cenzon totochtin* are the spirits or entities that inhabit people who are drinking, causing them to things under the influence of *pulque* that they would normally not do. One of the most iconic images of the rabbits (Figure 9.7) from the *Florentine Codex* Book Two is of them singing, probably intoxicated.

In addition to the Song of Ayopechtli, the collection of sacred songs from the *Primeros memoriales* also contains a song invoking the *Cenzon totochtin*. This text and its counterpart included in the *Florentine codex* have caused confusion because they appear to have been published with one of the folios inverted. Seler, Ángel Garibay Kintana, and Miguel León-Portilla have all addressed this issue.

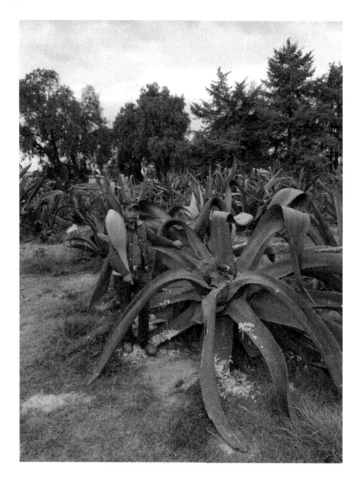

Figure 9.6 *Tlachiquero* and gourd next to scraped maguey plant 2019: Creative Commons.

Patrick Johansson has worked through the issues and created a Spanish-language matrix based on the two versions of the song, which we will use in this analysis (91–92). His research also indicates that some of the proper names that had been identified as places are actually names of some of the *Totochtin* involved in the discourse of the song. A close reading of my English translation will help illustrate this.

The first stanza consists of a series of vocalizations that are used to call the listeners' attention. The vocalization may have been accompanied by drumming and dancing as many of these texts were. "*yyaha, yya, yya ayya, ayyo oviya,/ ayya yya, ayya yya, yyo/ viya, ayya yya ayya yya yyo viya*" (91).

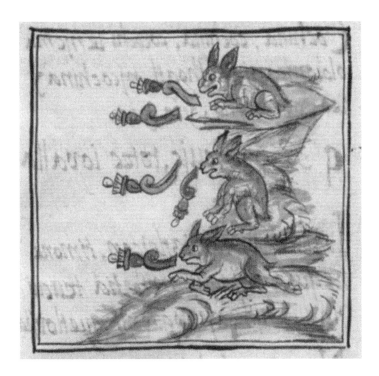

Figure 9.7 *Florentine Codex* Book 2, folio143v
https://www.wdl.org/en/item/10096/view/1/406/
https://wiki2.org/en/Centzon_T%C5%8Dt%C5%8Dchtin#/media/
File:Historia_general_de_las_cosas_de_nueva_Espa%C3%B1a_
page_406_1.png.

Then, like the previous song, the place of the action is identified here as Coliuacan. "Coli[u]acan/*lugar de veneración/a casa del maguey-hombre a/ yyo ayya yya yyo*" (91) and followed by more vocalizations. While at the time of this composition, an actual city called Coliauacan existed, Johansson makes the case that this place is the mythical Coliuacan of Nahua origin stories, placing the beginning of the cultivation of *aguamiel* and *pulque* in ancient times. I agree with Johansson's identification and with the ancient origin of the drink. The song situates the place of veneration in the home of the maguey-man in Coliuacan (91).

The following section introduces the divinity, "Tezcatzon," as the "god of the twentieth row." The conversation of the translation of *tecpantli* has been controversial. It can mean "in the palace," but Johansson explains that this could also have a connection with a process of counting people (or rabbits, or maguey cactuses) in lines of 20 (82). Johansson cites Remí Siméon's definition of *tecpantli* as an adjectival form signifying "to count people twenty by twenty up to four hundred: *centecpantli* [one *tecpantli*], twenty; *ontecpantli* [two *tecpantli*], forty; *etecpantli* [three *tecpantli*], sixty; *macuiltecpantli* [five *tecpantli*], one hundred; *chicunauhtecpanti* [nine *tecpantli*], one hundred and eighty; etc. (81 *para contar las personas de veinte en veinte hasta cuatrocientos: centecpantli* [one *tecpantli*], veinte; *ontecpantli* [two *tecpantli*], cuarenta; *etecpantli* [three *tecpantli*], sesenta; *macuiltecpantli* [five *tecpantli*], cien; *chicunauhtecpantli* [nine *tecpantli*], ciento ochenta; etc.)"

Johansson remarks that "This definition of rows of twenty up to four hundred as the term integrates perfectly in a semantic constellation of 400 rabbits that circulate around *pulque* [production and consumption] (81) *Esta definición de "hileras de veinte hasta llegar a cuatrocientos" para el término se integra perfectamente a una constelación semántica de 400 conejos que giran en torno al pulque).*" 20 rows of 20 is a perfect field of 400 that neatly describes the *Cenzon totochtin* (400 rabbits) associated with *pulque* and the maguey plant.

Previously, we had seen Mayahuel as "Noble Woman of Eight-in-a-Row" or perhaps "of the eighth row" possibly identifying her in the 160th position of the maguey planting. Now we have one of her rabbit sons, Tezcatzon, identifying as "god twentieth row." As Mayahuel serves as the personification of the maguey plant, Tezcatzon is the personification of the *aguamiel/pulque* liquid in the song of his 400 brothers and sisters. In this stanza in Johansson's matrix, Tezcatzon, the liquid, is *tlacihqueado*. We remember that the *tlachiqueros* are those in charge of planting, cultivating and harvesting the maguey plant. They remove plants from the wild, transplant them in the rows, pierce them and cut the hearts from the leaves when the plant is ready, scrape the sides so that the sap runs, extract the liquid several times a day and nurture the *pulque* while it ferments in larger vats or jars. Johansson has selected the term *tlachiqueado* to describe the action in this section. In this context, the *tlachiquero's* works the maguey to make it "cry," as we saw in the earlier incantation from the *Tratado*. In trying to understand the connection between this song and the *pulque*-making process, I suggest a possible translation of Johansson's matrix into English could be: "Tezcatzon divinity eighth row/ is *tlachiqueado* (being scraped and worked by the *tlachiquero*)/ Is he crying yet?/ Avia/ Not yet, not yet. (91) *Tezcatzon dios hilera de veinte/ Es tlachiqueado/ Ya llora ya/ Avia/ Así no, así no).*"

As Johansson explains, it takes some time for the liquid *aguamiel* to run freely into the maguey's cavity. It seems that this section

invoking Tezcatzon presents the early attempts to make the sap run—
to make the divinity cry—and they are not yet successful. Then,
another round of *tlachiqueando* "the divinity is *tlachiqueado/ el dios
está siendo tlachiqueado*" produces the exclamation "*ye*," which
Johansson identifies as an exclamation surprise or excitement,
followed by "he cries now/ *Huía* [another exclamation of surprise or
excitement] (91 *yye, llora ya/ Huía.*)" Johansson explains that "[t]he
exclamation of the god corresponds metaphorically here to the seeping
of the scraped maguey: the *aguamiel* (91 *El llanto del dios corresponde
metafóricamente aquí al rezumo del maguey raspado: el aguamiel.*)"

The next section is identical to the previous one except the voice
calls the divinity "Axalco divinity of the twentieth row (92 *Axalco dios
hilera de veinte*)" rather than Tezcatzon. Similar statements about the
work to produce *aguamiel* follows: "The divinity is being
tlachiqueado/ He is crying already/ Not yet, not yet. The divinity is
being *tlachiqueado/* He is crying already/ Now he is crying (92 *El dios
está siendo tlachiqueado/ Ya llora ya/ Así no, así no/ El dios está siendo
tlachiqueado/ Ya llora ya.*)"

It appears that the *tlachiquero* has succeeded in making the maguey
cry. The next section reframes the *pulque*-making process. First, the
place of the divinity Tezcatzon (Tezcatzonco) is called "place of the
warrior heart and already the divinity created the rabbit [made the
intoxicating beverage?] (92 *Tezcatzonco, lugar de tu corazón a
guerrero y ya/ Al conejo creó mi dios).*" Then the voice shares "I will
cut it; I will perforate it [the heart of the maguey]/ [from?] Mixcoatl's
mountain [a place where maguey grew wild?] in Colhuacan [the
ancient city] (92 *Yo lo cortaré, yo lo perforaré/ Mixcoaltepetl,
colhoacan.*)"

The final stanza appears to cover the final steps of production: "I
have my throat [the *tlachiquero* has the gourd to extract *pulque*]/ I
mistreat [disrupt?] the little mirror, the little mirror [the shiny surface
of the *aguamiel*?]/ Come and distill [ferment?] the white skin of the
mirror [the *aguamiel*] in pulque. (92 *Tengo garganta ya/ Maltrato iyao/
Al espejito, espejito/ Ve a destilar en pulque la piel blanca del espejo*).
This is the time in which the *tlachiquero* removes the pool of *aguamiel*
collected in the hollow of the plant. This is a well-documented process
in Mexican photography. Here we have an image of a *tlachiquero* from
1908 extracting the sweet liquid from the plant. Johannson suggests
that the "*garganta*" in the song is the gourd used by the *tlachiquero*
as a straw to remove the liquid (92). I agree that the image of the
"throat" "mistreating" the "little mirror" does represent the removal
of the liquid, now flowing freely. As we can see from this photograph,
tlachiquero could be described as suckling the liquid from the "breast"

that is the gourd. The images of Mayahuel nursing babies (and some-times animals) while seated within or emerging from the massive agave can also be visually connected to the removal of *aguamiel*.

The final line exhorts the listener to "Drink *pulque*! *a ho a* [excla-mation]/ (92) *Bebe el pulque a ho a*)." As we have seen, the origin, production, and consumption of *pulque* form an important aspect of Mesoamerican life, complete with rules and rituals as well as charac-ters that cultivate the beverage and consumers who use it in a variety of ways. Importantly, all along the process, the entities that contribute to the success of *pulque* brewing are recognized for their efforts, demonstrating how connected the agricultural and industrial processes are with everyday life and sacred practices.

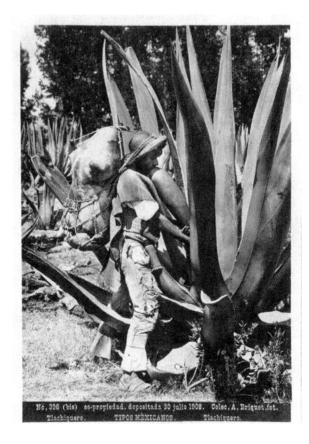

Figure 9.8 *Tlachiquero* collecting *aguamiel* with gourd 1908.
Public domain from getty.edu.

Despite their efforts, the missionaries were unable to eradicate *pulque* from the lives of their charges, although there was a time in the twentieth century when beer was more popular. Recently, *pulque* has seen a resurgence of popularity and now high-end *pulque* boutiques are popping up throughout the Distrito Federal and across the country. *Pulque* is mixed with tropical fruit and other flavors. It has become the drink of choice for the nightclub scene. Drink *pulque*!

Bibliography

Atlas de las plantas de la medicina tradicional mexicana. "Maguey." Biblioteca digital de la medicina tradicional mexicana. http://www.medicinatradicionalmexicana.unam.mx/apmtm/termino. php?l=3&t=agave-americana

Escalante A., López Soto D.R., Velázquez Gutiérrez J.E., Giles-Gómez M., Bolívar F. and López-Munguía A. "*Pulque*, a Traditional Mexican Alcoholic Fermented Beverage: Historical, Microbiological, and Technical Aspects." *Frontiers in Microbiology* 7:1026, 2016. doi: 10.3389/fmicb.2016.01026.

Codex Magliabechiano. http://www.famsi.org/research/graz/magliabechian-o/img_page171.html *Codex Mendoza.*

Johansson, Patrick. "*Totochtin incuic Tezcatzoncatl*: Un canto para las primicias del *pulque* nuevo." *Estudios de cultura nahuatl.* 26 (1996), 69–97.

Rémi Siméon, *Diccionario de la lengua nahuatl o mexicana*, Mexico, Editorial Siglo XXI, 1977.

Ruíz de Alarcón, Hernando. *Treatise on the Heathen Superstitions That Today Live among the Indians Native to This New Spain, 1629.* trans. James Richard Andrews, and Ross Hassig. Norman: University of Oklahoma Press, 1984.

Sahagún, fray Bernardino de. *Florentine Codex: General History of the Things of New Spain.* 12 vols. and introduction, translated by Arthur J. O. Anderson and Charles E. Dibble. Santa Fe, New Mexico: School for American Research, 1950–1982.

———. *Primeros Memoriales Part 2: Paleography of Nahuatl Text and English Translation.* Paleography by Thelma B. Sullivan, Completed and revised with additions by H. B. Nicholson, Arthur J. O. Anderson, Charles E. Dibble, Eliose Quiñones Keber and Wayne Ruwet. Norman: University of Oklahoma Press, 1997.

Seler, Eduard, editor. *Los cantos religiosos de los antiguos mexicanos.* Ciudad de México Universidad Nacional Autónoma de México Instituto de Investigaciones Históricas (Cultura Náhuatl: Fuentes, 13), 2016.

10

Como agua para chocolate: Like Food for Emotion, Like Illness/Injury for Transition/Transformation

Debra D. Andrist

In Laura Esquivel's *Como agua para chocolate*,[1] both novel and film versions, space and time create reality that resonates for most readers and viewers, yet the details of cooking, eating, illness, and madness appear to transcend scientific and medical principles, squarely situating this work in the genre of magical realism. In Esquivel's fiction, food is infused with the emotion of the cook and translates that emotion to those who consume it; healthy and pathological responses to food, environment and healing are indicative of character. Elements of paradox (joy and grief, heat and cold) and mimesis (in character and situation) in heighten pathos and emphasize the coded messages in pathology and healing. These narrative effects provide information to the astute reader or viewer about plot, character development, and narrative tone. The novel's physical consequences, viewed through a medical and scientific (biological, chemical) representation of the body by means of illness, injury, treatment, and death focus especially on the negative physical pathology and on the psychological effects that self-manifest in destructive social behavior.[2] Using a semiotic approach, this study explores examples of such situations in the novel and points to the central role of the magical (or mythical)/scientific (or medical) representations that develop plot and character.

The transitions/transformations that occur as a result of these magical/scientific aspects are clarified through the application of Alicia Suskin Ostriker's theories on women writers as revisionist mythmakers.[3] Ostriker theorizes that all women writers are foreigners to, or at least on the margins of, the traditional system of symbols. Women have to create everything anew; they create new myths because they have to recreate everything from the feminine point-of-view rather than from the masculine. This revision of myths especially stands out in the works of women writers like Esquivel who choose genres of the fantastic such as magical realism. Although Ostriker was not writing about Latin American magical realism but about poetry in English, she proposes three strategies that are telling in the context of *Como agua*: (1) transformation, or a radical change in physical representation; (2) writing in code, or concealment of the theme or message of the work by coding messages; and (3) mirroring/mimesis, in the exhibition or development of shared characteristics or behaviors, as if one character or event could stand for the other.

Tita's great-niece narrates the novel in a sort of flashback reading of recipes from Tita's cookbook-journal. The journal and recipes represent a codification or concealment of the theme or message of the work, according to the Ostriker model. An ingredient of the first recipe, onion, and the tears shed due to the fumes released when cutting them,[4] not only establish the leitmotif of tears, but also mirror the affinity between protagonist and narrator, whose response to onions is associated with Tita's: "*Mamá decía que [yo lloraba tanto al cortar la cebolla] porque yo soy igual de sensible a la cebolla que Tita, mi tía abuela/* Mom used to say that [I cried so much when I cut the onion] because I'm just as sensitive to onions as Tita, my great aunt" (3).

Salt, one of the chemical requirements of life and a staple in the kitchen, is emphasized as a component of tears, beginning with Tita's audible sobbing from the womb when Mamá Elena chops onion, and continuing with Tita's birth on the kitchen table amid a salty flood of tears (rather than amniotic fluid) which provides seasoning in the kitchen for a considerable period.[5] Thus, too, begin Tita's ties to the kitchen, to food itself, to cooking and its substitutions and to paradoxes. Mamá Elena's husband dies of a heart attack two days after Tita's birth, and Mamá Elena has no milk for her. While the stated message is that Mamá Elena is overwhelmed with grief and responsibility, the coded inference is distinct: the narrative later reveals that Mamá Elena's consternation may have resulted from fear of social exposure of her earlier infidelity. Her inability/unwillingness to nurture Tita, either physically or emotionally, is emphasized repeatedly and is mirrored in Rosaura, the eldest and the daughter most like Elena.

Nacha, ranch cook and Tita's substitute mother, rescues Tita: "*se ofreció a hacerse cargo de la alimentación de Tita [quien] se mudó a la cocina y entre atoles y tés [en lugar del mamar] creció/*she offered to take over feeding Tita [who] moved into the kitchen and between hot, corn-based beverages and teas [instead of sucking] grew up" (4–5). As a result of living vicariously through kitchen activities and food, Tita sees an equation where most observers would see a paradox: "*no diferenciaba bien las lágrimas de la risa de las del llanto. Para ella reír era una manera de llorar [hasta el punto de confundir] el gozo del vivir con el de comer*/it did not differentiate the tears of laughter from those of crying well. For her to laugh was a way to cry [to the point of confusing] the joy of living with that of eating" (5). Even Tita's childhood toys and games are paradoxical substitutions: she transforms the trademark sausage of the family ranch into imitations of balloon animals she has seen and makes a game of sprinkling water on the hot griddle to see it dance.

When Pedro announces his love to Tita one Christmas in the kitchen, Tita has already recognized his interest in the drawing room because of the heat she felts from his gaze, "quemándole la piél/burning her skin" (15). When Pedro agrees to marry Rosaura to remain near Tita, Tita feels a cold so intense and dry invading her body that her cheeks paradoxically burn and redden as they did under Pedro's gaze at the Christmas party (13). John Brown will later explain her joy and suffering in terms of his grandmother's theory of the internal matches (16–17), but for now, Tita can only suffer from the literal and metaphorical cold without understanding it. For many years, Tita tries to relieve her physical and mental suffering with an activity that implies warmth and manual occupation, "*tejir a gancho . . . sacó de su costurero una colcha que había empezado a tejer el día en que Pedro le habló de matrimonio . . . tejió y lloró, y lloró y tejió, hasta que en la madrugada terminó la colcha y se la echó encima. De nada sirvió*/to crochet . . . she pulled out an afghan from her sewing box that she had begun to weave the day Pedro told her about the marriage . . . she wove and cried, and cried and wove, until in the early morning she finished the afghan and threw it on top of herself. It was of no use" (18).

Throughout her life, Tita's efforts to find warmth will be in vain, but she continues to add to her *colcha*.

During the wedding preparations, she is forbidden to cry by Mamá Elena, but Tita sobs as she prepares Pedro and Rosaura's wedding cake and frosting (*fondant*) and even the *turron*/nougat (34), her tears blending with the batter.[6] The wedding sweets induce a bitter-sweet response among the guests, who weep for their own lost loves to the point of nausea and vomiting. Seen another way, consumption of the cake and other sweets prepared by the psychological-but-not-physical bride cause vomiting as a metaphor for the social rejection of Pedro and Rosaura's inappropriate marriage.[7] Paradoxically, Pedro whispers his continuing devotion to Tita at the wedding reception, and only months later does he finally consummate his marriage to his substitute-wife (39).

Following the wedding the paradoxical events and responses continue. Tita is severely beaten by Mamá Elena, partly because Nacha cannot corroborate her innocence in putting a vomitive in the wedding cake because, the reader is rather belatedly informed, Nacha is dead. Nacha dies the night before the wedding, yearning for her lost love, a yearning presumably inspired by her tasting Tita's *fondant* (34), which results in a headache and her death. Tita finds Nacha dead, with medicinal leaves on her temples and clutching a photo of her own lost love, a man chased away by Elena's Mamá (40), in another mirroring of circumstance. With Nacha gone, Tita, just suspected of poisoning the guests, becomes the official ranch cook. Substitute-wife, Rosaura, is not able to substitute as cook, though she tries her hand, and the entire family suffers indigestion. When Tita has been ranch cook for one year, Pedro offers Tita a sheaf of roses. In the moment of Tita and Pedro's joy, Rosaura cries with jealousy, and Mamá angrily warns Pedro and orders Tita to throw out the roses. Tita clutches the roses to her and the thorns pierce her skin, staining the roses redder with her blood, in a metaphorical consummation of her love with Pedro.

Rather than dispose of the roses, Tita decides to prepare a meal of quail in rose petal sauce, a literal and figurative reinforcement of the 'deflowering' metaphor already suggested. Now Tita's blood blends with the sauce recipe. A second metaphor is obvious when Tita only injures the first quail rather than dispatching it—to her horror (47–48). Tita relates the half-dead bird's physical pain to her own psychological suffering—the analogy of the broken bird to her broken heart—and she realizes that she must imitate her mother's forcefulness in killing but, out of mercy. Tita, determined not to cause them to suffer, is able to kill the birds decisively and finish the dish. Both the birds and Tita are implicated in the sacrifice of the innocent.

Overwhelming sexual arousal (felt as heat) in all the dinner guests is occasioned by consuming the dish. Notably, Mamá Elena complains that the dish contains too much salt![8] The passion that should have been physically consummated between Tita and Pedro, but which was dispassionately consummated between Rosaura and Pedro, will now be psychologically displaced upon the second sister, Gertrudis. This danger was noted (unscientifically) in the recipe: "*Se desprenden con mucho cuidado los pétalos de rosas, procurando no pincharse . . . pueden quedar impregnados de sangre [que] puede provocar reacciones químicas/* carefully detach the rose petals, taking care not to get pricked . . . they may be impregnated with blood [which] can cause chemical reactions" (45). Gertrudis sweats pink, rose-scented drops which evaporate into a cloud as she tries to cold-shower away the all-consuming heat. Crazed with passion, she is carried away, literally and figuratively, by a revolutionary soldier, to consummate her awakened, displaced passion. Their psychological pathology—the idea of being 'crazy with passion'—and the social pathology—aberrant behavior as a result of the passion—mimics the political pathology of the Mexican Revolution during which the novel is set. However, this atmosphere of pathology is beginning the process of curing other pathologies; in one sense, Gertrudis breaks free of the sexual repression of the ranch, and in another sense, as a revolutionary general, functions as a metaphorical physician who models a cure for a social ill: the subjugation of Mexican women. In other ways, personal apects of this 'pathological passion' will later be cured, not in the culinary sense of treating food to preserve it, but in the medical sense of recovering a healthy state of balance.

At this point, recovery is distant, and Tita's suffering is likened to the last food item on the tray, the one no one dares to take lest he or she be thought a glutton. Starved for warmth and wishing to be chosen, Tita compares herself to *un chile en nogada olvidado en una charola*/chile pepper in sauce forgotten on a tray, a rich and spicy delicacy that is left untried and is headed for the rubbish bin (57). Again, Tita sublimates her passion, throwing her energy into work. She crochets nightly, the unfinished project reflecting the unconsummated relationship, and her thoughts fixed in the consideration of heat in all its definitions. Tita translates her pain into creativity in the kitchen as well: "*De esta época de sufrimiento nacieron sus mejores recetas*/her best recipes were born during this period of suffering" (69).

The birth of Roberto as a turning point in Tita's suffering and development direct the reader to the figurative significance of Tita's creativity in the kitchen. The words "impregnated' (in the description of the rose petal sauce) and "being born" (referring to Tita's creation of her recipes) are significant in light of Tita's involvement with Roberto. Soon after, she delivers Roberto and swaddles him *como taco*/like a taco wrap (74) to calm and warm him.[9] Tita is preparing *mole*/chocolate peanut pepper sauce (with three kinds of peppers, pepper seeds, and onions) for the baptism and she rhythmically pulverizes ingredients in a *metate*/mortar & pestle. Attracted by the delicious smells from the kitchen, Pedro enters and is seized by passion as he can't take his eyes off the sympathetic movement of Tita's unfettered breasts as she rocks. In her typical way of thinking about life in terms of food, Tita considers how "*el contacto con el fuego altera los* *elementos [y] en sólo unos instantes [de mirarlos con passion] Pedro había tranformado los senos de Tita, de castos a voluptuosos, sin necesidad de tocarlos/*contact with fire alters the elements [and] in just a few moments [of looking at them with passion] Peter had transformed Tita's breasts, from chaste to voluptuous, without the need to touch them" (67). This transformation/stimulation may be a precursor of Tita's miraculous (but physically possible) lactation. When Rosaura cannot nurse/nurture baby Roberto (as her mother could not nurse/nurture Tita), and the wet nurse is accidentally killed in the Revolution, Tita is able to feed him from her own breasts.[10]

Tita and Pedro feel as if they are the parents of Roberto, and Tita takes Rosaura's place at the baptism party when Rosaura is too ill to attend. Mamá Elena notices their happiness and soon sends Rosaura, Pedro, and Roberto across the border (81–82), ostensibly for better medical care—but science fails. In San Antonio, Roberto dies, as Chencha says, because *"todo lo que comía le caía mal/*everything he ate didn't sit well with [his digestion]" [11] (99). Rosaura, like her mother, lacks Tita's sympathetic nature and cannot access the spiritual support that Tita gets from Nacha. Rosaura cannot cook and has never cared for a baby, so the move is predictably fatal to Roberto.

The news destroys Tita's sanity, and her mental breakdown signals another transition/transformation in her character. When the news arrives, Tita, her mother, and Chencha are making sausage. When her mother refuses to let her grieve, Tita explodes in anger, her mother strikes her, and Tita climbs up to seeks refuge in the dovecote, taking with her a young bird that she has been compulsively feeding. The dovecote is the only place Mamá Elena cannot reach her due to her fear of heights. Nearly catatonic and mute after spending the night there, during which her little bird dies from indigestion (a mirroring metaphor for Roberto), Tita refuses to come down, and her mother sends for Dr. John Brown to take Tita to the insane asylum.[12] John takes her away, her enormous, multi-colored woven afghan trailing from his carriage, but he cares for Tita in his own home. Tita has no work to do and never speaks but John tells Tita about his work and about his *Kikapú* grandmother (*Luz del Amanecer*/Light of Dawn), who had a theory about happiness and grief that allows Tita to understand her life with Mamá Elena and Pedro. The turning-point is broth—beef, not chicken soup![13]—delivered by Chencha, who is now the ranch cook. Chencha's ox-tail soup, hot both in temperature and spice (containing salt, onion and peppers) conjures up Nacha, bringing about emotional reconnect (124).

Tita's foresworn return to the ranch is occasioned by injury: the night Chencha returns from John Brown's house, the ranch is attacked,

Chencha is raped by the bandits, and Mamá Elena is paralyzed by a blow when she attempts to defend Chencha (130). Reentering the life where Mamá Elena is a kind of substitute for the child and childcare forbidden to Tita, Tita's care for her is now more labor-intensive than before: Mamá Elena, paralyzed, is truly 'as helpless as a baby.' Tita prepares broths to help heal her mother but Mamá Elena repeatedly detects a bitter flavor—the emotion of an unwilling cook. Elena dies as a result of repeatedly dosing herself with syrup of ipecac,[14] in fear of poison, effecting another narrative transition. In an effort to explain her unexpected lack of feeling over her mother's death, Tita turns again to food analogies:

> *Tita no sentía dolor ninguno. Hasta ahora comprendía el significado de la frase de "fresca como una lechuga," así de extraña y lejana se debería sentir una lechuga antes su repentina separación de otra lechuga con la que hubiera crecido. Sería ilógico esperar que sufriera por la separación de esa lechuga con la que nunca había podido hablar ni establecer ningún tipo de comunicación y de la que sólo conocía las hojas exteriores, ignorando que en su interior habían muchas otras escondidas./* Tita didn't feel any pain. Not until now had she understood the meaning of the phrase "fresh as a lettuce leaf," how strange and distant a lettuce leaf should feel before its sudden separation from another lettuce leaf with which it had grown [as a complete head of lettuce]. It would be illogical to expect it to suffer from the separation from that lettuce leaf with which it had never been able to speak or establish any kind of communication and of which it only knew the outer leaves, ignoring that inside there were many others hidden. (137)

Among her mother's things, Tita discovers that her mother's parents had forbidden her to marry José and that he was shot and killed the night they planned to run away. José is the illegitimate son of a *mulata*,[15] and he becomes the father of Gertrudis after Elena's forced marriage to Juan de la Garza. Juan learns of Gertrudis' parentage when he goes to the tavern to celebrate Tita's birth and suffers a heart attack.[16] When he dies several days later, Tita becomes the family's last daughter and thus, according to tradition, cannot marry. Perhaps in an effort to restore her honor in society and to expiate her guilt over the extramarital affair, Elena remains an unremarried widow; she sacrifices Tita's innocent life, mirroring a substitution for her own errors.

During the funeral, Pedro and Rosaura, who is about to give birth, arrive at the ranch to discover that John and Tita intend to marry.

Esperanza is born but Rosaura again can't nurse and Tita refuses to nurse her and raises her on *tes*/teas and *atoles*/hot corn-based beverages, as Nacha had done with Tita (5, 146). When Rosaura suffers complications with an imbedded the placenta,[17] she is unable to have more children though John saves her life with surgery. This pathology and its cure provide another transition/transformation and create a new issue: Rosaura intends to sacrifice Esperanza just as her mother sacrificed Tita.

Following Esperanza's birth, heat imagery abounds, with both Pedro and Tita "boiling," *como agua para chocolate* (151). Pedro is angry and irritable due to Tita's plans to marry John. Tita is upset over Rosaura's plans to imprison Esperanza in caretaking. One day Tita relieves the growing tension with a cool shower (recalling Gertrudis' shower episode). She abruptly realizes that the water is growing warmer: *"De pronto empezó a sentir que el agua se entibiaba y se ponía cada vez más caliente hasta empezar a quemarle la piel*/suddenly she started to feel the water warm up and get hotter and hotter until she started to burn her skin" (154). She opens her eyes and discovers Pedro on the other side of the shower planks watching her with eyes that "glow" (*brillan*) in the dusk. The incident figuratively scalds Tita, making her angry, rather than inflaming her with passion (154–155). Before dinner is served, in a tense atmosphere, John asks Pedro for Tita's hand, they discuss details of the wedding and John presents Tita with a ring. The glittering diamonds remind Tita of the brilliant light in Pedro's eyes earlier in the evening. Late that night, Tita is alone in the kitchen putting away dishes when Pedro, who had concealed himself, throws Tita on Gertrudis' abandoned bed where *"la hizo perder su virginidad y conocer el verdadero amor*/he took her virginity and caused her to know true love" (159). Their lovemaking creates a visible show of fireworks, *"un resplandor extraño*/a strange glow," where *"[v]olutas fosforescentes se elevaban hacia el cielo como delicadas luces de bengala*/phosphorescent spirals rose skyward like delicate flares" (159). Rosaura and Chencha see the fireworks and Chencha identifies the display as the spirit of Mamá Elena returned from Purgatory. The irony is explained by the narrator: fear of Mamá Elena now provides *"la oportunidad ideal*/the ideal opportunity" for Pedro and Tita's lovemaking (160).

Though Rosaura, having gained weight and developed digestive problems, asks for Tita's help in recovering Pedro's affection, a recovery or cure that will prove impossible. Rosaura reveals a radical change in her physical representation straight out of Ostriker:

> *Desde hacía unas semanas tenía graves problemas digestivos, sufría de flato y mal aliento. Rosaura se sintió tan apenada . . . que inclusive tuvo que tomar la decisión de que Pedro y ella durmieran en recámaras separadas . . . No se explicaba por qué desde que regresó al rancho había empezado a engordar tanto/* For a few weeks she had serious digestive problems, suffered from flatulence and bad breath. Rosaura felt so sorry . . . that she even had to make the decision that she and Pedro sleep in separate bedrooms . . . It was inexplicable why since she returned to the ranch she had started to gain so much weight. (169–70)

Rosaura's problems made visible in *"un voluminso y gelatinoso cuerpo/a bulky, gelatinous body"* temporarily capture Tita's sympathy but only until Rosaura reaffirms her vow to follow Mamá Elena's example, imprisoning Esperanza in caretaking.

Mamá Elena's spirit appears and confronts Tita for having had relations with Pedro (173) and curses Tita's unborn child. Tita believes that she is pregnant and soon confides in Gertrudis (189–90), who has returned to the ranch as a general in the Revolution and as the wife of Juan, the soldier with whom she ran away (179). Gertrudis reveals that a year before, she gave birth to a *mulato* child and that Juan has not forgiven her for the suspected infidelity; fortunately, Tita can reveal the truth of Gertrudis' parentage and resolve the problem (181).[18] For her part, Gertrudis arranges to discuss Tita's supposed pregnancy within earshot of Pedro (191). These events (in *"septiembre"* and *"octubre"*) bring to mind Ostriker's mimesis theory in that Gertrudis' experience in the world allows her to put herself in Tita's position and to act decisively for what she sees as Tita's happiness. Tita, because of her knowledge of their mother, is able to provide information that saves Gertrudis' marriage to Juan.

Whether Tita's pregnancy symptoms point to her true condition—or intend to symbolize a false-transformation in the form of stress-related amenorrhea—Elena's ghost validates the pregnancy when she accuses Tita and curses the child.[19] Having had enough of her mother's abuse, Tita rejects her mother with the words, *"la odio . . . las palabras mágicas para hacer desaparecer a Mamá Elena para siempre/*I hate you . . . the magic words to make Mama Elena disappear forever" (200). Tita finds that she is no longer pregnant—if she ever was: *"Los músculos de centro de su cuerpo se relajaron, dando paso a la impetuosa salida de su menstruación/*The center muscles of her body relaxed, giving way to the impetuous exit of her period" (200). The purgative confrontation restores Tita's physical—if not her emotional—equilbrium.

The "*imponente imagen*/imposing image" of light and heat that is Mamá Elena's spirit, however, is not quite exhausted and inflicts its final damage on Pedro. It "*se acercó a Pedro girando vertiginosamente, y con furia hizo que el quinqué más cercano a él estallara en mil pedazos. El petróleo esparció las llamas con rapidez sobre la cara y el cuerpo de Pedro*/it approached Pedro spinning dizzyingly, and furiously made the oil lamp closest to him explode into a thousand pieces. Oil quickly spread the flames over Pedro's face and body;" he runs along the patio, converted into "*una antorcha humana*/a human torch" (201). This horrifying scene has the paradoxical effect of restoring Tita's sympathies toward Pedro, and it makes public their relationship when Pedro rejects Rosaura's offer of comfort and clings to Tita (202–203). Tita uses traditional medicine: she treats Pedro's burns with egg whites and raw potatoes.[20] To heal his scars, she seeks the advice of Nacha who gets the answer from the aforementioned grandmother of John, *Luz del Amanecer*: the bark of the *tepezcohuite* tree for which she must send Nicolas to "*el mejor brujo de la región*/the best healer in the area" (202–203).[21]

The narrative moves to Rosaura's death, many years later (a year before Esperanza's wedding) and again works from paradoxical representations. As if Rosaura were a negative photographic image of Tita, her death is of the most opposite to the delicious food imagery and smells produced by Tita's cooking. Its nature is described as "*de lo más extraña*/the strangest.*" Pedro is distracted from his book one evening by the noise of Rosaura's passing gas, described as "estos desagradables ruidos/these disagreeable noises" (232). Pedro tells himself "*que no era posible que ese prolongado sonido fuera del producto de los problemas digestivos de su mujer*/that it was not possible that that prolonged sound was the product of his wife's digestive problems" and he wonders whether the "*estruendosos cañonazos la revolución se había reiniciado*/ thunderous cannons [of] the revolution had restarted" (233). He remarks (to himself) about "*un olor . . . nauseabundo*/a nauseating odor" which penetrates the rooms "*a pesar de haber tomado la precaución de [usar] un trozo de carbon encendido y un poco de azúcar*/in spite of having taken the precaution of [using] a piece of charcoal on and a little sugar" (233). He soon discovers Rosaura "*de labios morados, cuerpo desinflado, ojos desencajados, mirada perdida*/with purple lips, body deflated, disembodied eyes, lost [empty] look.*" John Brown pronounces the cause of death "*una congestión estomacal aguda*/ an acute stomach congestion" (233). As a medical aside, Rosaura's continuing condition and symptoms could indicate severe food allergies.[22]

Following Rosaura's death, Esperanza and Alex, John's son, are married on the ranch. This marriage, with Esperanza as alterego for Tita, is a kind of vicarious fulfillment for Tita and unites the two families in true love. Even more important, the marriage precludes, for all time, any future attempt to sacrifice the innocent in the de la Garza tradition. Esperanza and Alex can look forward to a healthy life because the illnesses of the relationships which preceded theirs have been cured.

Esperanza is emphasized as a mirror or fulfillment of potential for Tita when she describes her response to Alex's gaze on her body. She tells Tita that she feels "*como la masa de buñuelo entrando al aceite hirviendo/* like the donut dough entering the boiling oil" (239), a sentiment and a metaphor that resonates with Tita, who had used it to describe the effect of Pedro's eyes on her at the Christmas party the night he had declared his love: Tita "*comprendió perfectamente lo que debe sentir la masa de un buñuelo al entrar en contacto con el aceite hirviendo/*understood perfectly what the dough of a donut must feel when it came into contact with the boiling oil" (15). Tita describes the conversion of her breasts, from "*castos/*chaste" to "*volulptuosos/*voluptuous" under Pedro's gaze in similar terms. In all these instances, the emphasis is on the change that fire (heat) brings to "*elementos/*elements [ingredients]" (67). Like Tita, Esperanza is not the boiling liquid of *como agua*, but the low-temperature, 'inert' element—*chocolate, masa, buñuelo/*chocolate, [corn]meal, fritter—that is changed irretrievably and instantly upon contact with heat. This image of joining culinary opposites for an erotic outcome appears in the special dish Tita prepares for Esperanza's wedding, *chiles en nogada*, which blends of spicy/savory and sweet ingredients (228).

Two final scenes, both related to Esperanza and Alex's wedding, return to the theme of heat—and this time, the heat of passion provides a searing closure. When Tita and Pedro are finally alone, they begin to make love, but Pedro suffers a heart attack *del éxtasis/*of ecstasy (246), fulfilling the warning of the *Luz del Amanecer's* philosophy of the internal matches (117–18), as articulated by John to Tita after Roberto's death:

'*Si por una emoción muy fuerte se llegan a encender todos los cerillos que llevamos en nuestro interior de un solo golpe, se produce un resplandor tan fuerte que ilumina más allá de lo que podemos ver normalmente y entonces ante nuestros ojos aparece un túnel esplendoroso que nos muestra el camino que olvidamos al momento de nacer y que nos llama a reencontrar nuestro perdido origin divino. El alma desea reintegrarse al lugar de donde proviene, dejando al cuerpo inerte*' [sic]/ 'If by a very strong emotion we come to light all the matches that we carry inside us in a single blow, there is a glow so strong that it illuminates beyond what we can normally see and then before our eyes appears a splendid tunnel that shows us the path that we forget at the moment of birth and that calls us to rediscover our lost divine origin. The soul wishes to reintegrate to the place from which it comes, leaving the body inert'. [sic] (245–6)

Juliet-like, Tita then consumes the poisonous phosphorus matches and calls upon her memories of Pedro to kindle the fire that her "damp" matches and the breath and words of Pedro can no longer inflame.[23] Having achieved her own *extasis*, Tita joins Pedro in the tunnel of origin and returning. From Tita's passion for Pedro, the ranch catches fire and all is destroyed except the key to the story: Tita's cookbook-journal (246–247).

Esquivel's revisionist mythmaking creates a magical body of narrative over what is a realistic framework of scientific and traditional medicine in *Como agua para chocolate*. Food transforms, creating a radical change in physical representation through emotional response. Esquivel shows the alteration working in reverse as Tita's emotions inform her food. Physical and psychological consequences of these catalysts ensue, viewed through Esquivel's scientific and magical representation of the body, illness, injury, treatment, recovery, & death. These events of pathology, leading to cure or resolution, both conceal and reveal Esquivel's work. A part of this process is the characters' mimetic activity: they mirror or mimic other characters, exhibiting or developing identical or similar characteristics or behaviors, as if one character represents or substitutes for the other. Instances of illness, injury and madness follow a degree of medical and scientific protocol. These instances work to bring the novel's action to a denouement of equilibrium, to a restoration to health, paradoxically through processes of illness, injury, madness and heat. These transitions or transformations may be read productively as a narrative cures, not only for the characters and for the de la Garza family as a social entity, but for Mexican society and for the narrative that represents it.

Notes

1   Quotations from *Como agua* appear in the Doubleday Anchor paper edition (1989). Scientific (biological, chemical and medical) information comes from electronic resources and is generally presented without quotation marks in these notes. The name of the author(s) or keywords from the title appear at the end of the note and cross-reference the head-word for the citation in "Works Cited" (given at the end of the volume) under sub-head "Electronic Resources."

2 In spite of the fictional focus on negative behavior and destructive pathologies, the novel adopts a paradoxical view of these events, mingling grief and joy in some of its most shocking and harrowing scenes.

3 See <http://www.rci.rutgers.edu/~ostriker/home.htm>

4 Slicing the onion releases enzymes called allinases which break down substances like amino acid sulfoxides that are released from the onion cells. Amino acid sulfoxides form sulfenic acids, which rearrange themselves into a volatile gas. When the gas reaches the eyes, it reacts with the water in them, producing a mild form of sulfuric acid, irritating the nerve endings in the eyes and causing them to tear in an effort to neutralize the irritant. See Fitzpatrick.

5 Salt maintains the electrolyte balance at the cellular level. Human blood contains 0.9% salt, the concentration found in the (USP) sodium chloride compound commonly used to cleanse wounds (Salt Institute).

6 Tears help to relieve depression and stress because tears contain chemical compounds linked to depression and stress. Tears carry these compounds out of the body. See "Grieving and Mourning."

7 Only the *turrón*/nougat contains raw eggs (ten egg whites) (34). No eggs go into the cake filling (*relleno*) or *fondant*, but the 170 preserved eggs in the cake batter, if not "properly cooked," or if involved in "cross contamination" of substances or surfaces, could have resulted in salmonella food poisoning, whose effects include the symptoms experienced by the guests (nausea and vomiting). Sweets and eggs are among common modes of infection. See "Salmonella," 1. Of all the sweets, Nacha samples only the *fondant* (34).

8 The oils contained in rose petals undergo transformation, especially with heat and salt-related compounds. Rosewater was distilled by the Arabs at least as early as the ninth century (*Kitab Kimya' al-'Itr wa al-Tas'idat [Book of Perfume Chemistry and Distillation]* qtd. by Hayward. A by-product of rosewater production is said to great power: "It restores hearts that have gone and brings back withered souls." (See Hayward.)

9 Swaddling creates a slight pressure around the infant's body that seems to provide a sense of security or nervous system 'organization.' A newborn may sleep better when swaddled. See Lin-Dyken.

10 Although lactation can be induced without a preceding pregnancy, ir requires production of exogenous hormones, artificially intense or extended suckling, or both. See Creel, Monfort, Wildt & Waser.

11 When a child is abruptly weaned and put on cow's milk, diarrhea and vomiting may result from the change, due to allergic reaction or for digestive reasons. Without adequate treatment, dehydration may ensue. Death may follow quickly if there is no relief. See Krugman and "Dehydration in Infants".

12 Aggression and emotional disconnect (dissociative symptoms) can be symptoms of syndromes associated with stress such as acute stress disorder (ASD), which may arise in the first month following a traumatic event. See Gibson.

13 Chicken soup, long believed in traditional medicine to be of value in illness, is now known to help with at least respiratory problems, not because of the ingredients, but because of the vapor created by heating, so any kind of broth would have the same effect. See Diagnose-Me.

14 Ipecac syrup is a plant extract from the ipecacuanha shrub found in Brazil. Ipecac is a single-use drug used as a vomitive when one has ingested poison or overdosed on medication. Its misuse can cause severe medical complications (such as heart damage) and result in death. See Rader.

15 Mamá Elena's parents were undoubtedly scandalized both by José's illegitimacy *and* by his mixed race.

16 Stress may increase excretion, making the heart more sensitive to electrical abnormalities and leading to a rise in adrenaline which causes the blood to clot more readily. Since stress can constrict the coronary arteries, blood flow to the heart is reduced. See "Coronary."

17 *Placenta accreta* (and its variant conditions) describe a placenta that implants too deeply into the uterine wall to be expelled normally, and hemorrhaging results. As in Rosaura's case, the placenta can be surgically removed to stop the bleeding, and a hysterectomy (removal of the uterus) is necessary. See *Obstetric Hemorrhage*: "Placenta Accreta."

18 *Mulato* in Mexico is a social distinction. Here, it refers to skin color and hair type since the child has Mamá Elena's blue eyes and presumably her "fine" features (235). See Fülöpp's online esssay, especially references to Aguirre Beltran's "caste system." One explanation for this child's appearance is that Gertrudis' unexpressed genes found a match with similarly unexpressed genes carried by Juan.

19 There are many different reasons for lack of menstruation. The issue of "false pregnancy" is also complex. See "Delayed" (Health Journal) and "'False' Pregnancy," esp. the discussion of "blighted ovum."

20 A collection of home remedies advises: "For boils: Take out the inner skin of a raw egg and place on boil. For burns: Scrape the inside of an 'arsh' potato until it is a pulp and rub on the burn." See Gorin.

21 MIMOSA TENUIFLORA: "*Arbusto del sudeste mexicano, también denominado Tepez-cohuite [tepezcohuite]. Posee una importante acción regenerativa del tejido cutáneo y eleva el nivel de hidratación/* Shrub from southeastern Mexico, also called *Tepez-cohuite [tepezcohuite]*. It has an important regenerative action of the skin tissue and raises the level of hydration." See D'Arnal. The bark is sold in ointment form and in powder form today in *herberías*.

22 Food allergies, whose symptoms include tiredness, bloating, pain, diarrhea, and constipation, may damage to the intestinal tract over time and can lead to other illnesses such as Celiac disease, Irritable Bowel Syndrome, Chron's disease, etc. (See 'Food Allergies")

23 Refer to John's explanation of his grandmother's philosophy/metaphor, 116–118.

Bibliography

"Albert D'Arnal Dictionary." *Albert D'Arnal International.* < 24 June 2005.

"Amenorrhea: Absence of Menstruation Problems." *Women's Health.* <> 24 June 2005.

"Coronary Disease/Heart Attack." *Diagnose-Me.com.* <> 24 June 2005.

Creel, Steven L. Monfort, David E. Wildt & Peter M. Waser. "Spontaneous lactation is an adaptive result of pseudopregnancy." June l991. *Letters to Nature.* <> 24 June 2005. Access through a library membership or private subscription.

DeHaan, Martin R. *Chemistry of the Blood.* Grand Rapids: Zondervan Publishing, 1981.

"Dehydration in Infants can be Life-Threatening." *Vitrual Children's Hospital: Health Prose: A One-Minute Up-date for Your Health.* University of Iowa Health Science Center. <http://www.vh.org/pediatric/patient/pediatrics/prose/infantdehydration.html> 25 June 2005.

de Rojas, Fernando. *La Celestina.* [*La tragicomedia de Calisto y Melibea*] Humberto López Morales, ed. Barcelona: Planeta, 1980.

Fitzpatrick, Megan. "Crying for Onion Chemistry." Nov. 21. No. 44. *Chem. Ecology Education Center.* <> 24 June 2005.

"Food Allergies." *PhysiciansPlus Medical Group.* <http://www.docwong.com/health/foodaler.htm> 24 June 2005.

Fülöpp, Tomás J. "Latin America and the Concept of Social Race." *Vacilando*.org. <http://www.vacilando.org/index.php?x=810> 25 June 2005.

Gibson, Laura E. "Acute Stress Disorder: A Brief Description." National Center for PTSD Fact Sheet. *National Center for PTSD.* 24 June 2005. <>

Gorin, Sandra K. "Tip #170: Old Time Remedies" Aug 06, 1998 <> 24 June 2005.

Hayward, Michael R. "The Roses of Taif." Nov./Dec. l997. *Saudi Aramco World.* <> 24 June 2005.

"Healthy Grieving and Mourning to Release Broken Bonds." *CharmingHealth.com.* <http://www.charminghealth.com/self-help/healthygrieving.htm> 24 June 2005.

"Ipecac Abuse and Eating Disorders: Ipecac Abuse." *Rader Programs.* <> 24 June 2005.

Krugman, Scott D. and Howard Dubowitz. "Failure to Thrive." Sept. 2003. *American Family Physician.* <> 24 June 2005.

Lin-Dyken, Deborah. "Ask the Experts: What is Swaddling'? What are the pros and cons?" *BabyCenter.com.* <> 24 June 2005.

"'False' Pregnancy." *Med help Inernational and Maternal and Child Health Forum.* <http://www.medhelp.org/forums/maternal/archive/1389.html> 25 June 2005.

Marks, Jay. "Information on Intestinal Gas (Belching, Bloating, Flatulence)."

Medicine.net. Ed. Leslie J. Schoenfield. <> 24 June 2005.

"Medieval Medicine: Religion, Illness and the Practice of Medicine." 30 May 2004 <>

Miller, David A. M.D. "Obstetric Hemorrhage." *High Risk Pregnancy Directory.* <http://www.obfocus.com/high-risk/bleeding/hemorrhagepa.htm> 26 June 2005.

Ostriker, Alice. *Writing Like a Woman.* University of Michigan Poets on Poetry Series. Ann Arbor: UP, 1983.

Ostriker. "Alice Suskin Ostriker Webpage." <http://www.rci.rutgers.edu/~ostriker/home.htm> 24 June 2005.

"Salmonella." *Medical Information Organization.* <> 25 May 2005.

"Smoking and Curing Meats for Home Food Preservation: Literature Review and Critical Preservation Points. National Center for Home Food Preservation: Guide and Literature Review Series: *Smoking and Curing.* <http://www.uga.edu/nchfp/publications/nchfp/lit_rev/cure_smoke_fs.ht ml> 24 June 2005.

"Salt and Health." Salt Institute. <> 30 May 2004.

Spadaccini, Jim. "The Sweet Lure of Chocolate." ("Page 8"). *Exploratorium Magazine.* <> 24 June 2005.

11

Eucharistic Bread & Wine: A Concrete Sacramentality that Liberates

John Francis Burke

The title for this essay is taken from Tissa Balasuriya's work, *The Eucharist as Human Liberation* (1979). Balasuriya is a theologian from Sri Lanka, not Latin America. However, his work is an integral part of liberation theology which arises in Latin America in the 1960s, especially with Gustavo Gutiérrez work, *The Cry of the Oppressed*. Over the past six decades, this literature has been one of the vital streams for pursuing and realizing a faith-based justice. Liberation theology reinterprets scripture and Christian teaching from the perspective of those on the margin of society. Specifically, it seeks to transform political, economic, and social structures not only to enable the poor to have access to these structures, but to be integral contributors to an egalitarian community that pursues the realization of a common good. In turn, US Latinx theology, over the past four decades, has added to this liberation engagement of theology and politics from the standpoint of the diverse strains of the US Latinx experience.

As much as the Balasuriya's work is the inspiration for this essay's title, I will focus on how Latinx spirituality, both in Latin America and the United States, engages the Christian focus on the Eucharist and its implications for evangelizing a more just society. For those less familiar with the Christian tradition, the Eucharist refers to the consecration of the bread and wine into the Body and Blood of Christ in the Catholic Mass. I will also cover how different types of food are integral to Latinx community and family gatherings throughout the liturgical year. Again, for those less familiar with the Christian calendar, the liturgical year begins with Advent, usually in early December, and then over the ensuing year transitions to the seasons of

Christmas, Lent, Easter, Pentecost, Ordinary Time (usually from July through November) and culminates in the feast of Christ the King in late November.

The other substantive stream I will draw from is Latinx popular religion. Popular religion entails the spiritual practices of the people, some of which are sanctioned by the institutional church and others which are not. Examples would include home altars dotted by saints, both Catholic and indigenous, and celebrations such as *El Dia de los Muertos* (the Day of the Dead) on November 2nd. These cultural practices are often where one finds the heart and soul of Latinx spiritual and political practices. In many respects, they entail a critique of the formality and hierarchy found in the institutional church.

Latinx popular religion weaves in out of liberation theology. Whereas liberation theology still largely is articulated through theologians, popular religion manifests the actual spiritual practices of the people. Each approach complements that of the other approach. Liberation theology without a grasping of popular religion too easily becomes abstract and also ripe for manipulation by secular sources informed by the Hegelian-Marxist tradition. Conversely, popular religion without the element of critique provided by liberation theology too easily becomes a cultural affirmation of the political, socio-economic status quo in Latinx communities. In addition, popular religion, insofar as it is indebted to African and indigenous spiritual practices as much as those of European origin, has a post-Western sensibility. This dimension is valuable to the ongoing discourses in theology, philosophy, and the social sciences on how to conduct dialogue between cultures that does not intrinsically privilege European thought frameworks.

My presentation will be divided into five sections. The first section will discuss, in general terms, the connection of eucharistic celebrations to the pursuit of social justice. The second section will then turn to Latinx recasting of this connection. The third section will then annotate specific food part and parcel of Latinx spirituality. The fourth section will review specifically the detailed articulation by Ángel F. Méndez Montoya of an alimentary theology through the preparation and sharing of *mole*. The fifth section will then briefly review the implications Latinx sacramental spirituality has for engaging food production and distribution, the plight of farm workers, and the challenges of climate change. I do not claim that this essay provides any new primary research, but it does make a contribution to interdisciplinary discourse by connecting theological reflection to specific political practices and by sharing this "grassroots" spirituality with secular audiences in Latin American and Latinx Studies.

The Eucharist

The Eucharist is the central feature of the Catholic Mass. The Mass itself is an affirmation of the Holy Thursday gathering in which Jesus Christ shares bread and wine with his apostles. In so doing, he consecrates it into becoming his Body and Blood, anticipating the sacrifice of his own life for humanity, as subsequently he is scourged and crucified by the Roman authorities.

In the Mass, through such the consecration of bread and wine, Christ's followers become this Body: "the sacrament of the Body and Blood of Christ transforms us into the living Body of the church, the Body of the risen Christ in the world" (Gaillardetz 72). Although technically the Eucharist is one of the seven sacraments of the Roman Catholic tradition, sacramentality is much broader than these specific rituals. Sacramentality refers to tangible signs that reveal the presence of God in our daily lives and to the world around us.

In light of sacramentality, the transformation of bread and wine into the Body and Blood of Christ is incomplete if it is solely shared around the eucharistic table. The eucharistic celebration calls us to manifest the Body and Blood of Christ in the world: "[the liturgy of the Eucharist] is a sacramental event that invites the involvement of the entire gathered community, so that, locally and globally, God might transform through Christ the entire way human beings relate to each other" (Groody 226). Believers have a responsibility to engage and transform human relationships and structures not reflective of the Kingdom of God: the transubstantiation of bread and wine into the Body and Blood of Christ "sets in motion a series of transformations in us, which call us forth to renew and transform the world until God becomes all in all" (Groody 228).

Liturgical and political action, thus, are integral to each other. Unfortunately, the temptation among many Christians is either to be content with just doing liturgy and conversely, to be content just doing social justice. The first temptation Timothy Radcliffe terms Communion Catholics. These believers circle the wagons around the eucharistic table, seeing themselves as the protectors of sacred purity and in battle with a pagan world. The other camp Radcliffe terms Kingdom Catholics who are preoccupied with realizing God's kingdom of justice and peace outside the formalities of Christian worship (Radclifffe 165–78). By contrast, genuine eucharistic engagement skirts these two temptations by integrating liturgy and social action.

Mary Albert Darling and Tony Campolo articulate this integration through the metaphor of a garden: beware either "staying in the garden so much that we do not notice the needs outside, or not going into the garden at all because we are too busy responding to the 'voices of woe'" (Campolo 174). Simply staying in the garden and not pursuing the Kingdom of God in the world is to withhold the liberation promised in the Gospels. Conversely, Christians engaging in social justice in the world, without coming back into the garden for refreshment and renewal, will often experience burnout or reduce their pursuit of social justice into a secular ideology that leaves "no room for wonder, awe, fascination, and mystery" (Empereur, *Models* 44). As put by J. G. Davies, the sacramental interconnectedness between humans and the divine, as well as between believers, in the Eucharist is incomplete if it does not lead to political engagement:

> The eucharist is a political act because it in its turn makes a statement about human nature and about the principles and groundwork of human interrelatedness. So, it speaks of equality, of concern for reconciliation that is the opposite of individual and social action. It is intended to be an embodiment and expression of efficacious love and therefore of justice in terms of freedom and welfare. But to proclaim these things is vain unless there is a consistent effort to have them actualized in society at large and this requires their embodiment in a political programme. (Davies in Empereur, *Worship* 117)

Both the garden and the world are integral to the sacramental realization of eucharistic community. Sacramentality is not something petrified with the walls of churches but rather realizes its fullness in a seeking just relations in the world.

The Latinx Recasting of Eucharistic Community

However, what is the Latinx understanding and articulation of this integral sacramental nexus of liturgical worship and political action? Especially James Empereur and Eduardo Fernández, in their work, *La Vida Sacra* (2006) point to several dimensions, which I will supplement with the insights of others working in Latinx theology.

First, Latinx spirituality has both a tactile and literal sensibility about it. Given that Latinx "affirm the natural value of the bread, wine, oil, water in themselves", they grasp "the presence of Christ" in eucharistic sharing (Empereur, *La Vida* 25). Even a very Protestant American celebration like Thanksgiving is a holiday that many Latinx immigrants can embrace due to the fact that the food of US harvest time—"pumpkins, cornstalks, squash, and shafts of wheat"—connects to the agricultural life that so many of these immigrants previously did and in some instances, continue to do (Dahm 180–81).

Second, in Latinx theology there is a sense that the Eucharist is not just for the worthy, but that it is "food for the journey, that it is nourishment for those who are weak," and even for those who are not church goers (Empereur, *La Vida* 106). For migrants especially who have crossed the deserts of the US Southwest or have traversed the Gulf of Mexico in search of better opportunities, the eucharistic stress on food and drink is not just figurative but literal. For example, take the very popular hymn, "Be Not Afraid/No temas más." Lyrics in English such as "you shall cross the barren desert, but you shall not die of thirst," or "if you pass through raging waters, in the sea you shall not drown," in Spanish become literal especially for the migrant fleeing subjugation either in Mexico, Central America, or in the Caribbean region. A Spanish-speaker music minister in Houston once shared with me that she sang this song repeatedly in Houston when one of her friends or relatives was crossing the desert in the US Southwest.

Third, eucharistic celebration in the Latinx world is not just something one participates in at church, but can be realized through family relationships, friendships, and community gatherings. To reiterate, sacramentality is not just something one practices through specific actions such as weddings and funerals. No, sacramentality is already present in the world if we just pay attention to it. Popular religion is not trying to access God as someone distant, but rather involves "engaging in some human activity where the power of God is manifested" (Empereur, *La Vida* 203).

Fourth, given the relational quality of the Latinx engagement of sacramentality, *fiesta* is not just a party, but an anticipation of a new universalism in which people will engage in genuine relationships of equality (Burke 109–110). Life is something given by God to us and therefore, through *fiesta*, we give thanks for this gift: "*Fiesta* is the way the community understands itself as receiving and responding rather than doing or achieving" (Empereur, La Vida 228). Such celebration is very defiant of the hardship many poor Latinx endure. Indeed, prophecy and *fiesta*, as Groody notes, go together. *Fiesta*, without prophecy, too easily degenerates into bacchanalian revels and prophecy without fiesta too easily becomes a stern judgementalism (Groody 196).

Fifth, *fiesta* and the Latinx emphasis on relationships stresses a strong sense of communitarianism which is critical of the excesses of individualism, not just in US culture, but in the modern world view: "'The central pronoun for Hispanics is the we, *nosotros,* while for Americans, it is the I'" (Richard Rodríguez in Dahm 157). In Latinx relationships, one only comes to one's full personhood in community.

Conversely, others cannot get to know you without having some sense of your family (Matovina184). When I first moved to Texas, I was struck by how the mother of a Mexican-American I was dating would ask me how my parents were even though she had never met them. Overtime, I came to realize that what she was actually asking me was how were the relationships that fostered me and was I being attentive to them (Burke 100).

Sixth, the Latinx sense of community is also manifested in the rituals and objects that mediate the gap between the natural and the supernatural. As opposed to the more straight-laced, rigid, hierarchical church that ensues in the Catholic world after the Council of Trent (1545–1563), many missionary efforts in Latin America in the 1500s manifest a "baroque emphasis on symbol, ritual, and celebration" (Dahm 154–55). Consequently "nonverbal activities, such as processions, statues, paintings, music, and drama" are at the center not at the margin of Latinx spirituality (Dahm 155). Both Ricardo Ramírez' extensive illustration of the daylong celebration of the feast of Our Lady of Guadalupe in Las Cruces, New Mexico and Jeanette Rodríguez and Ted Fortier's recounting of the Yaqui celebrations of Holy Week in the Guadalupe reservation in Phoenix, Arizona are salient examples (Ramírez 155; Rodríguez 49–53). Especially at Christmas time, both *posadas* (processions that reenact the denial of shelter to Joseph and Mary as she was about to give birth to Jesus) and *pastorelas* (a Christmas dramatization of the fight between good and evil) vividly communicate the birth of a savior, born of humble estate, who will redeem the world.

Seventh, the practice of public ritual and the centrality of *mística* further annotate the Latinx aesthetic rendering of sacramentality. Virgil Elizondo, in particular, dwells upon the intense spirituality in the graphic Latinx dramatizations of the events of Palm Sunday and Good Friday in the Latinx tradition. Inscribed in these rituals is, he accents, "a deep and healthy acceptance that suffering and death form part of the mystery of life" (Elizondo 118), but it does not defeat human beings. In turn, in this *mística*, one feels God's presence "not only in moments of fervent prayer, but in one's daily living" (*The 1987 National Pastoral Plan for Hispanic Ministry* in Dahm 157).

Eighth and finally, the Latinx sacramental sense of relationships also leads to caring for God's creation. Latinx spirituality grasps the beauty of the earth. With this ecological sensibility, sacramentality is not just the relationship between God and humanity or the relationship of humans to each other, but also stresses sacred manifestations in the natural world. This sensibility comes very much from the indigenous peoples' stress that there is a sacred presence not just in plants and animals, as well as in us, but also in supposedly inanimate objects such as mountains. Even in formal church liturgy, the Christian message for Latinx is communicated as much by the visual colors and aural sounds of the gathering as is the formal proclamation of God in scripture. The aura of Our Lady of Guadalupe is not understandable apart from the indigenous elements that comprise her manifestation—roses, for example, the roses blooming out of season. Admittedly, much ecological destruction is ensuing in Latin America, such as the deforestation of the Amazon River basin, but the holistic aesthetics of Latinx sacramentality constitutes a counterculture to such structural sin.

Concrete Illustrations

Consistent with this broader sense of sacramentals, in Latinx celebrations throughout the aforementioned liturgical year, specific types of food play a central role.

Our Lady of Guadalupe: *menudo*

tamales, tostadas, posole, buñuelos: candy in *piñatas*

Christmas: placing Jesus on a bed of hard candy

Epiphany-Three Kings: *Rosca de Reyes*

Holy Thursday: unconsecrated bread shared after mass

Harvest Season/Thanksgiving: pumpkins/cornstalks, squash, wheat (Acculturation to US Cultural Practices)

Día de los Muertos: sugar candy skulls placed on the altar, *pan de muerto* (Bread of the Dead), gingerbread skulls & skeletons

At other celebrations not tied to a specific day, this food is commonplace:

Funerals: *caldo & pan dulce*

Weekly: extensive use of holy water

La Niña de Atocha (holy day): bread and water given to prisoners by a child. (Dahm 159–96; Empereur, *La Vida* 274, 279, 289)

These liturgical food practices are not universal in Latin America. Some are practiced in some places and not others. Some are more past traditions which in some places have been discontinued. Others, such as the harvest foods, entail an acculturation by migrants to their cultural dynamics of their host as opposed to the home countries. Some are particularly striking, such as the literal embodiment of death in food on the Day of the Dead or the ritual of *la Niña de Atocha*, whose basket of food and gourd of water remains full after having served food and water to the prisoners (Dahm 187). But in each instance, there is a sacramental presence that is very sensory, if not tactile. For example, although many Catholics bless themselves with holy water, Latinx believers literally douse their homes, their persons, and their family members and friends so as to share "more fully [in] God's blessings" (Dahm 184). Food in Latinx spirituality is not just to be shared after religious rituals are concluded, but is integral to liturgical practices.

Mole y más

Having established both the eight facets of the Latinx sense of eucharistic sensibility and having reviewed specific foods integral to Latinx liturgical celebrations, let us turn to the "alimentary theology" of Ángel Méndez Montoya (*Making, Theology*). Montoya, in great detail, elaborates upon the centrality of food to Latinx theological understandings. For him, the sharing of food in Latinx spirituality suggests "a eucharistic discourse perpetually open to yet more elaboration and responsive to the touching, tasting, and nourishment of God's superabundant giving" (*Theology* 10x).

Specifically, alimentation for Méndez Montoya means that a transformation ensues both in the preparation of food and among those who share the ensuing meal (*Theology* 3). For him, such undertakings respect longstanding traditions but also pursue new directions. From a Christian perspective, the accents we need to grasp "God's excessive nourishing all that 'is' with the alimentary vitality 'to be'" (Méndez Montoya, *Theology* 4). In turn, we are then called upon to nourish each other (Méndez Montoya, *Theology* 10).

In particular, Méndez Montoya focuses on the making of *mole* as a concrete illustration of alimentary theology. Going back to pro-Columbian times, he suggests human sacrifice was how the indigenous peoples fed the gods to continue "cosmic sustenance:" "To eat *molli* thus was a way of eating the gods who in turn would eat humans at the moment of death" (Méndez Montoya, *Making* 363). But the actual creation of *mole*, Méndez Montoya traces to an incident where Fray Pascual Bailón, a cook in a Mexican monastery, accidently put soap into the main meal for the day. In frustration, he then puts an exotic combination of spices into another pot in which he was cooking turkey. Feeling guilty about his angry reaction, Fray Pascual seeks God's intercession and receives it in the form of this new concoction—

mole poblano. Méndez Montoya adds to this day, many Mexican cooks pray to Fray Pascual, who is the patron saint of cooks (*Making* 361). Through this *mole* sensibility, Méndez Montoya's alimentary theology has six components.

First, alimentary theology encourages hybridization between multiple cultures and spiritual outlooks. These combinations, in turn, represent a resistance to colonization. Especially in colonial Mexico, experimentation with cooking was one of the primary ways women were able to express themselves. Méndez Montoya adds the "in-betweenness" (*Theology* 31) manifested in *mole* beseeches each of us to close the gap between one's self and that of the other. In this regard, Christ's incarnation suggests a mixing—a *mestizaje*—of divine and human realities. In turn, Méndez Montoya continues "the eucharistic body nourishes in its act of sharing and celebrating differences" (*Theology* 38). Human beings in eucharistic community are neither melded into one another, nor dwell in sheer difference. Instead, a "unity-in-diversity" unfolds: "the eucharistic body envisions all human beings and creation . . . as being different expressions of one, cosmic, heterogenous divine banquet" (*Theology* 42).

Second, Méndez Montoya accents the erotic and subversive dimensions of alimentary theology. In this regard, he turns to Sor Juana Inéz de la Cruz, a Mexican nun, who in the second half of the 17th century, was banished to kitchen by ecclesiastical authorities for writing provocative theological treatises. According to Méndez Montoya, she pursued her culinary activities "as a space of creativity and liberation" (*Making* 367). At the same time, given the repression women like Sor Juana have endured, the making and eating of *mole* constitutes both a sense of festive harmony and "pain, suffering, and struggle" (*Making* 367).

Third, Méndez Montoya contends, that Sor Juana's subversion captures the integral relationship between *sabor* and *saber*—that aesthetic experience is essential to "the divine's self-communication and sharing" (*Theology* 48). In eucharistic terms, "*gustas*, becomes the medium and guide to the soul and the intellect (rather than the other way around) leading them to participation with God" (*Theology* 69). But this participation in turn, as previous mentioned, is incomplete without eucharistic communion leading to transformation of political, social, and economic structures that marginalize people: "Just as God feeds humanity, the partakers are called to feed their neighbor, and are challenged to transform a world of hunger, exclusion, and violence" (*Theology* 74).

Fourth, Méndez Montoya draws out the implications of Sophia— "the Wisdom of God" for alimentary theology. Building on insights from the thinker, Sergei Bulgakov, Méndez Montoya suggests eucharistic communion deepens our relationship with God (*Theology* 96). If humanity fell away from God in the Garden of Eden, he continues, "Sophia's fruit intimates a recovered sense of inner connection with God" (*Theology* 101). Indeed, he pinpoints how wisdom is referred in Proverbs and Ecclesiasticus, as manifesting "the sweetness of honey," exuding "perfume and flowered scents," and bearing fruit from the vine (*Theology* 101). Méndez Montoya especially stresses that being draw into closer relationship to God is not just a transcendent ecstasy, but that this communion should lead us to challenge a world whose food exchanges actually leave people starving (*Theology* 112).

Fifth, Méndez Montoya thus pursues what he terms "a divine-human *body politic*" (*Theology* 115). As opposed to the traditional rendering of politics as power relations, in alimentary theology, politics is nurtured by a "divine caritas, which is expressed with a radical gesture of kenosis, reciprocity, and concrete communal practices" (*Theology* 115). One example he gives of such community is the story of Exodus in which God gives manna to the people of Israel in the wilderness. This manna, by Méndez Montoya's reckoning, "is the call to share with one another and thus nurture the life of the community, particularly those in greatest need" (*Theology* 124). At the same time, he notes, this other is a stranger, not a dependent, who if properly welcomed, becomes "a gift of unity and transformation" (*Theology* 135).

Méndez Montoya's alimentary theology offers what he terms a new polis, grounded in the Mystical Body of Christ, that is characterized by participation and reciprocity. He reviews at length the Pauline emphasis on community meals in *First Corinthians*. These early Christian food tables make manifest "the liturgical gestures of giving thanks, blessing, breaking, and sharing of bread and wine" (*Theology* 139). Once again, tactile expression, is intrinsic, not superficial to this experience: "divine alimentation also involves higher and deeper lives of agapeic/erotic intimacy such as touching, tasting, eating, and drinking" (*Theology* 149). This tasteful sharing, he continues, indeed reflects the dyads of "self and other, the human and divine, spiritual and material, the individual parts and the whole" that are fully realized in "the in-betweenness that is the Body of Christ" (*Theology* 140). Méndez Montoya's new polis, thus, is a critique of political arrangements characterized by contractual atomized relationships (*Theology* 156).

Sixth and finally, Méndez Montoya concludes that food and the Eucharist are closely related. He stresses that the eucharistic communion manifests "a cosmic-divine banquet" in which hunger is transformed into satiety and "individualism into communal feasting" (*Theology* 159). He notes, in this regard, the Spanish verb, *convivir* combines both 'to live' with 'being with' (*Theology*, 160). Hence engaging the other, especially in terms of their hunger, creates a communal space of nourishment. The Eucharist not only entails God's offering in the form of food and opening up to others, but creates "a time and space of fellowship wherein physical and spiritual hunger will be no more" (*Theology*, 160). True to his exegesis on making *mole*, just as *picante* literally arouses our sensibilities, his spicy alimentary theology provokes us to call out when human communities exclude and refuse nourishment to others (*Making* 375).

Giving the sensory aroma of Méndez Montoya's alimentary theology that links divine-human communion ultimately to political socio-economic liberation its full due, his use of the term *polis* to describe this divine-human nexus is problematic. Indeed, this dwelling on harmony amid recognizing differences moves beyond politics as conventionally understood. Politics is a relationship between human beings that recognizes the fundamentally differences that lie between us. In this life, it can be an edifying power between people that is not unlike the harmonious community in Méndez Montoya's "new polis." Unfortunately, it can also be a "power over" or a "lording over" other people. Now, Méndez Montoya seeks in a prophetic way to call out and transform the latter forms of domination and I concur that the Christian eucharistic vision entails engaging and transforming unjust political, socio-economic structures. But in so doing, one is ultimately moving beyond politics to an alternative set of relationships reflective of divine harmony. Political relationships, at least in this life, retain a distance or tension between people and between groups that defies easy resolution through human means alone.

Food, Farm Workers, and Ecology

Building on the political engagement called for by the Latinx sacramental rendering of sharing food and nourishment, let us examine three concrete applications—food distribution, the farm workers movement, and climate change. With food distribution, the norms of an alimentary theology are implicit. In the case of César Chávez' mobilization of farm workers, the impact of Mexican Catholicism is quite explicit. Finally, the call to care for God's creation is made by an Argentinian, Francis I, who both in his theological writings and pastoral ministry has been a strong advocate for the preferential option for the poor, a major theme of liberation theology.

Food distribution is closest to the alimentary thrust of Méndez Montoya's argument. The connection between spirituality and food cultivation and distribution, is well-developed in Thomas O'Loughlin's *Eating Together, Becoming One* (2019), Norman Wirzba's *Food and Faith* (2019), and Mary McGann's *The Meal That Reconnects* (2020). Although none of these arguments are Latinx theology per se, in spirit and content they are consonant with an alimentary theology.

O'Loughlin focuses on how Christians cannot truly be a eucharistic people if their gatherings do not manifest ecumenism. He accents the eucharistic meal is not just the material through which transubstantiation happens, but in and of itself is "a reality within our human world that is also a mystery embracing the divine" (32). Therefore, we are called to invite, not reject, others to this eucharistic banquet. O'Loughlin contends that when we deny others access to the Eucharist in liturgy to others due to denominational differences, we end up subscribing to a sectarianism that is contrary to Jesus's institution of eucharistic table sharing (2019 120). Instead, he insists, we need to put into practice the heavenly banquet articulated in *Luke* 13:29 in which people come from every direction to gather "at table in the Kingdom of God" (151).

Wirzba, in turn, accents the conduct of eucharistic gatherings. He puts particular emphasis on the importance of service to others, hospitality, and community. In particular, he stresses eucharistic living entails that we "welcome, receive, and attend to each other's lives" (219). Building upon an insight from the Mexican-American theologian, Virgil Elizondo, Wirzba notes how Jesus broke bread with "strangers and outcasts" and therefore opposed "social systems of rejection and exclusion" (198). Echoing Méndez Montoya's outlook, such hospitality fosters a unity, not of uniformity, but in difference (224). He shares, for example, how Trinity United Church, an African-American faith-based community, through its farmer market and educational food center, not only teaches people how to eat in a healthier lifestyle, but actually to how to be a eucharistic community. In this regard, he concludes that dominant cultures have much to learn from peoples on the margins, for the latter "have the sense to accept and appreciate the significance of God's hospitality" (235).

McGann, finally, focuses specifically on food distribution. She distinguishes between understanding food as a gift versus food as a commodity (6). She argues the former is a consecration of our relationship to the world whereas the latter is a desecration of this relationship. In the early years of Christianity, she shows how Christian meals were connected to the Hellenic notion of symposia. However, she emphasizes, the Christians' recasting of symposia was not a fawning to the Roman emperor but rather manifested *resistance* to Rome through the new covenant created in Jesus' death and rising (36–53). McGann then divides her examination of the food crisis into an indictment of the prevailing food order and then what would be viable Christian alternatives based on eucharistic sacramentality. First, as much as meals should enable us to nourish each other, she shares that "food priorities such as taste, nutrition, variety, wholeness, and ripeness have been sacrificed to the economic goals of increased productivity, efficiency, and ultimately corporate profit" (69). Second, she adds, the more we create and use genetically-engineered crops, we destroy the soil as "an image of divine fecundity" (101). Third, although there is no reason anyone in the world should go hungry today, she chastises the "corporate food system" that fosters and exploits "social inequality and environmental instability" (112). In spiritual terms, McGann stresses hunger "leaves its victims disempowered, marginalized, denied a place in a society of shared goods, and ultimately denied God's precious gift of nourishment" (113). As opposed to such exploitation, McGann shares concrete examples constructive of genuine eucharistic engagement such as regenerative agriculture and organic cultivation. She also pinpoints how faith-based communities transform vacant lies into gardens or bring the homeless off the streets for sharing in liturgy and actual meals (156). In turn, she maintains *how* the bread and the wine used in eucharistic liturgy is cultivated in just as integral to eucharistic communion as the consecration itself: "The common loaf should bear the hands of the community members, who form the dough with love and care, from grain that is locally grown, related to the community's everyday   sustenance, with methods that honor nature's wisdom, and in fields where growers are given just wages and solicitous care" (196). She concludes, from a eucharistic perspective, we have to change a consumption-focused economy to one characterized by "giving and co-abiding" (201). Ultimately, she emphasizes, Jesus as realized in eucharistic sharing is not found above, but in the world around us (McGann 202; *LS* #236).

Part and parcel to the cultivation of food is the plight of farmworkers. César Chávez, in his mobilization of farmworkers, utilizes key facets of Mexican spirituality such as prayer, penitence, and fasting. He frequented Mass and saw work as a sacred matter (García 36). Indeed, his fasting ultimately cost him his life. But, besides being an act that drew public attention to the plight of farmworkers, Chávez, though fasting, sought to keep the movement itself true to the moral norms that were its compass. Indeed, in 1968, he concluded one of his most significant fasts by going to Mass and sitting side-by-side with Robert Kennedy, who at the time was running for president.

The famous 1966 pilgrimage from Delano to Sacramento manifests how Chávez was able to take central elements of Mexican spirituality and recast them into a protest march. In Mexico, penitents take pilgrimages all the time to holy sites, particularly Marian ones. These pilgrimages may take days. Chávez adopted this heritage to stage a march, during Holy Week, from Delano to Sacramento, culminating on the steps of State Capitol, to draw attention to the farm workers' plight. Banners in the march extensively featured Our Lady of Guadalupe and others prominently stating "Penitence, Pilgrimage, and Revolution."

In addition, farm worker mobilizers also drew upon the aesthetic dimension of Latinx spirituality, such as manifested in *posadas* and *pastorelas*, when they staged dramatizations of the workers' struggle with the growers. Such dramas were intended to sustain the workers' steadfastness to the cause and to bolster their spirits.

The 1960s farmworkers movements in the 1960s and 70s were actually much more successful out in California than in Texas due to stark differences in spiritual and political cultures. In the California case, in addition to the leadership of Chávez, the United Farm Workers mobilization benefited from the fact that the state had a history of organized labor, supported by Catholic social teaching. In addition, a liberal Protestantism indebted to the Social Gospel Movement provided a backdrop through which the farmworker mobilization could broaden its support to bring pressure on the growers to come to the bargaining table and negotiate (Watt 6–8).

Texas, on the other hand, was another cultural universe. There was no organizer comparable in status and skills like Chávez. Although there were supportive Catholic leaders such as Archbishop Robert Lucey in San Antonio, the Catholic Church in south Texas was much more traditional than its California counterpart and not terribly receptive to liberation theology. In addition, the Protestant spirituality that informed the dominant Anglo population was a rather pietistic faith that was preoccupied with saving souls, not a eucharistic understanding of the material needs of peoples (Watt 6–8). Any attempt in Texas to implement a liberation theology steeped in eucharistic sharing ran up against a traditional elitist culture whose articulation of Christianity was not only opposed to this vision, but quite ruthless and effective in suppressing it.

Finally, a sacramental eucharistic outlook suggests that we need to make a consciousness change to meet the challenges of climate change and global warming. Toward this end, Pope Francis I, in his encyclical, *Laudato Si* (LS), articulates what he terms an integral ecology.

Over the first half of his encyclical, Francis makes an indictment of the contemporary economic order. He pinpoints how the growth of migrants is directly related to the environmental degradation caused by the industrial order (LS #25). For example, many people, he shares, do not have access to safe drinking water (LS #28).

Francis takes the critique of consumerism and technocratic thinking that McGann criticized in terms of the food economy and applies it to dealings with the world's ecosphere. This global order, he bemoans, is oriented by a technocratic paradigm that is preoccupied with profit at the expense of what his predecessor, Benedict XVI, referred to as the grammar of creation (LS #109, CV #48). Francis challenges both the anthropocentrism and relativism that obstructs the giving of God's goodness (LS #122 & 123).

Consequently, Francis puts forth integral ecology as an alternative to the domination of the global economy—note the parallel to the early Christians opposing Roman imperialism. Humans, he insists, have a responsibility to be caretakers as opposed to consumers of nature. In sacramental terms, he points out nature is the "locus of his [God's] presence" (LS #88). We are called to engage nature as part of creation, and not just as an object to be merely used, or worse dominated (LS #82).

In practical terms, he accents that campesinos have a right to land (LS #94). Toward this end, he calls for, as did his predecessors, Benedict XVI and John III, the formation of a genuine world political authority that would ensure that a just economy and a just ecology characterize human relations (LS #75). In so doing, especially those from the margins of society would share in the earth's bounty. Francis' integral ecology, thus, emphasizes an interdependent relationship between human development, the preferential option for the poor, and care for creation.

In the end, Francis seeks a universal fraternity not unlike the eucharistic communities outlined previously: "Care for nature is part of a lifestyle which includes the capacity for living together and communion" (LS #228). He specifically states that the Eucharist provokes us "to be stewards of all creation" (LS #235). Consonant with this end, Empereur and Fernández, pinpoint the Latinx sensory rendering of spirituality grasps "the sacramentality of the world in the most insignificant pebble, the barren frozen ground, or the glories of a large colorful butterfly" (Empereur, *La Vida* 289). This tangible as opposed to abstract sensibility gives hope that we can heal the earth (Empereur, *La Vida* 289).

Indeed, at the culmination of *Laudato Si*, Francis suggests our personal growth is rooted the extent that we go out from to ourselves to live in communal relationships with God, with others, and with all creatures" (LS #240). Ultimately, he concludes, in nature and the universe, we encounter the "infinite beauty of God" (LS #243). This encounter beckons us to abandon our inclination to use and abuse the earth for our own selfish needs and instead to cherish and cultivate in mutuality with plants and animals the sacramentals in nature. This *metanoia* regarding our relationship to nature should provokes us to initiate environmental practices to stem global warming and climate change and to reduce our personal and collective carbon footprint.

Conclusion—*¡Provecha!*

My reflection has reviewed the Latinx recasting of eucharistic community; specific Latinx spiritual rituals in which food plays a central role; Montoya's alimentary theology; and finally, the connection of the Latinx liberating sacramentality to the ongoing issues of food production and distribution, farm worker conditions, and climate change. First, as opposed to just understanding eucharistic sharing as simply distributing the Body and Blood of Christ in a mass, in the liberation tradition, sacramentality is found not just within the doors of a church, but in caring relationships between human beings and in our relation to the natural world. Second, this social and nature-oriented sacramentality calls us to engage and transform unjust political, socio-economic human relations and shift our relationship with nature from being one of domination to one of mutual interdependency. Third, the alimentary sense of sacramentality in the Latinx tradition conveys that the disclosure of the divine is not something esoteric or abstract, but is at least partially grasped in the mutual sharing of food and drink. Finally, the Eucharist, especially in Latinx culture, is not just receiving a wafer or a cup of wine but sharing a meal in a way that not only challenges political socio-economic structural sin, but begins to realize the inclusive egalitarian relations, free of oppression, that will characterize the kingdom of God (or the kin-dom of God in the feminist construction). Indeed, this Latinx sacramentality that liberates is captured very well in the refrain of the hymn, "La misa es una fiesta/ La misa no termina": "*La misa es una fiesta muy alegre, la misa es una fiesta con Jesús. La misa no temina aquí en la Iglesia. Ahora la empezamos a vivir.*" Amén.

Bibliography

Balasuriya, Tissa, OMI. *The Eucharist as Human Liberation*. Maryknoll, NY: Orbis Books, 1979.

Burke, John Francis. *Mestizo Democracy: The Politics of Crossing Borders*. College Station, TX: Texas A&M Press, 2003.

Campolo, Tony and Mary Albert Darling. *The God of Intimacy and Action: Reconnecting Ancient Spiritual Practices, Evangelism, and Justice*. San Francisco, CA: Jossey-Bass, 2007.

Caritas in Veritate (CV): On Integral Development in Charity and Truth. 2019. http://www.vatican.va/content/benedict-xvi/en/encyclicals/documents/ hf_ben-xvi_enc_20090629_caritas-in-veritate.html

Dahm, Charles W., OP. *Parish Ministry in a Hispanic Community*. New York: Paulist Press, 2004.

Elizondo, Virgilio. *Christianity and Culture: An Introduction to Pastoral Theology and Ministry for the Bicultural Community*. San Antonio, TX: Mexican American Cultural Center, 1975.

Empereur, James, SJ. *Models of Liturgical Theology*. Bramcote: Grove Books Limited, 1987.

——, SJ. *Worship: Exploring the Sacred*. Washington, D.C.: The Pastoral Press, 1987.

Empereur, James, SJ and Eduardo Fernández, SJ. *La Vida Sacra: Contemporary Hispanic Sacramental Theology*. Lanham, MD: Rowman & Littlefield, 2006.

Gaillardetz, Richard R. and Catherine E. Clifford. *Keys of the Council: Unlocking the Teaching of Vatican II*. Collegeville, MN: Liturgical Press, 2002.

García, Mario. T., Ed. *The Gospel of César Chávez: My Faith in Action*. New York: Sheed and Ward, 2007.

Groody, Daniel J, CSC. *Globalization, Spirituality, and Justice*. Maryknoll, NY: Orbis Books, 2007.

Laudato Si (LS): On Care for Our Common Home. 2015. http://www.vatican.va/content/francesco/en/encyclicals/documents/papa-francesco_20150524_enciclica-laudato-si.html

Matovina, Tim. *Latino Catholicism: Transformation in America's Largest Church*. Princeton, NJ: Princeton University Press, 2012.

McGann, Mary E. *The Meal That Reconnects: Eucharistic Eating and the Food Crisis*. Collegeville, MN: Liturgical Press, 2020.

Méndez Montoya, Angel F. "The Making of Mexican *Mole* and Alimentary Theology in the Making." In *Creating Ourselves: African Americans and Hispanic Americans on Popular Culture and Religious Expression*, Eds, Anthony B. Pinn and Benjamín Valentín. Durham, NC: Duke University Press., 2009

——, *Theology of Food: Eating and the Eucharist*. Oxford, UK: Wiley-Blackwell, 2009.

O'Loughlin, Thomas. *Eating Together, Becoming One: Taking Up Pope Francis's Call to Theologians*. Collegeville, MN: Liturgical Press, 2019.

Radcliffe, Timothy, OP. *What is the Point of Being a Christian?* New York, NY: Burns & Oates, 2005.

Ramirez, Ricardo. *Power from the Margins: The Emergence of the Latino in the Church and in Society.* Maryknoll, NY: Orbis Books, 2016.

Rodriguez, Jeanette and Ted Fortier. *Cultural Memory: Resistance, Faith, and Identity.* Austin, TX: University of Texas Press, 2007.

Watt, Alan J. *Farm Workers and the Churches: The Movement in California and Texas.* College Station: Texas A&M University Press, 2010.

Wirzba, Norman. *Food and Faith: A Theology of Eating.* New York: Cambridge University Press, 2019.

PART IV

Sustenance & the Soul:
Representation Via the Visual Arts

Introduction to Sustenance & the Soul: Representation via the Visual Arts

Since food and drink are so tied in human experience to the senses, this part of the collection consists of observations about visual, i.e., artistic, representations of food and drink, both in studio art & in cinema.

A. PAINTING

Enrique Mallén, founder of the *On-line Picasso Project*, the world's most comprehensive site for all things Picasso, has written extensively on nearly every aspect of Picasso's life and work. He has collaborated on every volume of *Hispanic Worlds* with chapters filled with fascinating and original insights. For this collection, Mallén has contributed two new chapters, adding more historical context to Picasso's artistic career and personal life in terms of food & drink in *What's Cooking with Picasso: Conjuring Up Food in the First Year of Occupation* [by the Nazis during World War II] and a focus on Picasso's still lifes in *The Devouring Eye (I) of Picasso*.

My chapter in Part IV, *Sustenance for the Soul & Spirit: Frida & Fruit*, was inspired to segue from Mallén's work on still lifes by Picasso, but also particularly by my interest in art per se, especially by women. My on-going amazement at the commercialization known as *Fridamania*, which seemed to take off in the U.S. not long after I began to research Frida Kahlo's life work during my Mexican university time at *Instituto Tecnológico/Monterrey* in the early 1970s, when Frida was still known chiefly—unreasonably—outside Mexico as Diego Rivera's wife, also played a role. The scholarship, as well as exhibitions in museums large and small, in the interim years have corrected that denigration. This is quite apart from the on-going commercial *Fridamania*, which could be construed (by me, at least) as "tacky," given her talent and production—but I do think she personally would have enjoyed it immensely, having been a conscious and self-acknowledged "drama queen" in life, as the contemporary term portrays.

Food & drink are very frequent themes, topics and content for many, many women artists, whether visual or literary, who traditionally have focused on so-called "women's work," like food & drink preparation and presentation, not only since they are such integral parts of women's experiences, but also in order to create work viewing-acceptable to the (overwhelmingly misogynous) public of their times. However, rather than reprint any of my numerous previous studies in print and presentation on such work, as the studies are not specifically dedicated to food and drink, I simply acknowledge just a couple of these artists. Remedios Varo, the Spanish-born Mexican surrealist artist, represented "women's work and topics," as well as food, not infrequently in various guises. For a few, she painted baby food in *Celestial Pablum*, 1958, a reference in "The Semiotics of Hispanic Womanhood," a chapter in *S/he: Sex & Gender in Hispanic Cultures*, the third book in this series (189); the self-explanatory *Resurrected Still Life*, of a whirling dining table, 1963; and *Vegetarian Vampires*, which, according to at least one art critic, interprets her liquid lunches with a painter girlfriend,1962. Both of the latter are mentioned in "The Female Body & Control Via Transformation," in *The Body: Subject & Subjected*, the first book in this series (62–3). A Latina (self-identified prior to the now-preferred term, Latinx) artist, Carmen Lomas Garza's bilingual children's books about culture and pride, e.g., *In My Family/En mi familia*, prominently feature food & drink in nearly every work.

B. CINEMATIC

A reprint from the fourth book in the *Hispanic Worlds* series, *Family, Friends & Foes,* Haiqing Sun's "Family, Friends & Fighting" compares the cinematic version of Mexican Laura Esquivel's 1990 magical realism novel, *Como agua para chocolate/Like Water for Chocolate,*[1] and the Chinese film, *Eat Drink Man Woman*, which came out in the U.S. in 1994. In their own contexts, both movies revolve around food & drink, in the first case, the culinary results of a victimized daughter/protagonist pressed into duties as the family cook in rural Mexico and, in the second, a chef in urban China and his familial relationships.

Had the film, *Truly Texas Mexican*, by Adán Medrano, aforementioned in Part II, Food & Drink & Physical Space, my chapter on the kitchen and dining room, on preparation and presentation, been the sole subject of a chapter, as it easily could have been—and not so tied to establishing the food/drink identity aspect that it fit better as a lead-in to the chapter in which it was cited—it certainly would have appropriately appeared in Part IV B, in the cinematic. Thus, a visual recall of this film by the reader, perhaps via an on-line (free) viewing on Amazon.com would round-out the concept of the cinematic representation of food & drink.[2]

What's Cooking with Picasso: Conjuring Up Food in the First Year of Occupation

Enrique Mallén

In the current environment of quarantines, isolation and shortages, the mind wanders to similar trying periods in history. I am reminded of the situation Pablo Picasso found himself in during the German occupation of Paris. It was June 14, 1940 when *Wehrmacht* troops entered the capital. It happened almost silently. The city had already lost 60 percent of its population and, aside from army vehicles, its streets were almost empty. Soldiers took up positions in front of ministries, while senior officers installed themselves in the city's best hotels, starting with the *Crillon* in the *Place de la Concorde* and soon also the *Meurice*, *Lutetia*, *Raphaël* and *George V*. The German command, the *Militärbefehlshaber in Frankreich (MBF)*, set up its headquarters in the *Hôtel Majestic*, close to the *Arc de Triomphe*. The *Luftwaffe*, in turn, took over the French Senate. Abiding by old principles put to the test during previous years, Germany set out to sap the morale of the French population by bringing them around to the victor's views and, at the same time, alienating them from the authorities that had previously governed them. In practice, this initial policy was aided by the docility of the defeated government and its tendency to go the occupying forces one better but it was often undercut by rivalries within the Nazi camp. At first, Picasso's output did not reflect the new circumstances he was forced to live under, although slowly he would allow the realities outside the studio to enter his creative world. One must consider that, as a foreigner in an invaded country and a supporter of Republicans in Spain, he was already cast as a prime enemy.

Even before the German invasion, shopping and eating out in Paris had become increasingly difficult. Although there were not yet shortages in the shops, what Parisians could legally buy and when they could buy it grew impossibly complicated: in addition to just three days when meat could be purchased, the sale of *apéritifs* was banned on Tuesdays, Thursdays and Saturdays; and the sale of chocolate in shops and restaurants was outlawed on Tuesdays, Wednesdays and Fridays, to give a few examples.[1] In this context of restrictions, Picasso wrote the poem, *Le repas*: "first course carries tears in a heap of sand and is made to crack between the teeth by men and women chosen as among the most beautiful."[2] At one point, formal rationing was instituted in Paris.[3] Its purpose was to ward off inflationary prices and panic; but instead, the system eventually created endemic food shortages and malnutrition, owing partly to an unequal distribution and availability of provisions to the population. Critical foods like bread, meat, cheese and milk were rationed, with the daily amount being rationed decreasing as the war continued.

Already in works the artist executed in March, such as *Buste de figure féminine*,[4] the sitter appears to be made out of kneaded dough. His figures were reduced to spherical or conical component parts, which, loosely connected, were only recognizable as human beings at all by a few economically inserted elements, such as breasts or eyes.[5] Janis notes that,

> Picasso never works directly from the model. His portraits are of persons remembered. They portray, through the instinct and vision, through the delicately balanced co-ordination of eye, mind, hand, and heart, a new realism reaching into the deepest recesses of man's inner nature . . . Characterized by the extreme eccentricity and psychopathic distortions of their personalities, the likenesses are visibly stamped with their traumatic scars.[6]

Pablo once said: "People keep speaking of naturalism as the opposite of modern painting. I would like to know if anyone has ever seen a natural work of art. Nature and art are totally different and can never be the same thing. We use art to express our idea of what nature is not."[7] As McCully wrote, "he no longer interpreted nature, but made it."[8] Nevertheless, Picasso succeeded in maintaining a balance between naturalism and abstraction. Neither of these two principles ever occurred without the other. He did not paint exclusively natural pictures nor completely abstract ones.[9] The gouache *Buste de femme*,[10] executed in subtle shades of grey against a delicate beige background, for instance, may be read as a highly sculptural portrait of Dora Maar. Like many of his most extreme abstractions, it could actually exist in the three-dimensional world. She is presented as a construction in three sections. Her face is balanced on a balustrade that serves as her mouth and neck, behind which her hair falls like a theatrical curtain. The head gives way at the bottom to the elegant arcs and soft forms of two large and pointed breasts that could also act as a sculptural plinth.[11] Works such as this might have served as substitutes for real sculptures, which were unfeasible in his temporary quarters in Royan.[12]

Although owners of food shops purchased their supplies from the fruit and vegetable market in *Les Halles* and from stocks held in Paris mainline railway stations, Parisians found shortages in some parts of the city, notably of coffee, milk, wine, some tinned goods and pasta.[13] The German authorities imposed a 9 p.m. curfew so that throughout the night the only lights visible were the ghostly blue streetlamps and the torches carried by pedestrians. Factors such as curfews, food shortages, air raid drills, a lack of automobiles and the "repedestrianization" of the modern city turned it into an eerie warren of sinister places, avoided by the majority of anxious citizens.[14] Probably the first major adjustment following the Occupation had to do with automobile transportation. Parisian owners of large cars (in particular, models from 1938, 1939 and 1940) were ordered to take them to the Vincennes hippodrome, on the outskirts of the city, for evaluation and "purchase" by the authorities. Buses were transformed from gasoline power to wood and charcoal power (*gazogène*), which was provided by large containers atop the vehicles. The bicycle—soon *de rigueur* for anyone not walking—became even more prevalent and in the occupied zone, every one of them had to be registered.[15]

Picasso stayed locked up in his studio most of the time in Royan. Named a degenerate artist, he would not be allowed to show his canvases in one-man exhibitions during this period. In fact, his wartime output was hardly ever seen outside his workplace.[16] He was frequently visited by Nazi soldiers, who seemed more intrigued by his reputation than concerned with any possible subversive activity. Picassos could still be found for sale, as it appears that public art life in occupied Paris was more plentiful than might be assumed;[17] but the ones sold were almost entirely resale items, offered at auction or in galleries by desperate collectors or dealers.[18] On August 20, he wrote *larga procesión*: "long processional of eyes of walking on the tips of toes . . . the crust of bread only just taken from the oven."[19] Around this time, a Paris police report confirmed that the conditions in the city were deteriorating but, contrary to Pétain's assertions, it concluded that the Germans were mainly responsible for the prevalent shortages: egg deliveries were few and far between, milk could be delivered only in the afternoon, cheese was in short supply.[20]

As the Occupation lingered, Parisians began to feel alienated, disconnected from their familiar environment, emotionally detached. One of the ironies of an occupied city was that, while it brought its citizens closer together physically, it separated them psychologically.[21] According to Mlle. Rolland, the situation for foreigners even in the small town of Royan had become untenable. They were exposed to the suspicion of the Germans, as well as to the xenophobia of some of the French, especially those who seemed to be accommodating themselves easily to the Occupation.[22] Therefore, Picasso asked Marcel to take him and Sabartés to Paris on August 24, bringing also Kazbek and some of the paintings he had completed.[23] Dora traveled by train at the same time, while Marie-Thérèse and Maya would remain behind in Royan.[24]

Everybody sought someone else to blame for the growing shortages and rising prices. Shopkeepers accused the farmers and wholesalers of hoarding and of price manipulation; shoppers accused the shopkeepers of profiteering; collaborationists blamed the Jews. Vegetables became rare: leeks, carrots, turnips, cabbages and potatoes were in short supply.[25] The Vichy government officially introduced an extraordinarily complicated system of rationing. It was hopelessly inadequate as a solution to the issue of scarcity.[26] Picasso's poem from September 18, *vu matin*, included many references to food items: "clouds oozing drool on the sky's liquid bricks stinking up the sheets of the vines . . . the blue's harp sprinkled over the batter . . . cheese crusts . . . butter grass caress of fingers . . . a rain of dead birds hits the wall and bloodies the room with its laughter."[27] The next day, he continued with "autre matin": "while sliding its paunch into the room rips its skin at the butter saw of the plaster's frigid lips . . . drops of blood flowing from its ripped out feathers . . . heaped in a corner for this feast."[28]

At one time, he had meant to go back to live at rue de La Boétie and use the rue des Grands-Augustins studio only to work. The smaller flat was easier to heat after all, although it was at the top of a tall building, exposed to the icy winds and with no warmth coming up from the lower floors any longer, but it was two miles from his studio. With few buses or subway trains, no taxis and no gas for his own car, that took a lot of his time walking from one to the other, which was even unpleasant due to the weather and the odious presence of German soldiers.[29] So, on October 11, he closed his apartment for the duration of the war, living exclusively in his studio, the vast proportions of which enabled him to resume sculpture.[30] He installed a magnificent stove, but as shortages increased, there was no fuel for it. He refused special supplies of coal from German visitors, reportedly saying: "A Spaniard is never cold."[31] When he and Dora could no longer bear the low temperatures, they sought refuge at well-heated restaurants like *Café Flore, Les Deux Magots* or *Le Catalan*.[32] In this, he was different from many other Parisians, who could only afford to eat at home with what they acquired with ration cards, supplemented by extras bought on the black market and what they could get from relatives in the countryside.[33]

By early 1941, the Germans had built concrete fortifications at all key junctions and before important buildings throughout the city. Massive bunkers were constructed under the streets and rail stations. They had also set up warehouses everywhere, especially near major train stations, in which to store the items they had "appropriated" from Jewish and "foreign" families. German outposts were in almost every quarter and neighborhood. Every district had an office of the Occupation authorities or an apartment building that had been totally or partially requisitioned.[34] The severe weather conditions continued, making it even harder to find food. A Paris resident, Paul Léautaud, wrote: "Almost 40 centimeters of snow in Fontenay. Nothing to eat. Not even bread . . . All day long and into the evening the wind howled, getting everywhere in the house; spent my time shivering with cold despite my clothes, and my hands frozen despite keeping on the move."[35] Lengthy and slow lines in an occupied city reinforced the idea of being a prisoner, of having one's will continuously thwarted. The occupiers knew that lines were a means of control—of one's time, one's space, one's desires.[36] A *Time* magazine reporter witnessed a riot at a queue of people. Waiting in line for their meager rations at a food store, they had become overexcited and began throwing rocks. German authorities watching nearby tried to stop the mob but the rock-throwing continued. As punishment, the Germans banned potato distribution for 40 days. With the imposition of the food rationing system instituted in September, tensions ran high. People began to feel the pains of hunger and desperation set in.

In the heart of the cold winter, Picasso jotted down on the pages of a simple notebook a play in six acts: *Désir attrapé par la queue*.[37] Written in a few days, it represented his views on the Occupation: "Light the lanterns. Throw flights of doves with all our strength against the bullets and lock securely the house demolished by the bombs."[38] His characters were fixated on three things: cold, hunger and love, and their attempts to avoid the first two and satisfy the third inevitably ended in disappointment. Tragic farce or clownish tragedy, the piece adopted a Rabelaisian and macabre tone. We find the same kinship with the dada and surrealist spirit that had earned him the admiration and encouragement of Breton, Éluard and Hugnet in the 1930s. A mixture of eroticism, scatology and gluttony, the play had a cathartic effect on him. Directed by Albert Camus and dedicated to the memory of Max Jacob, it would be read a few months before the Liberation on March 19, 1944 in the apartment of Louise and Michel Leiris in the presence of top figures of the French intelligentsia.[39]

The play has been called a "gastro-poietic account of the Occupation." As one German report noticed, "the entire Occupation was "a question of the stomach" [*Magenfrage*].[40] Two of the main and recurring themes of the play, hunger and cold, flowed directly from the severe conditions most of the population had to endure, increased rationing coupled with a very harsh winter. The artist responded to the privations with the exaltation of daily life and the celebration of vital functions, pleasures derived from rare food items mingling with those of sex.[41] Purely visual images were possibly outnumbered by those which appealed to other senses, such as taste or smell: the fumes of potato chips suffocate the actors at the end of the fourth act and *La Tarte* melts "into the fragrant architecture of the kitchen," attracting *Gros Pied* (Picasso's alter ego) by "the sweet stink of her tresses."[42]

As new ration cards were put into circulation in February, the black market made up for shortages. Pablo was going through a rough time as everyone else. He had hardly painted since August when he had returned from Royan and seemed to be looking for a way to express the horrible environment by other means. Writing became a sort of refuge for him.[43] On February 11, he started composing the surrealistic *Mourlot Text* with *tout le fatras immonde*. The entire work would be completed by September 16. He would later say:

> There are stacks of poems sleeping here. When I began to write them, I wanted to prepare myself a palette of words, as if I were dealing with colors. All these words were weighed, filtered and appraised. I don't put much stock in spontaneous expressions of the unconscious and it would be stupid to think that one can provoke them at will.[44]

The verbal imagery includes such phrases as "unclean jumble," "open wound showing its teeth," "torn piles," "foundation of bones planted on the clay," "fragments of shattered windowpane," "agitated clocks," "distressed lamentations of flowers crushed under the wheels," all of which are suggestive of death and destruction. They may have been alluding to scenes he had heard described about German advances elsewhere in Europe.[45] This same month, the Paris-based clandestine journal sponsored by the PCF, *La Pensée libre*, published its first issue running to ninety-six pages. It was spearheaded by three of the party's intellectuals: Jacques Decour, Georges

Politzer and Jacques Solomon.[46] On the opposite side of the spectrum, Marcel Déat, with the backing of Heinrich Otto Abetz, the German ambassador to Vichy France, created the collaborationist party *Rassemblement national populaire (RNP)*, based at 128, rue du Faubourg Saint-Honoré. Some of its members came from the *Mouvement social révolutionnaire (MSR)* led by Eugène Deloncle, who had founded the pre-war right-wing terrorist group *La Cagoule*.[47]

> "The Occupation was intolerable; people barely survived," Baer has written.
>
> Some have called it a time of Purgatory . . . All is gloomy, dark, and cold. One might also describe this period as a long winter that lasted four years . . . This cold drove people into themselves, into a total silence. People lived under the leaden lid of a stormy, icy sky . . . Streets were empty, the intersections full of boards covered with German Gothic lettering. Curfew, glacial winter and fear were the only items on the menu. You never knew what might happen to those you loved. No one talked . . . silence and suspicion were the watchwords . . . Poor Picasso! No doubt he was a little bit paranoid during those years. But what beautiful paintings he made out of that real but imagined persecution.[48]

Living and working in his cavernous studio, Picasso immersed himself in his work, living a much quieter life, removed from the pre-war artistic and bourgeois society of which he had been a part. He turned to his immediate surroundings as subject matter, resulting in a hauntingly powerful series of still lifes.[49] As O.F. Bollnow noted, "our humanity is determined by the way we act within specific, lived-in spaces . . . When the individual no longer can take comfort from the predictability of movement, another set of anxieties is created."[50] It is precisely that feeling of anxiety that is alluded to in the poem *la casserole*:

> the open mouths flying to the windows . . . the leaves violently squeezed into a crowd thick in the four corners of the white-washed wall . . . its dress perfumed by its involuntary incense accuses it pushes it into confessions tortures it castrates it and throws it all ground up onto the sky behind the acidic clouds . . . the nails driven into the back of the various four walls of the room completely forced and slapped onto the air . . . between the fingers of the darkness and the light tightly squeezed dying of fear in the most wretched corner.[51]

Probably to get his mind off things, Picasso concentrated on certain artistic problems which can be traced back to the cubist years as in *Nature morte au boudin.*[52] A dull light shines from a funnel-shaped ceiling lamp onto the table surface where a large dagger-like knife lies in front of a rolled-up blood sausage. They are joined by two artichoke stems, a corked bottle of wine and an open wrapping paper with a piece of cheese behind it. He opted for a monochrome statement in different shades of gray with certain lightening due to a dirty white on a partially translucent brownish background. From the open drawer of the table, a set of knives and forks protrudes as if wanting to free themselves.[53] The tilted-up perspective brings objects in the background closer to the picture plane and to the viewer but also threatens to spill them out of the picture. There is an underlying menace in the apparently innocent, even hospitable, presentation of food and cutlery at that table.

In a rare comment on his own work, he said that this painting has "an atmosphere like Philip II, dark and dismal . . . The knives and forks are like souls out of purgatory." It is appropriate that Picasso should have used the word *purgatory* to describe some aspects of the painting because most of his works from the wartime years suggest that he found the Occupation exactly that—a life that was put on hold, without change and without hope. The allusion to the sixteenth-century king might be explained as a reference to a reign coinciding with the Counter-Reformation, a period of cruel repression. He may have also been thinking of Parisians, destined to suffer interminably in occupied Paris.[54] The German grip on the city affected many aspects of French culture but nothing was hit harder than its cuisine. Food was an essential part of national identity. Adapting to a less plentiful and lower quality fare proved difficult. A correspondent for the magazine, *Le Gerbe,* wrote: "Eating and, more important, eating well, is the theme song of Paris life. In the street, in the metro, in cafes, all you hear about is food. At the theater or movies, when there's an old play or movie with a huge banquet scene, the audience breaks into delirious cries of joy."[55] Despite their difficulties, people courageously dealt with their circumstances, nicknaming their system of improvisation *le système D*, from the verb *se débrouiller* (alternatively *se démerder*). The poem, *chasuble de sang*, included allusions to the same animism of things we observe in the painting:[56]

> chasuble of blood thrown over the naked shoulders of the green wheat shivering between the wet sheets . . . the wall painted in ochre flapping its big apple-green mauve-white wings tearing its beak against the panes . . . the uncombed hair of the landscape spread out under

the sun . . . the hanging tongue of the plough stuck to plowing sweating.[57]

Children occupied an unexpected place during this period and, in their own manner, they mirrored the harshness of the times. As innocent as they are cruel, they express, like animals, the same type of unconscious or blind violence as Picasso's portraits of women. This is the case of the disturbing *Jeune garçon à la langouste*[58] painted in June. Sitting cross-legged, sneering, he is half-undressed, his sex prominently exposed. With his toothless and idiotic smile, his round and pink face, he evokes a reaction of disgust mixed with sympathy. The toddler harks back to the dwarves of Diego Velázquez or the *Bobo*/fool in Bartolomé Murillo, as Bernadac notes.[59] A feeling of uneasiness emanates from his upset anatomy. The prey he holds in his hand like a funny rattle denotes a sense of cruelty. Lobsters were a rare commodity, so its presence also rings sarcastic. Only Nazi officers were offered such delicacies at restaurants like *Le Prunier*.[60] Overall, there is a very unchildlike quality about this child. He actually resembles Picasso—the black, slicked-down hair; the dark, piercing eyes, and the broad nose—which highlights the sarcastic intentions behind the crustacean.[61]

On July 8, Picasso painted the oil *Nature morte au bouquet*[62] with the motif of a vase on a table in front of a window that he had first explored in Saint-Raphaël in 1919. In contrast to those still lifes, done in a curvilinear style, the artist here turned to the more angular synthetic cubism. The chromatic accents are embedded in the clearly articulated black structure of the picture, the brilliant spots being the deep carmine-red of the table with the yellow lemons in a green bowl and the red-edged flowers in the blue glass vase. The picture possesses a severe reticence typical of other wartime still lifes. It was not only Picasso's studio that gained in importance as a safe retreat. The Parisian apartment figures prominently in many recollections of the Occupation. It was more than a place of expected physical comfort, it was also a shelter from confusion and uncertainty. Hearing and seeing whatever was going on outside from the relative security of their window helped alleviate the ever-present sense of claustrophobia that characterized daily life during the Occupation.[63]

At the end of the July, he completed the oil *Femme à l'artichaut*,[64] which shows Dora Maar's features. She sits in an armchair holding the artichoke in her right hand like a scepter. The long-stalked vegetable is an unusual motif and invites speculation as to its possible meaning. Some have compared it to a mace, a spiked club used as a weapon in the Middle Ages, or to a Spanish *garrote*. The monumental scale of the sitter is daunting, although the throne is a simple wicker chair and plain clothes have replaced the expected royal robe.[65] The strong deformation of her face and body and the transformation of the fingers of her left hand into a claw gives the woman an ambivalent role, both as perpetrator and victim of violence. The wide-open eyes, especially the one on the nasal appendage, seem to reflect a sense of horror or shock, belying the smiling mouth. One finger of the hand holding the artichoke seems to be pointing, perhaps in reproach. It may stand for Pablo's attitudes about the continuing German execution of hostages.[66] The palette of dark greens, grays, and browns reinforces the lugubrious mood. The somber, dissonant colors make this portrait a symbol of human cruelty. Out of the depths of despair, however, the artist was able to extract reasons for hope.[67] Like the French national symbol of Marianne, the female figure embodies the people and, despite the eradication of her dignity, she still exhibits some form of resistance. The spirit of militancy manifests itself in the provocative-casual posture with the legs crossed, in the tectonic plates of the clothing section and in the claw-raking hand.[68]

As for all others who remained in Paris, the deprivations of life in the city hit Picasso hard. Food shortages and rationing of all kinds of materials were rife. Although he was wealthy enough to be able to afford to purchase goods from the black market and had friends who assisted him in acquiring art supplies such as plaster, paper and even the highly sought-after bronze, he was largely forced to make do with whatever was available. Pages of the city's daily newspapers, for example, were used as support for studies, saving his precious canvases and paper stock for more developed ideas. Brassaï photographed Pablo painting on such an improvised palette paraphrasing Breton's idea that the work should be "next to the daily newspaper." He scribbled portraits of deformed, animalistic and absurd portraits on the pages of collaborationist papers like *Paris-Soir*. Leaving the text visible, these "palimpsest works" spoke of the repressive environment during the Occupation. An avid reader of newspapers, he indulged, through these dark idol-like figures, in a sort of "reinvention of portraiture."[69] Dora continued to be his primary model, her dark features and striking presence dominating endless "portraits," as Picasso responded to life under the oppressive regime.

Notes
1   Drake 2015, 37.
2   Rothenberg & Joris 2004, 190.
3   The decrees had been approved on September 1 and October 14, 1939 (Bernard 2019, 107).

4 *Buste de figure féminine.* Royan. 2-March/1940. Oil on paper mounted on canvas. 64 x 46 cm. Private collection, Zurich. OPP.40:005.
5 Buchholz & Zimmermann 2000, 56.
6 Janis & Janis 1947. n.p.
7 Walther 2001, 53.
8 McCully 1981, 215–218.
9 Walther 2001, 42–43.
10 *Buste de femme.* Royan. 3-March/1940. Gouache on paper laid down on canvas. 65,5 x 47 cm. Christie's. #539, 6146, 06/30/99. OPP.40:488.
11 Christie's 1999, cat. no. 539, 6146.
12 Barr 1946, 224–227.
13 Drake 2015, 66–67.
14 Rosbottom 2014, xxix.
15 Rosbottom 2014, 112.
16 FitzGerald 1998, 113–116.
17 Nash 1998, 25–26.
18 FitzGerald 1998, 118.
19 Rothenberg & Joris 2004, 222.
20 Drake 2015, 109.
21 Rosbottom 2014, 15.
22 Goggin 1985, 61.
23 Daix 1993, 263; Nash 1998, 214; Nash 1998, 214; Gasman 1998, 65; Bernard 2019, 108. Others date the return later to August 25 (Goggin 1985, 6, 60; Gohr 1988, 12; Morris 1993, 155; Mahler 2015, 184; Dagen 2009, 489; Álvarez, et al. 2019, 33; Limousin, et al. 2019, 143; Tosatto, et al. 2019, 104); to late August (Penrose 1981a, 332); to the end of August (Spies 2011, 188; Cowling 2016, 162; Caruncho & Fàbregas 2017, 116); or later to October (Milde 2002, 401).
24 Bernard 2019, 108.
25 Drake 2015, 126.
26 Drake 2015, 124–125.
27 Rothenberg & Joris 2004, 223–224.
28 Rothenberg & Joris 2004, 224.
29 O'Brian 1994, 351–352.
30 Bernard 2019, 110. Others date the move earlier to September (Baldassari 2006, 239; Mahler 2015, 184); simply to October (Milde 2002, 401); or even more generally to autumn (Gohr 1988, 12; Daemgen 2005, 33).
31 Cabanne 1979, 332.
32 Nash 1998, 217; Baring 2017, 201.
33 Riding 2010, 106.
34 Rosbottom 2014, 111.
35 Drake 2015, 169.
36 Rosbottom 2014, 190–193.
37 Written January 14–17, 1941 (Penrose 1981a, 334; Gohr 1988, 12; Baldassari 2006, 311; Dagen 2009, 489; Bernard 2019, 130).
38 Frechtman 1962, 57–60.

39 Tosatto, et al. 2019, 126–127.
40 Rosbottom 2014, 291.
41 Maldonado 2019, 40–43.
42 Penrose 1981, 337.
43 Tosatto, et al. 2019, 126.
44 Cited in Ashton 1972, 130.
45 Goggin 1985, 81.
46 Riding 2010, 273; Drake 2015, 310.
47 Riding 2010, 119; Drake 2015, 182.
48 Baer 1998, 85, 96.
49 Christie's 2018, cat. no. 15, 15469.
50 Rosbottom 2014, 162.
51 Rothenberg & Joris 2004, 243–244.
52 *Nature morte au boudin.* Paris. 10-May/1941. Oil on canvas. 92,7 x 66 cm. Tony and Gail Ganz Collection. OPP.41:002.
53 Ullmann 1993, 258.
54 Goggin 1985, 86–89; Boggs 1992, 268.
55 Cited in Taylor 2012.
56 Spies 2011, 233.
57 Rothenberg & Joris 2004, 248.
58 *Jeune garçon à la langouste.* Paris. 21-June/1941. Oil on canvas. 130,5 x 97,3 cm. Musée Picasso, Paris. OPP.41:013.
59 Bozo, Richet & Thiébaut 1979.
60 Tosatto, et al. 2019, 140.
61 Goggin 1985, 99–100; Ullmann 1993, 343.
62 *Nature morte au bouquet.* Paris. 8-July/1941. Oil on canvas. 92 x 73 cm. Emil G. Bührle Foundation Collection, Zürich. OPP.41:248.
63 Rosbottom 2014, 168–172.
64 *Femme à l'artichaut.* Paris. 31-July/1941. Oil on panel. 195 x 130 cm. Museum Ludwig, Köln. (Inv ML 01291. OPP.41:449.
65 Ullmann 1993, 302–304.
66 Goggin 1985, 162–163.
67 Nash 1998, 34.
68 Meyer 1988, 104.
69 Tosatto, et al. 2019, 127.

Bibliography

Álvarez, Athina, et al. "Chronologie." *Dossier de Presse. Dora Maar.* Agnès Benayer. ed. Paris: Centre Pompidou, Direction de la Communication et des Partenariats, 2019, 1–38.

Ashton, Dore, ed. *Picasso on Art: A Selection of Views, Documents of Twentieth Century Art.* New York: Viking, 1972.

Baer, Brigitte. 1998. "Where Do They Come From—Those Superb Paintings and Horrid Women of 'Picasso's War.'" *Picasso and the War Years: 1937–1945.* Steven A. Nash, ed. New York: Thames & Hudson, 1998, 81–98.

Baldassari, Anne. *Picasso–Life with Dora Maar: Love and War 1935–1945*. Paris: Flammarion, 2006.

Baring, Louise. *Dora Maar. Paris in the Time of Man Ray, Jean Cocteau and Picasso*. New York: Rizzoli, 2017.

Barr, Alfred H., Jr. *Picasso: Fifty Years of His Art*. New York: Simon & Schuster, 1946.

Bernard, Sophie. "1939–1945. Picasso au cœur des ténèbres." *Au cœur des ténèbres 1939–1945* Guy Tosatto, et al., ed. Grenoble: Fine editions d'art. 2019, 61–287.

Boggs, Jean Sutherland, ed. *Picasso and Things*. Cleveland: Cleveland Museum of Art, 1992.

Bozo, Dominique, Michèle Richet & Philippe Thiébaut. *Picasso, Œuvres reçues en paiement des droits de succession*. Paris: La Réunion des musées nationaux (RMH), 1979.

Buchholz, Elke Linda & Beate Zimmermann. *Pablo Picasso: Life and Work* (Art in Focus) Konemann, 2000.

Cabanne, Pierre. 1979. *Pablo Picasso: His Life and Times*. New York: William Morrow & Co; Morrow Quill Paperbacks, 1979.

Caruncho, Daniel R. & Anna Fàbregas. *Biografía ilustrada de Pablo Picasso*. Barcelona: Dos de Arte Ediciones, 2017.

Christie's. *Impressionist and Modern Art Evening Sale*. London: Auction catalogue 15469, February 27, 2018.

Cowling, Elizabeth, ed. *Picasso Portraits*. London: National Portrait Gallery Publications, 2016.

Daemgen, Anke. "Picasso. Ein Leben." *Pablo. Der private Picasso: Le Musée Picasso à Berlin* Angela Schneider & Anke Daemgen, eds. München: Prestel, 2005, 14–44.

Dagen, Philippe. 2009. "Chronology." *Picasso*. Philippe Dagen, ed. New York: The Monacelli Press, 2009, 483–92.

Daix, Pierre. *Picasso: Life & Art*. New York: Icon Editions & New York: Harper-Collins, 1993.

Drake, David. *Paris at War (1939–1944)*. Cambridge, MA: The Belknap Press of Harvard University Press, 2015.

FitzGerald, Michael C. 1998. "Reports from the Home Fronts: Some Skirmishes over Picasso's Reputation." *Picasso and the War Years: 1937–1945*. Steven A. Nash, ed. New York: Thames & Hudson, 1998, 113–22.

Frechtman, Bernard. *Desire: A Play by Pablo Picasso*. New York: The Citadel Press, 1962.

Gasman, Lydia Csató. "Death Falling from the Sky: Picasso's Wartime Texts." *Picasso and the War Years: 1937–1945*. Steven A. Nash, ed. New York: Thames & Hudson, 1998, 55–67.

Goggin, Mary Margaret. *Picasso and his Art during the German Occupation: 1940–1944*. PhD Dissertation. Stanford University. Ann Arbor, Michigan: University Microfilms International, 1985.

Gohr, Siegfried. "Chronologie der Jahre 1936–1945." *Picasso in Zweiten Weltkrieg: 1939 bis 1945*. Siegfried Gohr, et al., ed. Köln: Museum Ludwig, 1988, 11–13.

Janis, Harriet & Sidney. *Picasso: The Recent Years: 1939–1946*. New York: Doubleday & Company, Inc., 1947.

Limousin, Isabelle et al., eds. *Picasso et la guerre*. Paris: Gallimard, 2019.

Mahler, Luise. "Selected Exhibitions, 1910–1967." *Picasso Sculpture*. Ann Temkin & Anne Umland, eds. New York: The Museum of Modern Art, New York, 2015, 304–11.

Maldonado, Guitemie. "Une piece, des circonstances. Le desir attrape par la queue ou la vie au present." *Au coeur des ténèbres 1939–1945*. Guy Tosatto, et al., eds. Grenoble: In Fine editions d'art, 2019, 40–45.

Mallén, Enrique. *Online Picasso Project*. http://picasso.shsu.edu. Sam Houston State University, 2020.

McCully, Marilyn, ed. *A Picasso Anthology: Documents, Criticism, Reminiscences*. London: Arts Council of Great Britain in association with Thames and Hudson; Princeton, NY, Princeton University Press, 1981.

Meyer, Franz. 1988. "Picasso und die Zeitgeschichte." *Picasso in Zweiten Weltkrieg: 1939 bis 1945*. Siegfried Gohr, et al., eds. Köln: Museum Ludwig, 1988, 91–105.

Milde, Brigitta, ed. "Biografie." *Picasso et les femmes / Picasso und die Frauen*. Ingrid Mössinger, et al., eds. Köln: DuMont, 2002, 396–403.

Morris, Frances. *Paris Post War: Art and Existentialism 1945–55*. Tate Gallery: London, 1993.

Nash, Steven A., ed. *Picasso and the War Years: 1937–1945*. New York: Thames & Hudson, 1998.

O'Brian, Patrick. *Pablo Picasso. A Biography*. New York: W.W. Norton & Company, 1994.

Penrose. Roland. *Picasso: His Life and Work*, Berkeley: University of California, 1981.

Riding, Alan. *And the Show Went On*. New York: Alfred A. Knopf, 2010.

Rosbottom, Ronald C. *When Paris Went Dark: The City of Light Under German Occupation, 1940–1944*. New York: Back Bay Books, 2014.

Rothenberg, Jerome & Pierre Joris, eds. *The Burial of the Count of Orgaz & Other Poems*. Cambridge, MA: Exact Change, 2004.

Spies, Werner. *The Continent Named Picasso. Werner Spies: The Eye and the Word—Collected Writings on Art and Literature, The Gagosian Edition*. Vol. 5. Thomas W. Gaehtgens, ed. New York: Abrams, 2011.

Taylor, Alexandra. "Part IV: France: Food—Adapting to the Ration System." (February 18, 2012). https://tayloralexandra.wordpress.com/2012/02/18/part-iv-france-3-food-adapting-to-the-ration-system/

Tosatto, Guy, et al., eds. *Au coeur des ténèbres 1939–1945*. Grenoble: In Fine editions d'art, 2019.

Ullmann, Ludwig. *Picasso und der Krieg*. Bonn: Karl Kerber Verlag, 1993.

Walther, Ingo F., ed. *Pablo Picasso: 1881–1973*. New York: Taschen America Llc., 2001.

13

The Devouring Eye (I)
of Pablo Picasso

Enrique Mallén

Art is often said to be the result of conflict—no call for art in Eden."
(cf. O'Brian 1994, 280)

To understand Picasso's approach to portraiture and still lifes, one must first take into consideration the very close relationship he had with his environment. Even during the most abstract stages of Cubism, the artist maintained the preeminence of the physical domain in his art.

There is no "abstract art," he would say, "You must always start with something. Afterwards you can remove all traces of reality. There's no danger then, anyway, because the idea of the object will have left an indelible mark. It is what started the artist off, excited his ideas, and stirred up his emotions. Ideas and emotions will in the end be prisoners in his work. Whatever they do, they can't escape from the picture. They form an integral part of it, even when their presence is no longer discernible."[1]

In the so-called synthetic phase of Cubism, Picasso started introducing real elements such as stenciled letters in the composition. The reason for that is that letters not only have an independent existence, but they can also introduce an extrinsic, autonomous element into the picture. Soon after, he included more durable materials, such as wood, cardboard, etc. With them, Picasso managed to insert the actual texture of matter into his art. As Daix explains, this constituted the ultimate abolition of illusionism in painting since, by adding these extraneous elements, the work itself had become an object, independent and autonomous.[2] Despite the physical preeminence of these compositions, soon a conflict broke out between the reality of actual materials and reality re-created in art. The objects he incorporated into his still lifes served as a vehicle to communicate deep feelings inside of him. Through them he projected his own persona. To that extent they were metaphorical, rather than referential. Picasso himself was unequivocal about his use of metaphors: "I want to tell something by means of the most common object: for example, a casserole, any old casserole, the one everyone knows. For me it is a vessel in the metaphorical sense, just like Christ's use of the parables."[3] This notion of using artworks as a sort of parable is crucial to the point raised in this essay.

His concentration on still lifes can be traced back to the canvases he had executed during the summer of 1906 in Gósol, a remote village in the Catalán Pyrenées. Prior to this, the artist had not been attracted to them as an independent genre, but from now on they were to occupy a firm place in his work. *Nature morte aux vases (Le porron)*,[4] for instance, shows evidence of Picasso's growing interest in revealing the interrelation of the objects on the canvas. In this simple composition, while each object exists within its own spatial zone, it is also subordinate both to the rationale of confrontation and interaction. In another still life, *Nature morte au tableau*,[5] we find again objects of everyday use made in the typical shapes and from the materials of the region. Richardson wrote about these compositions: "These are the first glimmerings of Picasso's anthropomorphic concept of still life as a metaphor not just for sex but for all manner of conflicts and confrontations—a concept that will later help the artist to contrive a code that will divulge and at the same time conceal his secret desires."[6] The inscription "Les pregunt[s]" suggests the influence of Gauguin, whose Tahitian pictures very often carried similar texts, the most famous example being *D'où venons-nous? Que sommes-nous? Où allons-nous?* of 1897. The extra-pictorial references that such inscriptions suggested appealed to Picasso, who doubtless enjoyed the layer of intrigue it lent his work.[7]

Confrontation at a metaphorical level is even more emphatic in *Nature morte aux vases*.[8] This small gouache also painted at Gósol seems full of tantalizing contradictions. While the brown pottery jug, with its bloated body and inadequate handle, is rendered calligraphically, the glass *porrón*, awkward in its transparency is drawn with considerable energy. The objects, although obvious in themselves, are subtly related to each other and Picasso was conscious of certain possible sexual associations—the jug with the body of a woman, the porrón with virility.[9]

Picasso's Gósol paintings are of extreme importance and foreshadow the confrontational nature of his masterpiece from the following year, *Les Demoiselles d'Avignon*,[10] and his experiments leading to Cubism.[11] Robert Rosenblum explains how Picasso's production during his time in Gósol would redirect the course of his artistic development: "The serene and earthy equilibrium, often described as 'classical,' that marked much, though hardly all, of this summer productivity might appear to be the last gasp of traditional order before the detonation of 1907. But far from being buried forever in the rubble, the wide and experimental range of paintings, drawings, and sculpture from the Gósol months launches a wealth of fresh ideas that would be amplified in the new era inaugurated by the Demoiselles and would have many afterlives in Picasso's post-Cubist career."[12]

Conflict is also at the heart of an important still life from 1907, *Nature morte à la tête de mort*.[13] While here we see, once again, a conflict between the different objects in the composition, there is also a clear desire on the part of the artist to project his own self onto that confrontation. The dating of the work is open to debate. Originally assigned to the fall of 1907 by Zervos, its date of execution has been recently extended to the summer or fall of 1908, based on the hypothesis of Theodore Reff that the work is a *memento mori* for Picasso's friend, Karl-Heinz Wieghels, who hanged himself on June 1, 1908 in the *Bateau-Lavoir*, where both he and Pablo painted and lived.[14] The painting may have been a general commemoration for artistic genius, in particular, for Paul Cézanne, who had died in 1906 and for whom there were two important memorial exhibitions in Paris in 1907. While Cézanne certainly received more recognition towards the end of his life, both he and Wieghels were considered outcasts earlier on in their artistic careers. So, the painting may represent Picasso's own fear of being rejected, as *Les Demoiselles d'Avignon* had been met with overwhelming disapproval. In the background, from the finger-hole of a dull brown palette, spring five brushes, as if they were twigs. Propped against that landscape is a simple but glaringly gilt mirror, which reflects one of Picasso's voluptuous nudes of 1907. In the foreground, a skull is placed beside a pile of books against which a pipe rises as if it were a pen on an inkstand. The painting symbolizes an artist's world. It is restless and anxious, only barely resolved as the forces of the left half are balanced by those of the right, essentially the skull against the mauve triangle descending from the navel of the nude. The skull introduces the drama of death, thus contrasting with the nude which, although painted, is still symbolic of life.[15]

I propose that Picasso's still lifes are an intuitive manifestation of the mental confrontation with an "Other" explored by Georges Bataille and Jacques Lacan at a psycho-analytical level.[16] Bataille is above all a thinker of liminal conflict. The self—what he calls the "sovereign" being—is for him "suspended on the edge of the abyss," hanging at the border in eternal opposition with that existential "Other"—death—but never actually falling, except, of course, in his/her terminal demise. Life, in fact, is defined by Bataille as "existence striving to reach its limits," but never surpassing them, i.e., the being of the subject cannot be found beyond its limits as that would imply his/her complete dissolution. S/he confronts death while preserving life. To that extent, the principle of insufficiency is the guiding thread of impossibility that leads the subject to the heart of the labyrinth where all s/he finds is "absolute insufficiency."[17]

Bataille's thought occupies an unstable position between, on the one hand, a conception of life and transgression which finds its source in a Dionysian experience of excess; and, on the other, a view of death and work solidly grounded, via Kojève, in Hegelian dialectics.[18] But unlike in Hegel, contraries do not merge into one another in Bataille; they remain in a relationship of extreme tension. His writing embodies this tension. It is a writing of anguish (*angoisse*), a writing of the self (*moi*) almost at the point of destruction. Even to see, to know, to understand, opens up a tension in which blindness, non-knowledge (*non-savoir*) and incomprehension are immediately on the horizon. To write (*écrire*) at all is to maintain desire, thereby invoking the anguish of the cry (*cri*)—and the laughter (*rire*)—before death.

Lacanian psychoanalysis follows a similar quasi-dialectical conception of identity which relies on the confluence of three orders: the Real, the Imaginary, and the Symbolic.[19] This tripartite intersection constitutes the entirety of human mental life, whether in a cumulative way or in the various effects it produces. An individual is determined in, through and by these three orders.[20] Moreover, the structure they comprise is far from static; but rather, the orders constantly interact, defining each other and themselves in contradistinction to one another. In other words, they are disparate, but simultaneously interdependent for their definition.

In the psychological development of the individual according to Lacan, once the ego begins to recognize that it is separate from a totality (the Real), it starts to feel anxiety, which is caused by a sense of something lost. A consequence of its awareness of a separation from the Real is a demand to make that "Other" a part of itself—in other words, to reintegrate itself with its original source—something, on the other hand, impossible to achieve. Indeed, this unfulfillable desire ultimately, only as a constant reminder of loss or lack. The demand of the Imaginary does not proceed beyond a dyadic relation between the self and the object the ego wants to make a part of itself. The so-called "mirror stage" corresponds to this demand in so far as one misrecognizes in the mirror image a stable, coherent, whole self, which, however, does not correspond to the true self (and is, therefore, impossible to realize).[21] Picasso's still lifes are precisely such an attempt to make the "Other" in his surroundings a part of himself. In these compositions, he projected his Ego through anthropomorphic objects that defined aspects of his own persona and which, through their confrontation, served to outline the mental conflict faced by the developing self.

A third order, the Symbolic is all about language and representation. Once an individual enters society's established systems of representation and accepts their rules and dictates, s/he is able to deal with others through the intermediary structures available. Nevertheless, when one enters the cultural socio-symbolic sphere, there is a part that still refuses to be entertained, an excess or "accursed share" that is experienced as the "missed encounter," what Lacan calls the Real. The Real is that inaccessible aspect that haunts psychic life: "the essential object which is not an object any longer, but this something faced with which all words cease and all categories fail. An encounter with the Real is an encounter with the point where the coherency of a moment is pierced and the symbolic support of one's identity begins to give way; hence the Real is closely associated with Lacan's Death Drive.[22]

The Imaginary order is identified as the realm of unarticulated (but articulable) identifications and idealizations which are the building blocks of fantasy and the Ego. It is the most basic level of self-conception, and therefore, a precursor to subjectivity.[23] In short, the Imaginary order is a realm of spurious but necessary identifications with entities in the world by which the individual ceaselessly attempts to shore up his own identity. In Picasso's case, this confrontation applies at two different levels. First, the artist defines his persona metaphorically through the objects in his surroundings that he includes in the still lifes. These objects in turn establish their character by means of a conflict with the other items in that same composition. The Imaginary order deals predominantly with confrontation and identification.[24]

While in earlier canvases the object's main role had been to make us aware of the space around them, in *Atelier avec tête et bras de plâtre*,[25] we are presented with an anomalous heap of objects that do not belong to the same domain, that appear to come from places far removed from each other. What we see is an attempt at setting up a congenial spirit among elements that actually repudiate each other, that apparently have nothing in common.[26] The painting's underpinning remains cubist, but aspects of its facture and color and, above all, its imagery point to a new surreal dimension in Picasso's art. The square in the middle of the composition (apparently Paulo's toy theater) destroys any pretense of a coherent relationship of objects in space and undercuts the three-dimensionality suggested by the plaster bust which appears to float rather unrealistically above the table.[27] Years later he would explain to Penrose: "We [Cubists] wanted to go deep into things. What was wrong with [the] Surrealists was that they did not go inside; they took the surface effects of the subconscious. They did not understand the inside of the object or themselves."[28] The deep significance of objects is made manifest in the already mentioned bust. Critics like Meyer Schapiro found in it a certain resemblance to the cruel emperor Caracalla;[29] and Lydia Gasman saw in it as an apocalyptic vision of a fierce king.[30] Picasso was probably aware of the Roman emperor's orders that led to the assassination of his brother, Geta, with whom he had ruled after the death of their father, Septimius Severus. Equally mystifying are the related broken plaster casts of arms, one clutching a classical scroll, the other clenching its fist; and the pages of the opened book containing hieroglyphs which could be references to the threatening underworld of the Real.[31] As he said to Françoise Gilot much later, "I want to draw the mind in a direction it's not used to and wake it up. I want to help the viewer discover something he wouldn't have discovered without me."[32] Once the ego eliminates the "Other," it loses the opponent it needs to outline its own existence. According to Bataille, the mutual opposition is the necessary condition of a negative rapport where two individuals realize their singularity while they break the privileges of the "same" by using the heterological power of disintegration or even alterity.

The Imaginary finds itself caught between the Real and the Symbolic orders. The chief difference with the former is that it is available to the symbolization provided by the latter. However, as soon as it is articulated in conscious symbols, it is exposed to the structuring imperative of the symbolic order and it ceases to exist.[33] The process of identification typical of the Imaginary is also related to the trauma of the mirror stage whereby the initial narcissism (the inability to differentiate between oneself and any external entity) is fractured. The result is a new capacity to perceive differences between self and other, inaugurating the complementary quest to return to a pre-Imaginary merger of self and other. In pursuit of this impossible goal, the individual develops fantasized identifications seeking reassurance by imaginatively neutralizing differences, identifying in the process with an imago or ideal ego. In short, the Imaginary is a realm of spurious but necessary identifications with entities in the world by which the individual ceaselessly attempts to shore up his own identity.

From what I have summarized above, it follows that the human subject is always split between a conscious side—the part of the psyche that is accessible—and an unconscious psyche—that is, a "continuous series" of instinctual drives and forces which remain inaccessible. The cost of human consciousness and knowledge is that instinctual drives remain unknown, i.e., that which is most basic to being human, is what is most alien. We are what we are, on the basis of something that we experience to be missing from us, our unconscious desires that can never be satisfied. We experience this "something missing" as a lack or hole that we desire to close, to fill in or replace with something. For Lacan, this lack is desire. Desire is what cannot be satisfied even when our demands are met, as our needs themselves are converted into desires that can never be satisfactorily fulfilled. Unconscious instinct manifests itself by the way it insists on filling a "gap" in the psyche, that has been left by the very thing the subject feels is lacking in him/her, that is the unconscious i.e., the unconscious attempts to fill in the gap of the unconscious. Therefore, the Lacanian subject is de-centered and marked by an essential split, essentially lacking and alienated. Possessed of a hole, an empty center Lacan called *beance*.

Another still life, *Mandoline et guitar*,[34] evokes the scenery of his Juan-les-Pins studio by incorporating shorthand signs for sea, sky, and stars into its background. Picasso here hints at live water animals using oval organic forms like the left guitar which undergoes a metamor-phosis as its extended neck turns into a fish's tail with the repositioned sound hole suggesting its gills.[35] We observe a tendency on the part of objects in general to become transformed into living organisms, softly molding themselves into each other to form a whole.[36] The entire composition, though, could also invite an anthropomorphic interpre-tation. It is possible, for instance, to see the table with its spilling burden of objects as a grotesque carnival mask staring lewdly back at the spectator, the sound-holes of the two instruments as eyes, the bottle as a nose, the space between the table-legs as a bared, toothy mouth. In an alternative reading, the covert sexuality of the painting may be brought to the fore by projecting on it the contours of an odalisque reclining invitingly on a tumbled bed—the guitar and bottle forming her body from head to buttocks, the mandolin her hips and legs.[37] Equally, one may read the composition as two female figures, one corresponding to the mandolin, the other to the guitar, linked by a third figure, the bottle. Under this interpretation, one can view the array of objects in erogenous terms. Cowling, for instance, likens the strings of the mandolin and guitar to "a woman's hairy genitals and/or her anus" and "the bottle as a man's genitals and its eye-like base as his anus." There is no doubt that Picasso's still lifes of this period were indeed sexual metaphors, although they did not yet abound in genitalia puns and other encoded references as they soon would.[38] Everything in this still life is intended to allure the viewer, to trigger his/her desire for the "Other," to move him/her to see himself/herself reflected in the hiding/unveiling carnival mask. The odalisque projects an appealing "Other" that entices the viewer, an effect that is further emphasized by the sexual confrontation of guitar and bottle, transformed into sexual organs.

The fluid and reversible metamorphosis that we see here at play could be read as a parable of Lacan's three orders. Like a perpetually thwarted dialectic, they define themselves in purely negative relationships to each other, yet never they come to a point of synthesis at which each is subsumed by the others to produce a clearly integrated whole. In this configuration, no two qualities or postulates can be coupled or contrasted without a mediating third. Everything that exists "ex-sists"—has its being in relation to that which lies outside it.[39] Each defines itself in a negative relation to the other two orders, generating its positive attributes primarily by excluding some aspect of one or both of the others. That is, each relies for its internal consistency on the constant and unwavering exclusion of the other two, producing a definitional logic of (b)orders and their impossible/inevitable transgressions. The interaction of the three orders produces the analyzable human subject even as their encroachment upon each other generates a variety of more or less serious disruptions in that same subject. Thus, the presence of an incommensurable "other" against which it can set itself is the fundamental condition for each of the orders to maintain not only its consistency but its very existence. Although each of the orders fights for its supremacy by attempting to annihilate the conditions of its own existence (i.e., the other two orders), the tensions, pressures, and cross-order "cuts" produced by this conflict must remain in order to constitute the subject.

Concerning the still life *Tête de bélier*,[40] it has been argued that the artist accentuated the apprehensiveness of the composition by endowing the ghostly octopus and the scorpion fish with menacing eyes, while rendering those of the ram closed, dead.[41] Meanwhile, the open mouths of the fish and the spiky sea urchin resemble a *vagina dentata*. Everything looks ready to bite, cut or sting. Gasman notes how teeth stand out as the most unfailingly aggressive in Picasso's pictorial symbolism. They are also connected with his pictorial imagery of ritual sacrifice, making this is the scene of an exorcism, a protection against a feminine "Other."[42]

In the still life *Buste et palette*,[43] the vibrancy of local color and sun-drenched atmosphere is intentionally misleading. Set in an intricately paneled interior that opens onto brilliant blue skies, it displays his accustomed repertoire of guitars, mandolins, bottles and fruit bowls laid on luxurious patterned cloths. However, mixed with these familiar objects we find once again a fierce Roman bust staring directly out of the picture and with a strong contrast of light and shadow across its features. A palette stands erectly on edge, as if snapped to attention as do the set of brushes to its left. Although their dark brown handles lie on the tablecloth and parallel its diagonal stripes, their thickly painted bristles seem more three-dimensional than the flat, black shadow cast across the sculpture they lean against. Rather than mere utensils for an artist to wield, these traditional attributes seem to be presented as defensive weapons against the threatening bust.[44] They are a way for him to confront the threat of the Real with his tools of the trade that serve to construct the Symbolic persona.

While I have so far focused on Picasso's still lifes, it is unquestionable that parables of confrontation with an "Other" is also visible in figure compositions. The artist often reified the characters he portrayed, so that, in their object-like presence, they served as the needed "Other" in which to project his own personality. The intense decomposition and recomposition of the embracing couple in Le baiser,[45] for instance, cause the two figures to spread over the entire canvas as they attempt an impossible fusion into a whole.[46] Viewers are forced to disentangle what they see.[47] The symbols combine, but are interchangeable by their very displacements: eye, mouth, sexual organs merge into each other. The flat shapes are dislocated and freely reassembled like parts of a puzzle, limbs and organs turned upside-down.[48] On the left, we can hardly identify the figure of the man, his target-like eye, and his phallus-shaped nose. The mouth, which can also be read as an eye or the female sex, is shared by both figures, welded together by a pattern of horizontal bars and interpenetrating organs. The woman's head, shown both in profile and from above, is thrown back. The man clasps her with one arm around her neck and with the other pins her arms behind. Her feet seem to be lifted off the ground, the toes spread in ecstasy or in an effort to resist. Rosenblum interprets this as a representation of the conflict between instinctive sexual urges and the fetters of marriage, a clash between Pablo and Olga.[49] As Cowling asserts, the embrace looks literally devouring, the figures to be violently struggling and grappling; the interlocking of arms and hands at the center of the composition suggests ferocious biting and mauling; the toes of the naked profile foot look like giant nails driving viciously into the flesh.[50]

If Picasso always had a deep intuition of how his psyche was outlined through an unresolvable opposition to an "Other," this came to the fore more strongly during the Spanish Civil War. "I have not painted the war because I am not the kind of painter who goes out like a photographer for something to depict," Picasso later stated. 'But I have no doubt that the war is in these paintings I have done. Later, perhaps the historians will find them and show that my style has changed under the war's influence. Myself, I do not know."[51] In the oil *Nature morte: poissons et poêle*,[52] the oysters and lemon introduced a hint of domesticity to the picture,[53] but even in the peaceful countryside of Le Tremblay-sur-Mauldre where he painted this canvas, his anxieties about the war in Spain took a conspicuous position and informed the goggle-eyed fish corpses strewn about in disarray in the composition. Although he brought the fish to life through his playful use of color, their jagged, blade-like forms add a deliberately disturbing angularity to the painting.[54] At that time, he was also embroiled in a bitter dispute with his wife, Olga Khokhlova. After finally separating from her, the artist established a home with his young lover, Marie-Thérèse Walter, and their recently born baby, Maya. This was not enough to assuage his conflictive nature, though, and soon after he started a third relationship with the enigmatic and intellectual Dora Maar. It is therefore to the artist's personal life that one must look in order to discover the rationale behind his chosen subject. "I paint the same way some people write their autobiography," Picasso once explained.[55] The combination of concern for his family in war-torn Spain and the multiple conflicts at home led to a period of psychological turmoil and introspection in the artist Not surprisingly, the oysters and lemon that on the surface add a hint of eroticism and romance to the picture, are counteracted by the goggle-eyed faces which speak of direct confrontation.

The fluidity of metamorphosis in Picasso is nowhere clearer than in his relationship with the photographer, Dora Maar. As Baldassari notes, her first distinctly recognizable incarnation in his oeuvre had been as a female Minotaur, a character the artist had often identified with himself. On his return to Paris in May 1936, Pablo had renewed contact with the beautiful photographer.[56] Staring at the sun, carrying death like a Medusa, Dora appears as half-animal, half-human—a monster of sorts who shares with the painter the power that attends upon all freaks of nature.[57] This occurred on June 3–4, as Picasso prepared an etching as an accompaniment to the collection of Éluard's *Les yeux fertiles*.[58] It consists of an illustration using Kodatrace paper of his poem, *Grand Air*. The poet wrote the text on the plate and the following day Picasso embellished it. We see Dora reflecting back rays of light from her open hand, battling with the sun that she succeeds in blinding and putting out.[59]

The situation in his home country was getting the best of him as he wrote *spleen du quart de Brie*. In ancient Greek and medieval humoral medicine, it was believed that the spleen was responsible for making "black bile," one of the four humors that needed to be kept in balance to stay healthy. If a spleen made too much black bile, it would make someone sad or depressed. On this day Kahnweiler wrote to Max Jacob: "Picasso is saddened, saddened, depressed. The events in Spain worry him."[60] In two poems he wrote the following day, *l'une anonyme à l'autre* and *les pensées suceuses de formes*, he referred to a certain mental and emotional distancing: "sucking thoughts of forms within sucking forms of thoughts strength without muscles mouth full of blood of forms sucked from thoughts."[61] His suffering was reflected in the woman's split head in *Portrait de Dora Maar*[62] from November 11. As Palau notes, "the forehead apparently truncated, implacably marks a dividing line between the two halves of the face, the left half being all but submerged in the shadows. Of the two hands, the right one is a paw with three prongs, hard, schematic, while the other, the left, is painted with a fluid technique, apparently imprecise, as is the set of brushstrokes that form the background. Those hands, which had performed a kind of striptease to emphasize their nudity and had been one of the initial reasons for the painter's attraction to Dora, were now being mocked or at least distorted."[63] His fears would be equally projected through her in the drawing *Dora Maar à la coiffe*[64] from two days later. As the critic commented, "we again see her, face on . . . with her eyes a little scared, seemingly looking inward on herself, her eyes betraying a hint of fright on account of what was happening to her."[65] Since their first meeting, Picasso had been enchanted by her perceptiveness, and she came to be the mirror of the emotional and intellectual anxieties awakened in him by the war.

On January 17, 1937, thousands of Nationalist troops, assisted by Italian and Moorish soldiers had begun their assault on the Republican-held city of Málaga. As the siege was going on, he painted the oil *Portrait de la marquise de cul chrétien*,[66] an irrevocable indictment of the Nationalists and a defiant show of support for the Republicans. Against a garish yellow background, the main protagonist of this powerful painting is a strange, hybrid figure pictured craning out of a balcony, her outstretched, raised arm immediately reminiscent of the fascist salute. Adorned with an aristocratic and ostentatious feather-plumed hat decorated with what appear to be crosses, and brandishing, in her claw-like hand, a Spanish flag, the identity of this frenzied, fearsome woman becomes clear from the words emblazoned on the upper left of the composition. In stark black lettering, Picasso wrote: "*Retrato de la marquesa de culo cristiano*

echándoles un duro a los soldados moros defensores de la virgen."
With this inscription, he was directly indicting the supporters of
Franco's army: monarchists, Carlists and the wealthy, conservative
classes as well as the clergy.[67] If up until this point, his art had been
essentially autobiographical, deeply subjective and based entirely on
his own vision of the world, from now on his work became a symbol
of resistance against the forces of oppression that swept across
Europe.[68]

If his reaction to the attack on Málaga had initially been garbed in
allegory, just a few days later he projected his feelings of anger and
confusion on Dora herself in *Poupée et femme se noyant.*[69] The scene
depicted is unreal. The figure is immobilized like a mannequin on an
upright, tripod prong aimed menacingly at her sex, while she tongue-
kisses a black-masked, putrid sun (Bataille's *soleil pourri*).[70] Her dress
is fashionably decorated, her feet are in high-heeled laced shoes, and
she wears a chain of flowers or large pieces of jewelry around her neck.
But her feet hang down passively, while she holds a triangular banner
displaying two raised arms. Rays emanate from the dark sun,
spreading over the landscape like a rain of fire. In the sea, one can see
the head and pleading arms of a drowning man calling for help in vain.
This explains the banner sign which might be warning of potential
danger. The doll-like figure, therefore, is aware of the disaster that
occurs in her immediate vicinity. However, standing at the edge of the
water and sentenced to immobility (her feet do not reach the ground),
she is unable to help the poor man.[71] This reflects Picasso's own frustration at reading about the massacre in his hometown, unable to do
anything. He described her state of mind again in *Portrait de Dora
Maar pensive.*[72] As Mary Ann Caws states, "On [her] singularly
expressive face Picasso could read every international event as in a
newspaper."[73]

On May 24, 1937, Picasso executed the first of a series of weeping
women in *La femme qui pleure (Étude)* that often display the features
of Dora Maar.[74] As Arnheim notes, "the streaming tears have been
solidified into expressive objects. They supply the immobile head with
the tracks of downward movement, appropriate to the subject. They
also lacerate the skin with shocking grooves."[75] Her flared, nostrils
recall those of an animal. Indeed, her nose and mouth resemble the
snout and the open beak of the two devils on the far right of the
Isenheim Altarpiece, and her stare brings to mind the demonic glinting
eyes which hypnotize the spectator. So, although she is terrorized like
the wretched saint, in her panic she has become as monstrous as the
devils that assailed him.[76] With her tear-shaped eyes, the weeping
woman became an emblem of the sufferings inflicted on Picasso's

compatriots, and by extension on him.[77] She would become the icon of his dark output, which Dagen has described as a "cycle of metamorphosis of mourning."[78]

If the *Guernica*[79] mural had taken up the challenge as a "a monument to disillusionment, despair, destruction," to quote Breton's words in 1939, these female victims, described by Barr as "postscripts," followed it as "the artist's lament."[80] Often interpreted as a cruel distortion of Dora's personality, they also reflect Pablo's own inner anguish: "[He] believes that art is the daughter of sadness and pain," Sabartés had written. "He believes that sadness forces meditation and that pain is the essence of life."[81] By concentrating on the head and generalizing it, he focused on grief as an absolute. His principal instruments to represent it was extreme facial distortion, underpinned by brutal contrasts of tone and color. His favorite metaphors included the furrowed brow; pupils and eyelashes drawn as a crown of thorns; eyes and noses as tear-drops; running tears as needles or nails; eyelids as capsizing boats spilling out tears; ears as wing-nuts; noses as animal snouts; teeth as fangs; tongues as daggers, etc.[82] Poetic texts from this period document a similarly pathological-depressive worldview that accepts no positive perspective, neither in the private sphere nor with regard to the expected historical developments.[83] Many items in poem *chair en décomposition* refer to Christian sacrifice, such as "the crown of thorns nest of twigs at the sound of the tambourine awakened by the miserable memory."[84] The victim could be himself or Dora. Because of her intense artistic sensibility, her poetic gifts and her ability to participate in suffering, she was especially qualified to resonate his own inner torments. The twining that started to take place here between them reveals the empathetic and projective nature of their relationship.[85] As she said later on: "All [Picasso's] portraits of me are lies. They are all Picassos. Not one is Dora."[86]

A few years later, during the German Occupation of Paris starting in 1940, Picasso found a new enemy in places far beyond his personal situation. He found it in the strange paintings, frightening and burlesque, such as *Nature morte aux poissons*[87], and probably *L'araignée de mer*[88], both teeming with fish and disturbing crustaceans. In the former, the claws of the crab balance the shape of the scales. It might represent Picasso himself, weighing up the qualities of his two very different mistresses, Marie-Thérèse (the rounded fish in the center) and Dora (the aggressive, sharp-faced fish).[89] The crab with its wistful eyes and active claws is curiously appealing and the green eels with blue shadows self-absorbed, but the two fish are clearly predatory. The pointed fish is ready to cut off the crab's claw, while the white rascasse with its frightening bracelet of teeth keeps the others at bay. This sense of conflict and confrontation is heightened by the sharp edges in the painting such as the chain of the scale or the teeth of the fish. All these animals are trapped in an adversarial purgatory, that liminal place between life and death, the go and the Real.[90] The compositions of eels of fish and soles express in a mode, again metaphorically and symbolically, the cruelty of the war, but more deeply evoke simply Picasso's quasi-dialectal view of human identity.[91]

During this time of curfews and blackouts, the apartment became an extension of the self. The Parisian apartment figures prominently in many recollections of the Occupation. It was more than a place of expected physical comfort, it was also a shelter from confusion and uncertainty. Watching and seeing what was going on from the relative security of apartments could alleviate the ever-present sense of claustrophobia that characterized daily life during the Occupation.[92] The poem *La fenêtre* from May 1 contained multiple references to seclusion:

> the window scratches the mantilla its screams chalked on the slate
> . . . the hand of the door leaning on the arm of the armchair held up
> by the pearls of the curtains . . . the frying-pan where the potatoes are
> jumping butterfly wings frying souls in the blood of grilled blood-
> sausage . . . a bucket full of black olives a bucket full of green olives
> two liters of oil . . . at the bottom of a saucepan some leftover apple-
> and-orange-sauce a bunch of radishes four knives . . . a big clay pot
> full of melted butter—fresh butter in a plate a few potatoes under the
> sink and a few leeks and onions.[93]

Malnourishment, unpredictable regulations, conflicting rumors and false news reports, the absence of more than a million men locked away in German stalags, suspicion of neighbors—all combined unhealthily and the Parisians responded by shutting themselves down, physically and mentally.[94] The outside would become an "Other" that one had to confront to keep one's footing.

Probably to get his mind off things in such horrible circumstances, Picasso concentrated on certain artistic problems which may be traced back to the cubist years as in *Nature morte au boudin*[95] from May 10, 1941. A dull light shines from a funnel-shaped ceiling lamp onto the table surface on which a large dagger-like knife lies in front of a rolled-up blood sausage. They are joined by two artichoke stems, a corked bottle of wine and an open wrapping paper with a piece of cheese behind it. He opted for a monochrome statement in different shades of gray with certain lightening due to a dirty white on a partially translucent brownish background. From the open table drawer, a set of knives and forks protrudes as if wanting to free themselves.[96] The tilted-up perspective brings objects in the background closer to the picture plane and to the viewer, but also threatens to spill all the objects out of the picture. There is an underlying menace in the apparently innocent, even hospitable, presentation of food and cutlery on the table. In a rare comment on his own work, he said that this painting has "an atmosphere like Philip II, dark and dismal . . . The knives and forks are like souls out of purgatory." The poem *chasuble de sang* from three days later included allusions to the same animism of things we observe in the painting:[97]

> chasuble of blood thrown over the naked shoulders of the green wheat shivering between the wet sheets . . . the wall painted in ochre flapping its big apple-green mauve-white wings tearing its beak against the panes . . . the uncombed hair of the landscape spread out under the sun . . . the hanging tongue of the plough stuck to plowing sweating.[98]

It is appropriate that Picasso should have used the word *purgatory* to describe some aspects of the painting, because most of his works from the wartime years suggest that he found the Occupation exactly that—a life that was put on hold, without change, and without hope. The allusion to the sixteenth-century king might be explained as a reference to a reign coinciding with the Counter-Reformation, a period of cruel repression. He may have been thinking of the Parisians, destined to suffer in occupied Paris.[99] The German grip on the city affected many aspects of French culture, but nothing was hit harder than its cuisine. Food was an essential part of national identity. Adapting to a less plentiful and lower quality fare proved difficult. A correspondent for the magazine *Le Gerbe* wrote: "Eating and, more important, eating well is the theme song of Paris life. In the street, in the metro, in cafes, all you hear about is food. At the theater or movies, when there's an old play or movie with a huge banquet scene, the audience breaks into delirious cries of joy." By taking away their cuisine, the German occupier was robbing the French of their persona. Despite their difficulties, people courageously dealt with their circumstances, nicknaming their system of improvisation *le système D*, from the verb *se débrouiller* (alternatively *se démerder*), which could be translated as "muddling something up" or "making confusing." This brings to mind Bataille's concept of the limit.

Bataille's philosophy of transgression implies the preservation of the limits of the subject so that the "sovereign" can experience and endure death in life. The fluctuant, reversible movement forwards towards the flame of self-dissolution and its retreat backwards, towards life and the limits it involves, epitomizes Bataille's notion of existence. His conception of being remains "suspended" in an unstable, fragmentary, undetermined, reversible position between these two ontological alternatives. The character of the Minotaur, who would become essential to Picasso's personal mythology as a fragmented self, could be seen as typifying the figure of this fluctuant subject. It is perhaps for this reason that Bataille, along with André Masson, came up in 1933 with the idea of naming Albert Skira's new journal, *Minotaure*, after the Classical monster. The publication was intended to affect a rapprochement between Bataille and Breton, had been illustrated with a portrait of a Minotaur by Picasso.[100]

"Sovereign" existence is an experience of freedom. Not only does it express the strain between a free existence and imposed hierarchy, but it also articulates the tension between a disordered experience and an ordered concept. Bataille was fascinated with the way in which violence breaks down the integrity of the body or of things, and in the way it challenges limits. Inner experience comes from an awareness of the impossible (the impossible being both that which one experiences and that which constitutes that experience). It is an experience which is rich beyond comprehension, beyond being captured within the concept of experience. It transports one to an elusive beyond where all forms of external authority are dissolved. It is a finite experience that promises nothing outside itself. The result of this experience which explores itself to its limits is a contestation of those limits, of the language, of the subject, and whatever limits try to constrain this experience.

Contrary to Lacan, Bataille does not want to maintain a separation between the Imaginary and the Symbolic; he wants merely to nourish the tension between their boundaries. Bataille's theory of communication deconstructs, or at least displaces, the paradigm of identity. Since communication happens on a shared line of flaw, of wound where two individuals escape their "homogeneity," flow into each other, Bataille's anthropology of communication partakes not only of a subversion of the Law in breaking privileges of identity but also implicitly poses a definition of individuals escaping their identity. Here the debate focuses on the "identitary" status of the "loss" of singularities, of identities. Does it represent an absence of differences? Probably, but in a manner where the paradigm of difference merges singularities by substituting itself for the paradigm of identity. As Dragon explains, difference, within Bataille's anthropology of communication, is not to be found in the open structure of individuals during their attempt to interrelate but in an inner jump through the wound to reach the void.[101]

The same day he had written the poem, *chasuble de sang*, he made the gouache *Tête de femme au chapeau*[102] where the complex face gains in expressiveness through the artist's manipulations.[103] For him, everything feminine was both an object of desire and a fearful adversary. Following his private iconography of evil, he chose monstrously alienated female characters, the embodiment of mischief and calamitous powers. Woman became an incarnation of the "Other."[104] Bataille's conception of the subject walks a thin line between self-dissolution and self-preservation. Unlike Nietzsche, he does not posit "an excess of being" at the basis of human life, but rather a "principle of insufficiency." No element is ever complete or sufficient, and because of this insufficiency, every being is in an open relation to an "Other." The most powerful example of the principle of insufficiency is precisely language, which imposes itself on the speakers and puts them in a necessary relation to the "Other." This relation can never be fully mastered or controlled, thus destroying any hope that the subject can exist as a self-sufficient individual. Moreover, the relation between beings has no more sufficiency than the beings themselves, being defined by endless multiple oppositions. Yet paradoxically it is because of the instability of these relations that the subject can feel the illusion of being autonomous.

Picasso, like Bataille, recognizes himself only through an "Other" who maintains him as a stranger to himself. His practice of representation is to arrange objects and people in conjunction with a heterogeneous resonance and, by doing so, to introduce an outside, a radical alterity into the game. His interaction with the "Other" produces his own self even as its encroachment generates a variety of more or less serious disruptions in that same self. In short, the presence of an incommensurable "Other" against which to set himself is the fundamental condition of Picasso's very existence—and everyone else's, according to Bataille and Lacan. The intelligent Dora Maar saw right through the painter's many depictions of her. She pointed out to James Lord in 1940: "All [his] portraits of me are lies. They are all Picassos. Not one is Dora."[105]

Notes

1   Quoted in Zervos 1935, 176.
2   Daix 1965, 91–94.
3   Quoted in Gilot and Lake 1964, 74.
4   *Nature morte aux vases (Le porron).* Gósol, End-May–15-August/1906.

Oil on canvas. 38,5 x 56 cm. The State Hermitage Museum, Saint Petersburg. OPP.06:036.

5   *Nature morte au tableau.* Gósol, 22-June–15-August/1906. Oil on canvas. 82 x 100,4 cm. Gregory Callimanopulos Collection, NY. (Inv P350). OPP.06:094.

6   Richardson 1991, 441.

7   Christie's. #50, 1722, 11/08/06.

8   *Nature morte aux vases.* Gósol, Summer/1906. Gouache & watercolor on paper. 32,5 x 37,5 cm. Private collection, Europe. OPP.06:116.

9   Boggs 1992, 48.

10 *Les demoiselles d'Avignon.* Paris, June~July/1907. Oil on canvas. 243,9 x 233,7 cm. The Museum of Modern Art, NYC. (Inv 333.1939). OPP.07:001.

11 Sotheby's. #31, L17002, 03/01/17.

12 Rosenblum 1997, 263.

13 *Nature morte à la tête de mort.* Paris, Summer~Fall/1907. Oil on canvas. 116,3 x 89 cm. The State Hermitage Museum, Saint Petersburg. (Inv 9162). OPP.07:008.

14 Reff 1980, 5–33.

15 Boggs 1992, 54–55.

16 Bowie 1991; Evans 1996; Felluga 2002; Klages 2007.

17 Noys 2000, 16.

18 Lawtoo 2005, 4.

19 Ross 2002.

20 Bowie 1991, 91.

21 Ross 2002.

22 Pound 2008, 10.

23 Evans 1996, 82–83.

24 Bowie 1991, 91, 194; Pound 2008, 10.

25 *Atelier avec tête et bras de plâtre.* Juan-les-Pins. Late-June/1925. Oil on canvas. 97,9 x 131,1 cm. The Museum of Modern Art, New York. (Inv 116.1964). OPP.25:002.

26 Palau i Fabre 1999, 448–449.

27 Rubin 1972, 120–122.

28 Richardson 2007, 285.

29 Cited in Gasman 1981, 768, n. 3.

30 Gasman 1981, 768.

31 Boggs 1992, 218.

32 Gilot 1964, 60.

33 Evans 1996, 82–83.

34 *Mandoline et guitare.* Juan-les-Pins, End-July/1924. Oil & sand on canvas. 140,7 x 200,3 cm. The Solomon R. Guggenheim Museum, NYC. (Inv 53.1358). OPP.24:006.

35 Richardson 2007, 268.

36 Palau i Fabre 1999, 428.

37 Cowling 2002, 460–469.

38 Richardson 2007, 268–269.
39 Bowie 1991, 194.
40 *Tête de bélier.* Juan-les-Pins, Summer/1925. Oil on canvas. 80 x 99,1 cm. The Norton Simon Museum, Pasadena, CA. (Inv P.1978.6). OPP.25:024.
41 Cowling 2002, 460–469.
42 Richardson 2007, 294.
43 *Buste et palette.* Paris–Monte Carlo–Juan-les-Pins. Spring–Summer/1925. Oil on canvas. 54 x 65,5 cm. Museo Nacional Centro de Arte Reina Sofia, Madrid. (Inv AS.06524). OPP.25:023.
44 FitzGerald 2001, 116–117.
45 *Le baiser.* Juan-les-Pins. [Late-June]/1925. Oil on canvas. 130,5 x 97,7 cm. Musée Picasso, Paris. OPP.25:003
46 Palau i Fabre 1999, 447.
47 Warncke & Walther 1991, 365–367.
48 Daix 1993, 190–194.
49 Bernadac 1991, 80–83.
50 Cowling 2002, 469–482.
51 Picasso cited in A. Nash (ed.), Picasso and the War Years 1937–1945, New York, 1998, 13.
52 *Nature morte: poissons et poêle.* Le Tremblay-sur-Mauldre, 8-December/1936. Oil on canvas. 50 x 61 cm. Christie's. #44, 7599, 06/24/08. OPP.36:216.
53 Christie's 2015, cat. no. 17, 10378; Christie's 2010, cat. no. 32, 7831.
54 Christie's 2008, cat. no. 44, 7599.
55 Picasso, quoted in Richardson 1988, 17–48.
56 Cabanne 1979, 288.
57 Baldassari 2006, 116–117.
58 Christie's 119, 7712, 04/08/09.
59 Baldassari 2005, 245; Baldassari 2006, 115, 309.
60 Palau 2011, 301.
61 Rothenberg & Joris 2004, 125.
62 *Portrait de Dora Maar.* Paris. 11-November/1936. Oil on canvas. 66 x 53,3 cm. Sotheby's. #85, 11/08/95. OPP.36:188.
63 Palau 2011, 266.
64 *Dora Maar à la coiffe.* Paris. 13-November/1936. Brush & ink, wash & pencil on paper. 40,5 x 31,5 cm. Sotheby's. #35, L14002, 02/05/14. OPP.36:189.
65 Palau 2011. 270.
66 *Portrait de la marquise de cul chrétien.* Paris. 19-January/1937. Oil on canvas. 38 x 46 cm. Joe Lewis Collection. OPP.37:227.
67 Goggin 1997, xiii.; Christie's 2017, cat. no. 56A, 15004.
68 Christie's 2017, cat. no. 56A, 15004.
69 *Poupée et femme se noyant.* Paris. 28-January/1937. Pencil on paper. 40,2 x 31,5 cm. Galería Guillermo de Osma, Madrid. OPP.37:224.
70 Nash 1998, 16.

71 Ullmann 1993, 73.
72 *Portrait de Dora Maar pensive.* Paris. 28-January/1937. Pencil & stump on paper. 31 x 40,2 cm. OPP.37:061.
73 Caws 2000, 103.
74 La femme qui pleure (Étude). Paris. 24-May/1937. Pencil, lead pencil & gouache on paper. 29,2 x 23,2 cm. Museo Nacional Centro de Arte Reina Sofia, Madrid. OPP.37:099.
75 Arnheim 1962, 86.
76 Cowling 2002, 589–603.
77 Nash 1998, 18.
78 La Vaccara 2014, 6.
79 *Guernica.* Paris. 11-May–4-June/1937. Oil on canvas. 349,3 x 776,6 cm. Museo Nacional Centro de Arte Reina Sofia, Madrid. (Inv DE00050). OPP.37:001.
80 Tosatto, et al. 2019, 64.
81 Baring 2017, 196.
82 Cowling 2002, 589–603.
83 Ullmann 1993, 63.
84 Rothenberg & Joris 2004, 121–122.
85 Baldassari 2006, 163–165.
86 Baring 2017, 35.
87 *Nature morte aux poissons.* Paris. 19-March/1940. Oil on canvas. 60 x 92 cm. Scottish National Gallery of Modern Art, Edinburgh. (Inv GMA.1070). OPP.40 ; 478.
88 L'araignée de mer. Paris. 19-March/1940. Oil on canvas. 65 x 92 cm. Private collection, Madrid. OPP.40; 496.
89 Buchholz & Zimmerman 2000, 70–71.
90 Boggs 1992, 266.
91 Tosatto, et al. 2019, 123.
92 Rosbottom 2014, 168–172.
93 Rothenberg & Joris 2004, 244–246.
94 Rosbottom 2014, 164.
95 *Nature morte au boudin.* Paris, 10-May/1941. Oil on canvas. 92,7 x 66 cm. Tony and Gail Ganz Collection. Formerly Victor W. Ganz Collection, NY. OPP.41:002.
96 Ullmann 1993, 258.
97 Spies 2011, 233.
98 Rothenberg & Joris 2004, 248.
99 Goggin 1985, 86–89; Boggs 1992, 268.
100 Baldassari 2005, 241.
101 Dragon 1996, 33.
102 *Tête de femme au chapeau.* Paris. 13-May/1941. Gouache on wood. 60 x 40 cm. Fundación Almine & Bernard Ruiz-Picasso para el Arte. OPP.41:067.
103 Goggin 1985, 90–91.
104 Ullmann 1993, 218–219.
105 Baring 2017, 35.

References

Arnheim, Rudolf. *The Genesis of a Painting, Picasso's Guernica.* Los Angeles: University of California Press, 1962.

Baldassari, Anne, ed. *The Surrealist Picasso.* New York: Random House, 2005.

——. *Picasso—Life with Dora Maar: Love and War 1935–1945.* Paris: Flammarion, 2006.

Baring, Louise. *Dora Maar. Paris in the Time of Man Ray, Jean Cocteau and Picasso.* New York: Rizzoli, 2017.

Barr, Alfred H, Jr. *Picasso: Fifty Years of His Art.* New York: Simon & Schuster, 1946.

Bernadac, Marie-Laure. *Picasso Museum Paris: The Masterpieces.* Paris: Prestel, 1991.

Boggs, J. S., et al. *Picasso and Things.* Cleveland: Cleveland Museum of Art, 1992.

Bowie, Malcolm. *Lacan.* Cambridge, MA: Harvard University Press, 1991.

Breton, André. "Océanic." (1948), reprinted in Breton, *La Cité des champs,* Paris: Sagittaire, 1953.

Buchholz, Elke Linda & Beate Zimmermann. *Pablo Picasso: Life and Work* (Art in Focus). Konemann, 2000.

Cabanne, Pierre. *Pablo Picasso: His Life and Times.* New York: William Morrow & Co; Morrow Quill Paperbacks, 1979.

Caws, Mary Ann. *Picasso's Weeping Woman: The Life and Art of Dora Maar.* New York: Bulfinch Press, 2000.

Christie's. *Impressionist & Modern (Evening Sale).* Auction catalogue 1722, November 8. New York, 2006.

——. *Impressionist & Modern Art (Evening Sale).* Auction catalogue 7599, June 24. London, 2008.

——. *Old Master, Modern & Contemporary Prints.* Auction catalogue 7712, April 8. London, 2009.

——. *Impressionist/Modern Evening Sale.* Auction catalogue 7831, February 2. London, 2010.

——. *Impressionist/Modern Evening Sale.* Auction catalogue 10378, February 4. London, 2015.

——. *Impressionist & Modern Art Day Sale.* Auction catalogue 15004, November 13. London, 2017.

Cowling, Elizabeth. *Picasso: Style and Meaning.* London; New York: Phaidon. 2002.

Daix, Pierre. *Picasso.* New York: Praeger, 1965.

Daix, Pierre. *Picasso: Life & Art.* New York: Icon Editions & New York: Harper-Collins, 1993.

Dean, Carolyn J. *The Self and Its Pleasures: Bataille, Lacan and the History of the Decentered Subject.* Ithaca: Cornell University Press, 1992.

Dragon, Jean. "The Work of Alterity: Bataille and Lacan." *Diacritics,* Summer, Vol. 26, No. 2, 1996.

Evans, Dylan. *An Introductory Dictionary of Lacanian Psychoanalysis*. New York: Routledge, 1996.

Felluga, Dino Franco. "Modules on Lacan." 2002. https://www.cla.purdue.edu/english/theory/ psychoanalysis / lacanstructure.html.

Fink, Bruce. *The Lacanian Subject: Between Language and Jouissance*. Princeton, NJ: Princeton University Press, 1995.

FitzGerald, Michael C. *Picasso: The Artist's Studio*. New Haven: Yale University Press, 2001.

Gasman, Lydia. *Mystery, Magic & Love in Picasso, 1925–1938: Picasso & the Surrealist Poets*. Ann Arbor, Michigan: University Microfilms International, 1981.

Gilot, Françoise. and Carlton Lake. *Life with Picasso*. New York: McGraw-Hill, 1964.

Goggin, Mary Margaret. *Picasso and his Art during the German Occupation: 1940-1944*. Ph.D. Dissertation. Stanford University. Ann Arbor, Michigan: University Microfilms International, 1985.

Klages, Mary. "Jacques Lacan." 1997. http://www.Colorado.EDU/English/ENGL2012Klages/ 1997lacan.html.

La Vaccara, Ornella. "Dora Maar (1907–1997)." *Séminaire d'Histoire de l'art du XXe siècle. Les femmes artistes et collectionneuses dans la première moitié du XXe siècle*. 2014, 1–8.

Lawtoo, Nidesh. "Bataille and the Suspension of Being." *Lingua Romana*. Vol. 4 Issue 1 Fall, 2005.

Lechte, John. "Surrealism and the practice of writing, or The 'case' of Bataille." *Bataille: Writing the sacred*. Carolyn Bailey Gill, ed. London: Routledge, 1995, 117–132.

Mallén, Enrique, ed. *Online Picasso Project (OPP)*. Sam Houston State University, 2020.

Nash, Steven A., ed. *Picasso and the War Years: 1937–1945*. New York: Thames & Hudson, 1998.

Noys, Benjamin. *Georges Bataille: A Critical Introduction*. London: Pluto Press, 2000.

O'Brian, Patrick. *Pablo Picasso. A Biography*. New York: W.W. Norton & Company, 1994.

Palau i Fabre, Josep. *Picasso: Del Minotaur al Guernika (1927–1939)*. Barcelona: Ediciones Polígrafa, 2011.

Penrose, Roland. *The Eye of Picasso*. New York: New American Library, 1967.

Phillips, John. "Lacan and Language." 1999. https://courses.nus.edu.sg/course/elljwp/lacan.htm.

Pound, Marcus. *Žižek: A (Very) Critical Introduction*. Cambridge: Wm. B. Eerdmans, 2008.

Reff, Theodore. "Themes of Love and Death in Picasso's Early Work." In *Picasso in Retrospect*. Roland Penrose & John Golding, eds. New York: Harper & Row, Icon Editions, 1980, 5–33.

Richardson, John. "L'Epoque Jacqueline". In Michel Leiris, ed. *Late Picasso Paintings, Drawings, Sculpture and Prints, 1953–1972*. London: The Tate Gallery, 1988, 41–2.

Richardson, John. *A Life of Picasso, vol 1: 1881–1906*. New York: Random House, 1991.

——. *A Life of Picasso, vol 3: 1917–1932*. New York: Alfred A. Knopf, 2007.

Rosenblum, R. "Picasso at Gósol: The Calm before the Storm." *Picasso: The Early Years, 1892–1906*. Marilyn McCully, ed. New Haven, CT: Yale University Press, 1997, 261–276.

Rosbottom, Ronald C. *When Paris Went Dark: The City of Light Under German Occupation, 1940–1944*. New York: Back Bay Books, 2014.

Ross, Stephen. "A Very Brief Introduction to Lacan." Canada: University of Victoria, 2002.

Rothenberg, Jerome & Pierre Joris, eds. *The Burial of the Count of Orgaz & Other Poems*. Cambridge, MA: Exact Change, 2004.

Rubin, William S., Elaine L. Johnson & Riva Castleman. *Picasso in the Collection of the Museum of Modern Art*. New York: Museum of Modern Art, 1972.

Sotheby's. *Impressionist & Modern Art Evening Sale*. Auction catalogue L17002, March 1. London, 2017.

Spies, Werner. *The Continent Named Picasso. Werner Spies: The Eye and the Word—Collected Writings on Art and Literature, The Gagosian Edition*. Vol. 5. Ed. by Thomas W. Gaehtgens. New York: Abrams, 2011.

Tosatto, Guy, et al., eds. *Au coeur des ténèbres 1939–1945*. Grenoble: In Fine editions d'art, 2019.

Ullmann, Ludwig. *Picasso und der Krieg*. Bonn: Karl Kerber Verlag, 1993.

Warncke, Carsten-Peter & Ingo F. Walther. *Pablo Picasso 1881–1973*. New York: Taschen America Ltd., 1991.

Zervos, Christian. "Conversation avec Picasso," *Cahiers d'Art*, Paris, 1935, 176.

14

Sustenance for the Soul & Spirit: Frida & Fruit

Debra D. Andrist

Renowned for her iconic self-portraits with unibrow and indigenous costuming, referencing her physical & psychological tragedies and suffering, the Mexican artist, Frida Kahlo, was best-known as the wife (twice) of the Mexican muralist, Diego Rivera, during her lifetime and until decades after her 1954 death. Now better-known as something of a commercial cult figure whose image appears on everything imaginable, from clothing to dishware and beyond, Frida's unique talent and production was only professionally acknowledged in the art world a few years before her image and work were co-opted through public popularity.

Two 2021 artistic iterations of *Fridamania*,[1] far more professional & insightful than the now-common, strictly commercial, exploitation of Frida's image, focused on her still-lifes with fruit, thus directly relating to the theme of the collection of articles in *Sustenance for the Body & Soul: Food & Drink in Amerindian, Spanish & Latin American Worlds*. This is not to say that any suggestion of physical consumption of fruit plays into Frida's work; fruit as subject matter represents figurative sustenance for the soul and spirit. Somehow, the timing of the opening of the end-of-life-works-focus of both exhibitions, concurrent with the continuing horror of the suffering and death associated with the COVID-19 pandemic, given the overlay of illness and suffering that surrounded Frida's life, was even more appropriate, though unintended per se. However, the tie-in to the end-stage of her life, at first consideration, is not so obvious either. One of these two exhibitions, *Frida Kahlo: Five Works*, opened March 7, 2021 at the Dallas Museum of Art, along with the just-over a-year-long very real manifestations of the worldwide pandemic. Curator, Mark A. Castro, in Dallas, chose the five of Frida's works shown from lesser known [of Kahlo's] paintings she made later in life when her health was deteriorating and her art changed. Still-lifes were something she touched on throughout her career. . . But in those last few years she returned to them in greater number. Her themes remain: luscious fruits, love of Mexico, animals, Diego. But there are fewer radiant or tormented self-portraits. She told friends still-lifes sold well and were easier to do [since at this point, she was mostly bedridden].[2]

Biographer Frank Milner agrees. He posits that not only the documented marketability of Frida's still-lifes, possibly due to their smaller size and "less-complicated [required technique as well as] her wishes to gain more financial independence from Rivera" (72) may have persuaded her to focus more on this genre at this point in her life. Or, according to Hayden Herrera, author of one of the first comprehensive biographies of Kahlo in the English-speaking world, she was "in a hurry" to paint and sell works due to concern about being able to monetarily aid a then financially struggling Rivera (399).

Whatever Frida's possible external motivation for turning to still-lifes, Castro lets us know the oblique, overall, direct link to Frida's stage in life that motivated his choices for the exhibit. Her

later works are a kind of self-portrait, and Dallas conservation lab X-rays and infrared photography discovered for the first time how she worked. [For example] *Still-Life with Parrot and Flag* showed her changing the position of the bird's wing, and open fruit she'd initially painted intact. 'There was a process of refinement that she was going through,' Castro says. She moved from personal expression to 'focusing on how to make them work on a visual level.' Helpful information, as scholars go beyond Kahlo's life and hard times, to study her as a painter and intellectual . . . Castro felt this was the perfect time to exhibit [these works featuring fruit]. 'In this difficult period, people feel a strong connection to Kahlo's sorrows and triumphs.' Art helps us get through bad times, as making art did for Kahlo. 'Painting completed my life' she said.[3]

This quote from Frida is telling in more ways than one, since painting very many of the so-called "fruit" works literally did constitute and complete her work of the end of her life. An appropriate aside, too important to relegate to a footnote, is that the term in Spanish for still-life is *naturaleza muerta*/dead nature. Herrera calls attention to Frida's awareness of the irony in this term, as in 1952, she painted a work titled *Naturaleza viva/Live Nature* featuring "fruits and the way they are painted restless, even the title, written across the bottom of this painting, pulsates with life: the words are formed out of creeping tendrils" (398). Furthermore, both a formal explanation of symbolism in art, that it represents the visual equivalent of written allegory, reiterates what both curators and numerous art-critic sources featured in this essay claim.

> Allegory is often utilized as an extended metaphor of the ephemeral condition of life. The fruit, like human life, is intended to portray the transient nature related to our existence. Fresh fruit, represents fertility, vitality, youth, and abundance. When the fruit is in a state of decay, however, it characterizes the inevitable and undeniable mortality of our presence in the world.[4]

Castro continues relating the circumstances of this stage in Frida's life and artistic production,

> In Frida's last days while she was in her 50s, she painted lots of still-lifes. She was in such a horrible pain during this time that she was unable to go out of the house, and sometimes, even out of her bed. She usually uses the fruits from her garden and local market as the subjects of her still-life paintings. She would arrange the fruits on the table by her bedside and started painting. [As a long-time political activist] She also liked to add political meanings to her still-life paintings by adding flags, inscriptions or a peace dove to deliver some messages.[5]

Adriana Zavala, associate professor of art history and race, colonialism, and diaspora at Tufts University, [who] curated a 2015 exhibit at the New York Botanical Garden, which inspired the 2021 exhibit in San Antonio, Texas, featured later in this essay, concurs:

> An avid reader of philosophy, Kahlo knew that Mesoamerican people 'tended to believe in both the attraction of opposites and the interdependence of opposites: the sun and the moon, life and death, the underworld and the heavens.' While Kahlo's health continued to decline, she kept creating beautiful, vibrant works of art—an array of still-lifes of provocatively arranged tropical fruits. In *Still-Life with Parrot and Flag* [for example], a halved sapote is the focal point surrounded by mangos, guavas, prickly pears, an open cantaloupe, a ripe cherimoya full of seeds, and one banana. She was likely thinking about both the beauty and the fleeting nature of existence. 'I think that surrounding herself with the natural world was both because she

had an acute sense of her own mortality,' Zavala says, 'but it was also a way of understanding that that's the cycle of life.'[6]

Frida painted at least seventeen fruit-content-dominant still-lifes,[7] identified in order of appearance on the official website dedicated to her. The titles sometimes include specific fruits and the site usually features textual insights/history of the particular work. The fruits[8] that dominate Frida's paintings most frequently, not necessarily in numerical order of appearance, are watermelon, coconut, pitahaya, tuna (cactus), also known as prickly pear, banana, orange, papaya and cherimoya.

The fruit focus may depend on simply which fruits were most available to Frida from her aforementioned garden and/or a local market, due to what readily grows in or near the *Colonia del Carmen* neighborhood of *Coyacán* in Mexico City where her *Casa Azul* is located. Said garden is the theme of the other 2021 exhibit highlighted in this essay:

> The San Antonio Botanical Garden's exhibit, "Frida Kahlo Oasis," [which] features painstakingly re-created replicas of the iconic blue walls of *Casa Azul*, as well as of Kahlo's desk and easel . . . At the center of Frida Kahlo's home at the Casa Azul in Mexico City was a garden. Teeming with lush bougainvillea, fruit trees, cacti, and native plants like agave and yucca, Kahlo's garden was a creative refuge and a source of inspiration for her art. A lover of the natural world, Kahlo also surrounded herself with animals, including two pet spider monkeys named *Caimito de Guayabal* and *Fulang Chan*, parrots, an eagle, a deer, and a pack of *Xoloitzcuintli*, or Mexican hairless dogs.[9]

Frida's overall body of works and of thematic inclusions in her production are very Mexican-prevalent, e.g., her self-portraits in indigenous attire(s), along with animals like the aforementioned native *xoloitzcuintli* (Mexican hairless dog),[10] *ozomatli* (Mexican spider monkey)[11] and the *guacamaya* (macaw in Spanish, probably from one of the original maya languages),[12] as well as her state of mind/ deteriorating health could both, arguably, also be contributing factors on why she focused on still-lifes with these particular fruits (and animals) at this point in her production. Zavala from the 2015 exhibition agrees:

> In the forties in particular [the few painful years before her demise], Kahlo's paintings were full of plants, some more allegorical than

others, and still-lifes of the tropical fruits she found in abundance at markets in Mexico City. As Kahlo struggled with chronic illness and disability later in her life, she spent more and more time at home—and turned her artistic gaze inward as well. 'As she's experiencing more containment and enclosure at home, she's drawing inspiration from things that really signify her love of Mexican culture and her love of color,' Zavala explains.[13]

In any case, the fruits in her still-lifes are dominated by two of the four types of same, simple and accessory fruits, defined as

A simple fruit grows from a single ovary of a single flowering plant. For example, banana, grape, tomato etc. Aggregate fruits consist of mass drupelets and each drupelet is developed from several carpels of the same flower. For example, blackberry and raspberry. Multiple fruits form from carpels derived from multiple flowers. For example, pineapple. Accessory fruits are formed from adjacent tissues exterior to the carpel AND NOT from the floral ovary. For example, apple and pear.[14]

Given Frida's historical attention to aspects of what her works portrayed, she may have known, whether by research or experience and/or by intuition, both that several of these fruits were of Western Hemisphere origin. Some of those native and very common Mexican fruits that Frida painted follow the same concepts of fecundity as the fruit definitions, yet imply eventual death, e.g., the *pitahaya*, which is featured in in Frida's 1938 still-life of five pitahayas.

The pitahaya is a desert fruit with a melon-like taste that grows on rocks or in thickets. It is ovoid with a thick yellow skin that swells with excrescences and bulges. The inside is a mass of dense, translucent white flesh that contains many small black edible seeds. Kahlo loved pitahayas for their sweetness and juiciness. In many respects, Kahlo's depiction is realistic, even including two pitted rocks and round cactus to suggest the fruit's habitat. But the artist takes liberties and makes certain decisions that give her still life its special meanings. First, these pitahayas are decomposing; the healthy yellow skin has over-ripened to a garish red orange. The skins have burst open, and brown rot has set in. One has been sliced open to reveal what we would expect, the white flesh and black seeds. But the cuts are perfectly rounded rims. The sectioned fruits stare out with other-earthly eyes. Presiding over the fruits is a small, seated skeleton who holds a scythe that identifies it as the grim reaper—death itself. This figure is a calavera. It is associated with *El Día de los Muertos* (The Day of the Dead), Mexico's most popular holiday that commences for two days on November 1—All Saints Day in the Catholic liturgical calendar. Kahlo's still life is a meditation on death. Because of its watery freshness that can provide sustenance in the most barren of terrains, the pitahaya is known as the *fruit of the shipwrecked man*. But even this most life-giving of fruits is given to decay.[15]

Furthermore, the association of fruit with sexuality and fertility fits with the negative aspects of Frida's life's story, terrible physical and psychological problems due to the teenage bus accident which caused her horrifying gynecological injury and led to her later inability to carry Diego's child to term, as well as her philosophy of artistic content. Milner reminds us that

what Kahlo brought to this genre [still-life] was a robust and, at times extremely forthright, overlay of sexual suggestiveness . . . what is most striking, however, is the actual shapes of the fruits depicted: split open to reveal seeds or round, protuberant and ruddy, evocative of female genitalia . . . biomorphic allusiveness was a well-established part of Surrealist pictorial strategies . . . intended to unnerve spectators, to confront them with objects of hyper-real intensity the brought to the surface suppressed or subconscious sexual urgings. There is no doubt that this was Kahlo's intention. (72)

For example, watermelons, similar to *pitahayas* in appearance, figure frequently in her works and various sources repeat the associations of that fruit:

The watermelon, or watermelon, is a symbol of fecundity, because of the many seeds it contains. This is why, in Vietnam, watermelon seeds were once offered to newlyweds, together with oranges that have the same meaning. In the Hellenic world, it is the pomegranate seed that plays this role as a symbol of fertility.[16]

and

Watermelon. A watermelon is a large berry whose swollen roundness and vibrant red flesh connote fertility and sexuality. Fruit appears in myths from around the world. Often it is a symbol of abundance, associated with goddesses of fertility, plenty, and the harvest.[17]

In reference to her 1938 work which also features watermelon prominently, *Fruits of the Earth*, the dedicated website describes that

> This painting is the largest one among the several still-life paintings Frida Kahlo produced in her later [but not latest] life. The sky in the background was bright blue when first painted but she later repainted it and changed it to the dark gloomy sky to reflect her emotions . . . She likes to open or having wound on the fruits as she did in her self-portraits to opens or sounds on her own body. The fruits are also full of sexual indications as well as allusions to the cycle of life and death.[18]

Herrera reiterates Frida's active awareness and purposeful recognition of the/her cycle of life and death in her fruit still-lifes. "Significantly [the fruits] are sometimes bruised . . . she recognized their transience . . . as always when painting objects other than herself, Frida made her fruits look like her . . . cut open . . . making us remember her wounded self-portraits (397). One of the most graphically demonstrative of this motif of openness and/or wounds features watermelon, bananas and papaya in the 1939–40 versions of *The Bride Frightened at Seeing Life Opened*, again from the website:

> Like most of her work, there's a lot more going on than what appears on the surface. In a lot of Frida's paintings, the objects become Symbols. The bride is that little doll in the corner peeking from the open watermelon. The fruit is opened up. It's not two halves. The sexual overtones are quite evident. The male genitalia in the bananas and the female genitalia in the open papaya, and it all combines into a circle; a circle of the ying and the yang. When this particular painting was first made in 1939, it didn't include the little bride there on the left. The papaya wasn't split open. It didn't have these bright colors and the erotic undertones that make this an alluring, sexual still-life.[19]

FridaKahlo.com gives more insights into Frida's work as her state of mind and body, her physical and mental health, declined:

> In the latest years of Frida's life she painted lots of small-scale still-life[s] . . . Her prior still-life artistic creations of the 1930s and 1940s were filled with subtle or obvious sexual overtones. By the 1950s, when this still-life was painted, they had ended up all the more 'once again to nature' and 'some even convey a political message.' At that period of her life, Frida depended intensely on prescribed drugs to reduce her physical pain. Often, she takes drugs with alcohol, which

started to influence her capacity to paint with the accuracy and point of interest for which she was known. She is painting much smaller paintings with [fewer] objects like fruits. If you compare level of precision and accuracy in this painting to one done prior in the year (*Still-Life with Parrot and Flag*), you can see a perceptible contrast. On the off chance that you further contrast this painting with one painted in 1954 (*Still Life with Flag*), the distinctions are significantly more obvious.[20]

Similarly, though not of American origin and imported to the Americas via prehistoric trade routes,[21] another rounded fruit, rough husk on the outside, a little like the watermelon's rind but much harder to cut open, "meat" and "milk" hidden inside, released when it is hacked open, the coconut figures prominently in Frida's late-life still-lifes in the early 1950s.

In . . . [*Coconuts*], also in a similar painting painted that year (*Weeping Coconuts*) the coconut is given some personality like a human being and is sobbing. Presumably symbolizing her passionate state at the time or possibly an impression of her [self]pity over the loss of her capacity to paint in the exact way for which she was well-known. The quality, details and organization of this painting are to some degree reduced as it is in *Weeping Coconuts*. The shades are dull, not the common splendid striking colors that Kahlo would typically use. No flags, no commitments, no political message . . . just a common 'back to nature' still-life painting . . . probably painted only to kill the time.[22]

Each critic echoes the other about this "perceptible contrast." However, they do not agree that "killing time" was her motivation. Frida had become more and more dependent on drugs to diminish her pain, not to mention more and more concerned about selling work to help Diego with his financial difficulties. Herrera, one of many, documents this "perceptible contrast," saying,

The still-lifes Frida painted in 1951 and earlier are neat and precise in technique, full of refined detail and sly, suggestive wit. By 1952, her style had changed radically; the late still-lifes are not just animate but agitated. They have a kind of wild intensity, as if Frida were flailing about in search of something solid, a raft in a heavy sea of imperma-nence. Brushwork becomes looser; she has lost the exquisite precision of the miniaturist. Her characteristic small, slow, affectionate strokes give way to messy frenetic handling. Colors are no longer clear and vibrant but strident and grating. Modeling and surface texture are so summary that oranges lose their firm, appealing roundness, watermelons no longer look succulent.

Similarly, Milner observes the "only toward the very end of Kahlo's life do her still-life pictures perceptibly shift their meaning, losing their sexual resonance and becoming more directly evocative of nature itself" (72), as well representing the physical and mental states affecting her work.

A particularly evocative painting, the very last one that Frida made, is described on FridaKahlo.com as

> A vibrant conclusion to [her] short life . . . *Viva la Vida/Watermelons* features rich color contrasts, curves and angles, and a final message from the artist herself. Kahlo put the finishing touches on her watermelon-themed painting just a few days before her death in 1954. [She] inscribed "Viva la vida" on the central melon wedge at the bottom of the canvas, which translates as "Long live life," just eight days before she died. This may have been a straightforward statement as she neared death. It may also have been an ironic commentary on her pain-filled existence due to polio, a bus accident, and multiple surgeries. Watermelons have hard shells that protect the soft flesh inside. When you bite into the flesh, you experience cool, juicy sweetness. At its most elemental, a watermelon could symbolize the artist herself, who had to develop a thick skin to weather a life marked with physical pain, a troubled marriage to artist Diego Rivera and harsh criticism of her art. However, Kahlo shows in the painting that once her shell is cut open, it reveals an inner life that is vibrant, fresh and sweet. Also, the many seeds of the watermelons, like those of the pomegranate in Greek mythology, symbolize fertility as well as immortality. Once the fruit is gone, the seeds carry the promise of new life forward into eternity.[23]

Though Frida may not have been physically able to leave a human child to the world, she conceived her artworks and carried them to term, featuring fruit with seeds providing the promise of new life. Almost as if dying in childbirth, Frida birthed her iconic fruit still-lifes as allegories of her life at the end of her life.

Notes

1   The source which/who first coined this term is unknown, though Diana Vernon, from the online site, Fridamania: The Frida Kahlo Effect (theculturetrip.com) is credited in a google search. In keeping with this informal and ubiquitous tie-in to the term, the artist will be referred to

by her first name in this essay unless the source specifically uses Frida's surname.

2   5 FRIDA KAHLO WORKS—LESSER-KNOWN, MADE LATE-IN LIFE—NOW ON VIEW IN DALLAS: NPR
3   5 FRIDA KAHLO WORKS—LESSER-KNOWN, MADE LATE-IN LIFE—NOW ON VIEW IN DALLAS: NPR
4   https://www.markmitchellpaintings.com/blog/the-symbolism-of-fruit-in-art
5   5 FRIDA KAHLO WORKS—LESSER-KNOWN, MADE LATE-IN LIFE—NOW ON VIEW IN DALLAS: NPR
6   Márquez, Yvonne S. "Step into Frida Kahlo's Garden at a Lush New San Antonio Exhibit," *Texas Monthly*. May 17, 2021. Step Into Frida Kahlo's Garden at a Lush New San Antonio Exhibit –Texas Monthly.
7   *Viva la vida, Fruit of Life, Coconuts, Weeping Coconuts, Still Life with Parrot & Fruit, Fruits of the Earth, Living Nature, Pitahayas, Portrait of Luther Burbank, (Round) Still Life, Still Life with Flag, Still Life with Parrot & Flag, Still Life with Parrot, Still Life with Watermelons, Still Life, The Bride Frightened at Seeing Life Opened*, and *Tunas Still Life with Prickly Pear Fruit*. Frida Kahlo: 100 Paintings Analysis, Biography, Quotes, & Art.
8   "A fruit is the soft, pulpy part of a flowering plant that contains seeds. It is formed from the ovaries of angiosperms and is exclusive only to this group of plants." FRUIT DEFINITION: DISCOVER THE MEANING OF FRUITS, ITS TYPES AND FAQS (BYJUS.COM)
9   Step Into Frida Kahlo's Garden at a Lush New San Antonio Exhibit—Texas Monthly.
10 Xoloitzcuintle—Wikipedia.
11 Mexican spider monkey—Wikipedia.
12 guacamaya | Spanish to English | Zoology (proz.com)
13 Step Into Frida Kahlo's Garden at a Lush New San Antonio Exhibit—Texas Monthly.
14 Fruit Definition: Discover the meaning of fruits, its types and FAQS (byjus.com)
15 Pitahayas, 1938—by Frida Kahlo.
16 WATERMELON MEANING & SYMBOLISM | BROOCH PARADISE (BROOCH-PARADISE.COM)
17 Mar. 20, 2020. WHAT DO WATERMELONS SYMBOLIZE? (ASKINGLOT.COM)
18 FRUITS OF THE EARTH, 1938—BY FRIDA KAHLO.
19 The Bride Frightened at Seeing Life Opened—by Frida Kahlo.
20
21 usnh_0014.02.pdf (si.edu)
22 Coconuts, 1951—by Frida Kahlo.
23 Viva la Vida, Watermelons—by Frida Kahlo.

Bibliography

Cook, O.F. *History of the Coconut Palm in America.* usnh_0014.02.pdf (si.edu)

"Frida and Her Paintings." Frida Kahlo: 100 Paintings Analysis, Biography, Quotes, & Art.

"Fruit Definition." Fruit Definition: Discover the meaning of fruits, its types and FAQ (byjus.com)

García, Rupert. *Frida Kahlo.* Berkeley, CA: Chicano Studies Library Publication Unit, 1983.

"Guacamaya," guacamaya | Spanish to English | Zoology (proz.com)

Herrera, Hayden. *Frida Kahlo.* New York City: Harper & Rowe, 1983.

Márquez, Yvonne S. "Step into Frida Kahlo's Garden at a Lush New San Antonio Exhibit," *Texas Monthly.* May 17, 2021. Step Into Frida Kahlo's Garden at a Lush New San Antonio Exhibit–Texas Monthly.

Milner, Frank. *Frida Kahlo.* London: Bison Books Ltd., 1995.

Mitchell, Mark. "The Symbolism of Fruit in Art." July 16, 2016. Https://Www.markmitchellpaintings.Com/Blog/The-Symbolism-Of-Fruit-In-Art

Stamberg, Susan. "5 Lesser-Known, Late-In-Life Works by Frida Kahlo Now on View in Dallas," Mar. 8, 2021. 5 Frida Kahlo Works—Lesser-Known, Made Late-In Life—Now on View in Dallas: NPR.

Vernon, Diana. "Frida Mania: The Frida Kahlo Effect." Dec. 18, 2016. Fridamania: The Frida Kahlo Effect (theculturetrip.com)

Watermelon Meaning & Symbolism | Brooch Paradise (Brooch-Paradise.Com)

"Xoloitzcuintle" and "Mexican Spider Monkey," Wikipedia. Xoloitzcuintle—Wikipedia and Mexican spider monkey—Wikipedia.

CHAPTER

15

Family, Food & Fighting: A Comparative Study of the Mexican Film *Como agua para chocolate* and the Chinese film *Eat Drink Man Woman*

Haiqing Sun

While it primarily nourishes us physically, food gives us a sense of security—and of love—which is why one can understand values from different cultural perspectives of life. For a family, meals serve to connect the members and to contribute to their unity and communication. The quality of food in this sense can be a source of fame and/or a sign of social well-being and, for a nation,[1] can represent its traditional wealth. In countries like China and Mexico, which historically have suffered disasters of catastrophic ethnic nature,[2] food is part of the national patrimony and constitutes a refuge that helps to safeguard ethnic idiosyncrasy and imprints the image of a nation, or so-called racial group, on the daily necessities of the human being in the greater society.

In a certain sense, food is like a language, it represents a unifying force for a group of people. So, it's not unreasonable that the spiritual world is often associated with the image of food. In the same way, part of one's soul resides in the foods that nourish one daily over generations. Therefore, the cook, the creator of the typical dishes of a people, is not a simple "worker," but someone who carries in him/herself, besides personal wisdom, the cultural foundation of his/her group. It is this alliance between food and nation that characterizes the two films studied in this chapter, *Como agua para chocolate/Like Water for Chocolate* (1992) directed by the Mexican, Alfonso Arau, and *Comer, beber, amar/Eat Drink Man Woman*[3] (1993) by Ang Lee from

Taiwan. In both, culinary skill is a power associated with the particular culture and, at the same time, is mixed with a love story and with the possibility of a new life; Food works as well as a force that challenges, moves and reforms the everyday world. The two films can be examined as mutual reflections of an effort to reaffirm the values of a lesser-heard group in the cinematographic arena ruled by Hollywood and other Western countries since the beginning of the 20th century. That is, the strategies of representing cultural values in one film under the lens of the other will be more easily understood. The two directors provide us with vivid examples of how to exercise the power of speaking in a traditional culture through narrative techniques and games inherited from a modern film empire and thus, establish a dialogue between marginalized and dominant cultures.

The two films were produced in quite different scenarios and with quite different historical backgrounds. *Water for chocolate* based on the novel by the contemporary Mexican writer, Laura Esquivel, deals with privileged society in the rural environment of Mexico at the end of the 19th century and the beginning of the 20th century, with the Mexican Revolution as a socio-historical framework. Ang Lee's *Eat Drink Man Woman* takes its title from a Chinese saying: *yin shi nan nü* (饮食 男女), which means that food and sex are two basic desires of the human being. It tells the story of a middle-class family in the modern and cosmopolitan Taipei of the 1990s.

Reviewing *Like Water for Chocolate*, Janet Maslin says, "This film, a lively family saga that is centered on forbidden love and spans several generations, relies so enchantingly upon fate, magic and a taste for the supernatural." The same, in fact, may be said about the work of Ang Lee. The two films have several comparable aspects despite their different socio-historical backgrounds, such as history, central theme and social values, through which the viewer sees the presentation of experiences of spiritual nutrition under the different artistic perspectives of its directors. The plot of both films features a family of three daughters and a widowed parent, which, as Winnie Khaw notes, highlights "a portrait of the concerns of familial relationships and suppressed personal feelings in the foreground." The central theme both share is the "rebellious" love of the protagonists who are the cooks of the family. In addition, the narrative in each case is accompanied by a detailed representation of the customs and haute cuisine of the country. Both directors have tried to illustrate, through three-dimensional cinematographic art, the history of a tri-sensual art, with color, aroma and flavor, an art born of the enjoyment of the senses.

The presentation of the visual images of the food is more obvious than the presentation of the taste, since the latter does not depend on the visual aspect but on the communication with the audience through the narration. In both works, the history of the cook serves as a medium which transmits the flavors of life. The love difficulty is bittersweet, while domestic work guarantees basic nutrition and the banquet appears as the main aspect of both films: an event in which the richest dishes and the most intense conflicts in history coincide. Ang Lee has shown us that double function of the banquet in one of his previous films, *The Wedding Banquet* (1990), the first film that brought him international fame. It is a work about the crisis in a family around a homosexual child, during which the wedding with a rich banquet—a symbol of honor and happiness for parents—serves as a turning point for the fate of all the characters. The banquet accentuates the climax and offers an opportunity to reveal the emotional world of the protagonist and the conflicts between the characters during the development of the narrative. Meanwhile, the delicate relationship between people and power is interpreted through food, as this is something omnipresent that is smelled, digested and that everyone wants to share. In both films, the conflicts that take place at the table are finally struggles for power, a "food" for the ego, with which people must live in society.

The most obvious conflict in both plots is filial, between the parent and daughter(s). In *Como agua para chocolate*, Doña Elena, the widowed mother, sacrifices Tita, her youngest daughter; as the youngest, by tradition, Tita must remain, unmarried, at home to serve and care for her mother as the latter ages. Moreover, adding insult to injury, Doña Elena marries off her eldest daughter, Rosaura, to Pedro, Tita's would-be mate, which accentuates Tita's misery. Then, Tita, who, as a result of the tradition, is not permitted to determine her own fate, has to survive and claim what love she can, resorting to food and to the kitchen, where she is a conduit of culinary and family traditions. With her power to help and feed, she becomes the true mistress of the home. In *Eat Drink Man Woman*, Mr. Chu, the retired head chef of the Grand Hotel of Taiwan and father-widower, works alone at home, serving his daughters, all of them already adults. Even being the "king" of the kitchen and capable of preparing all the famous dishes, he has lost his sense of taste. In addition, he cannot get along with his daughters because each one has her own "worldview" and it is difficult to win them over to his with delicious food or the patriarchal rules of yesteryear. The death of his old colleague reveals the limits of existence and the importance of personal happiness, so Mr. Chu accepts reality and starts a new life. In both stories, conflicts in the family have roots in society where social norms impede the search for love by the protagonists.

In Tita's case, her "good habits" and obedience enslave her in the kitchen. In the case of Chu, the Coca-Cola and McDonald's-ized" city, so to speak, marginalizes traditional Chinese food and its artisans, isolating people of that age and outlook from the center of social life. However, both characters suffer from loneliness and are forced to rely on capturing any opportunity to express their lives via the creation of nutrition. Thus, it is seen that in both films, the production of sumptuous food contrasts with the difficulty-fraught love lives of Tita and Chu; food preparation is a refuge where the cook shares social values with the rest of the world. Although the social and/or personal "value" of either character is limited to prowess in the kitchen by public prejudice, not to mention personal complications, their souls are liberated right there with the food that feeds and inspires the rest. Moreover, both chefs use their culinary skills to convey the desire to love.

Food works as a channel of communication and strength of expression that helps the protagonists to give voice against prejudice and ignorance in their societies. In *Como agua para chocolate*, the communicative power of food is manifested via magical ingredients. An example is when the tears of Tita fall into the cake she prepares for the wedding of her sister, Rosaura, and her beloved, Pedro. Said tears serve as emotional leaven, which transforms the wedding not into a celebration of love but into the sad reminder of affective failure. Tita's tragedy is then re-interpreted with a tragi-comic scene in which all the wedding reception guests cry—and vomit—after sharing the cake, remembering their own past or present lovesickness, thus unconsciously sharing the pain of the protagonist. Thus, the culinary art is sublimated by a magical representation and forms a resistant voice that breaks the oppressive silence imposed on Tita by society. Another example of the sublimation of the food is the rose sauce prepared by Tita with flowers offered by Pedro, in which "not only his blood, but his whole being had dissolved [which] in this way penetrated the body of Peter. . . completely sensual" (quote from the movie). The magic of this dish is not limited in its function as a means of communication between Tita and Pedro. It also serves as the inspiration for love for her other sister, Gertrudis, who finds, with the mysterious scent of roses, her revolutionary-soldier love, and who starts her own heroic legend in a mission of social struggle. In the case of Gertrudis, the rose sauce conveys metaphorical and symbolic senses that synthesize the passionate physical love and philosophical revolutionary passion, since both deal with the desire for a better life for the common beings and both start at home with a romantic dish and end at home with a family banquet, for which Gertrudis returns in her new revolutionary identity.

In both films, in addition to the love story of the protagonists, the sisters' romance-route offers a subtle observation of the role of women in the social context and their notion of feminine dignity under multiple pressures. In Ang Lee's film, the love story of Chu and Jinrong, a young single mother and friend of the daughters of Chu, is accompanied by the preparation of a series of typical dishes. Unlike the Mexican film, the love between Chu and Jinrong does not carry any fantastic elements nor is it directly represented in the story dominated by the story of Chu's three daughters. The relationship between Chu and Jinrong is insinuated through the lunches that Chu cooks for Jinrong's little daughter. In the beginning, this girl brings the kind of simple and "standard" lunch that her mother prepares for her to her school, while the contacts between Chu and Jinrong are limited to dinners when the daughters of Chu invite her to enjoy the professional-standard dishes at their home. Then, the girl begins to take the cold leftovers that Jinrong brings home after dinner with Chu's family. Later, Chu starts to make "formal" lunches with rice, meat, vegetable and soup dishes for the girl and brings them warm to her class until he becomes a kind of informal cook for the girl's classmates. The richest banquet at the end of the film serves as the revelation of love between Chu and Jinrong, when everyone, even the audience, expects Chu to marry a woman his age according to social norms. The great richness of the meals forms a contrast with the silence and tranquility in the development of this love, while it effectively reflects the passion that finds no other outlet. It should be noted that, as in the Mexican film, the preparation of meals not only represents a love-passion but also reveals the protagonist's wisdom in the struggle for dignity, since both Tita and Chu manage to pass that important message on to their beloved without that third part, be it of characters or the audience, anticipating. It should also be noted that behind those romantic representations in the kitchen of both protagonists, there exists a great maternal-like culinary love, i.e., the will to care and protect, a basic tone of both filmic narrations.

On this same topic, it is notable that in both films the mother is an absent character from a traditional angle. In *Como agua para chocolate*, Doña Elena functions more as a patriarchal and conservative authority when she tries to dominate the future of her daughters using the traditional patriarchal approach and strictures. Tita's sister, Rosaura, marries Pedro and has a child, but she is not able to raise her son and has to resort to Tita's ministrations in order that the baby survive. In *Eat Drink Man Woman*, the mother died many years ago and is present only via a black- and-white photo hanging on the wall. Mr. Chu must act as mother for his daughters on the one hand and exercise patriarchal power on the other in order to maintain this small family unit. He is like Tita, to whom the control of the kitchen gives the strength to care for and protect; however, Chu shares the tortures of Doña Elena in *Como agua para chocolate*, secrets of ill-fated love, victimized by the power that he himself wields in the family. Apparently in both movies, maternal love manifests itself through the role of providing food. In the Mexican film, Tita raises her nephew (son of Rosaura and Pedro) with a magical ingredient, albeit very common, which is "a lot of love." Tita experiences tenderness when feeding the baby and thus, enjoys the biological maternal happiness that her society denies her. With this ingredient in food and life, at the same time that she feeds her family, Tita actualizes herself as a woman, i.e., she manages to play the role of daughter, sister, lover and mother, concurrently. The death of her nephew due to problems with his digestive system after moving away from Tita symbolically confirms the maternal function of the cook, for whom the concept of mother is interpreted metaphorically as the natural union of food and body.

In contrast, the story of *Eat Drink Man Woman* does not employ magical resources. Mr. Chu is called "Living Recipe" for the prestigious dishes he serves in the most luxurious hotel in Taiwan; however, he finds a new life via preparing the most ordinary dishes at home. Yet, like Tita, the most important ingredient for Chu is "a lot of love." At the beginning of the story, Mr. Chu's food is presented as a symbol of patriarchal authority: a dinner that the daughters are forced to eat at home every Sunday. Although the meal is very delicious, the daughters do not enjoy it since the dining room is not a space of communication but of conflict. As opposed to Doña Elena, in the end, Mr. Chu chooses a more flexible way to deal with the problems of his daughters, even when one gets pregnant before getting married, which is considered a big scandal in conventional communities. He helps to turn his dining room into a place of farewell when the daughters seek changes in lifestyle; they move, one after the other, in with their boyfriends. Tolerance and understanding are other ingredients in the offer of maternal love, which manifests in Chu, but is not in Doña Elena.

However, Chu's change of heart is not due to maternal love but rather to the influence of the modern social environment. His authority diminishes every day and his sumptuous food is not appreciated, which serve to highlight his loneliness as the master of an ancestral culture pitted against a young and thriving society. The old order of family that Chu wanted to preserve becomes, finally, a hindrance to his own life when he falls in love with Jinrong because, even today, while divorces among the young seem very common and acceptable, the second nuptials of the old encounter plenty of pitfalls: blame, public prejudice, even censure by their own children. Then, like in Tita's case, in Chu's story, culinary art not only serves as an expression of love but also conveys a strong sense of responsibility and capacity that the protagonist needs to win approval and be assured of his value to his family.

At the same time as his love story with Jinrong begins, Mr. Chu suffers a double crisis in his life: the daughters' challenges against his traditional authority and also the threat to his professional identity as chef-artist. The threat in large modern cities is embodied by the fast food which attracts more people every day, especially among the young people. His own daughter even works at a McDonald's-type restaurant! As a result, there are fewer people who appreciate true Chinese cuisine. Second, what worries him most in life is not his health but lack of companionship. In this sense, it is not exactly that Chu abandons social tradition at the end of story to marry again but that modern life has left him behind. For Chu's daughters, their father's food does not compete with sex, whereas, for Chu, the desire to love surpasses the fear of losing social approval. By helping Jinrong and her daughter, Chu regains the pride of husband and father and. at the same time, also recreates an environment in which his culinary art is appreciated in an intimate way. Unlike Tita, who has to choose between death or a life without love, in Chu's case, the social value coincides with the individual value, since his marriage, although surprising, is finally accepted among the all-important relatives.

In both films, the representation of food and culinary skills and instruments forms a greater visual attraction. But cooking, as a symbolic space that reflects the emotional world of chefs, functions differently. In *Como agua para chocolate*, Tita depends on the kitchen to show her love for her family and to protest injustice. In *Eat Drink Man Woman*, when looking for a new life, Mr. Chu abandons his kitchen-sanctuary. By marrying again, Chu decides to move and sell his house. At this moment, suspense dominates his great kitchen. In other words, the viewer realizes that the culinary aspect is not only a background of visual attraction but a character in and of itself—one that requires its own destiny in the plot. To whom and how can Chu leave it to the next generation?

In both films, the responsibility of inheritance is highlighted as a basis for the progress of culture. This represents the power of cohesion that guarantees the transcendence of love and fidelity of a people. In *Eat Drink Man Woman*, Jiachian, Chu's second daughter, a professional woman, buys the house that her father leaves. She inherits Chu's kitchen and, at the end of the story, she becomes a skilled cook of traditional food and the main connection between family members. Even so, the movie ends with a mystery. By tasting the soup prepared by Jiachian, Mr. Chu regains his sense of taste lost so many years ago. Who knows if the soup itself works a miracle or if it is his new life that restores his interest in food? But, most importantly, the kitchen is not lost or ruined. And, although Jiachian cannot master all the techniques of her father nor spend much time in the house, she plays the role of cook well, as that role manages to unite and communicate family values and affections. But the director sadly doubts if traditional cuisine, although it remains a symbol of security for a certain individual, may be where the power for social progress originates under modern conditions and Western influences. Such a sad possibility is suggested by the end of the story when Sunday dinner can no longer physically reunite the whole family.

In Arau's film there is much more concern about breaking up the family. While Ang Lee tries to fill his narrative with melancholy feelings, Arau frankly shows the tragic reality of loss, even despair of love, loss of life, traditional values and treasures in different aspects of daily life. In the narration of both films, there is a review of the irrecoverable family values through time and social changes—but Tita's family history reflects a step beyond Mexican history and the destinies of a people due to greater issues such as the Mexican Revolution. Food is represented as a poetic ingredient of history. Unlike Jiachian, Esperanza, Tita's niece, who is also the narrator of *Como agua para chocolate*, does not inherit her aunt's recipes simply as family treasures, but presents and shares them as a romance, in which death is a bitter ingredient, although essential. Therefore, one can extend the critical view towards the meaning of death in the two films, as well as in both Chinese and Mexican cultures. *Eat Drink Man Woman* presents the theme of death via a well-known Chinese attitude, that it is considered a threat and the deceased is mentioned with respect, silence and distance. It is insinuated in the story that Chu's deceased wife had been a woman of strong will whose frequent disputes with Mr. Chu about the education of his daughters have sown tense relations among other members of the family. But the influence of death is represented by the simple image of the black-and-white photo of said deceased wife, hanging in a corner of the house, symbolizing the precursors of the present conditions, despite the lack of an overt voice or discursive force.

In addition, the focus of the narrative is on Mr. Chu's search for a new life, while avoiding the interpretation of his existence under the shadow of the deceased. Sometimes the wife's voice is expressed by her daughters but the influence of her death as a direct cause of situations in this family does not appear explicit. Another death in history, that of a colleague from a heart attack, serves more as a warning sign and turning point in the development of the plot, since it pushes Chu to re-evaluate the quality of his present life beyond his reliance on conventional rules, so that he finally decides to marry Jinrong. Thus, it is seen that in Ang Lee's film, death is represented as an abstract concept, a symbol of nothing, and of fear and an opposition to positive aspects such as life, love, happiness and family. In *Como agua para chocolate*, however, the story is focused more on this topic. The death of Tita's mother during the politically chaotic period also serves as a point of return for the narrative and connects different plots in the development of the actions of the protagonists, since her death symbolizes the end of an era both politically for the nation of Mexico and in the family history. Unlike in *Eat Drink Man Woman*, Arau directly describes Tita's conditions beneath the shadow of her mother. Even after her death, Doña Elena continues to appear, as a ghost, who continues to exert her power over love and soul aloud within Tita's consciousness. Thus, death plays a living and aggressive role instead of being a pure symbol which enriches the interpretation of life and its crises. The contrast between the representations of the mothers who die in the two films is perhaps a not-so-subtle reflection of the attitudes of the two cultural entities towards their dead relatives and reminds us of the cultural differences between the two countries. In the Chinese tradition, respect and distance for the deceased is emphasized. This is seen, for example, in the observation (instead of celebration) of the "Clear and Illuminated Day" (Day of the Dead) in China, which is a day of silent rites by which each family memorializes their deceased in the media, privately visiting cemeteries with food and drink or performing simple rites in temples, all of which take place only among members of the same family. On the other hand, the celebration of the Day of the Dead in Mexico is totally festive, with bright colors and almost all inhabitants of towns, all their houses and places and all their deceased intertwined publicly. *El Día de los Muertos/Difuntos* is celebrated with decorations in cemeteries, altars with artifacts from the life of the deceased, meals at home and processions or parades in streets of cities and towns. Death is lived overtly in this case, i.e., it is treated as something alive, a part of life, just as it is represented in Arau's film, and it is incorporated, along with food, into a vital and magical experience.

Although the mother in both films is a crucial figure in the lives of the daughters, different representations of her image and her death show a difference of access to the values supported by the two cultures. In addition, in the absence of their mother, Chu's daughters continue to live out their anger and desires, while for Tita, the anger is extinguished but she lives with lasting bitterness, accumulates, and finally literally ignites, her duel against fate.

Both films depict the death of a cook: Mr. Wen, Chu's ever-friendly partner in drinking and eating, who, widowed and alone, grows old and dies quietly in the kitchen—his home and workplace, an event that warns Chu to look for a new life. But in *Como agua para chocolate*, Tita's death is a last resort in order to fight and protest, as it is a way to win in death where life has failed. The study concludes that, in both *Like water for chocolate* and in *Eat Drink Man Woman*, the heiresses of the culinary art—Jiachian and Esperanza—allow the kitchen to play a metaphorical role for both directors, in the sense that they interpret the value of the two cultures. Both heirs come to know and revive the value of food as spiritual wealth and cultural heritage. Similarly, both directors reiterate the cultural idiosyncrasy of their peoples through film, a means of representation whose time and space are limited but whose power to interpret and move is enormous: a legacy for the future.

Notes

1   Nation in this sense does not necessarily constitute a single political entity but may refer to any one ethnic or linguistic group which self-identifies within said entity.
2   These catastrophes may—or may not—have been orchestrated as (in)formal "ethnic cleansing" mechanisms by a greater—or lesser—but certainly, more powerful group(s), who avail themselves of the opportunity to choose scapegoats and/or to consolidate power. However, such catastrophes may be "natural" ones, like earthquakes, which decimate places where any ethnic group is concentrated.
3   The Spanish translation of the movie title from the Chinese is the equivalent in English of *To Eat, To Drink, To Love* but the perhaps more familiar translation of the title to English from the Chinese is *Eat Drink Man Woman* (no commas*)*.

Bibliography

Drink Eat Man Woman. Dir. Ang Lee. Con Hsiung Lung y Chienlien Wu. Guión de Hui-Ling Wang y Ang Lee. GE Film Production, 1993. 104 min.
Como agua para chocolate. Dir. Alfonso Arau. Con Ada Carrasco y Mario Ivan Martínez. Miramax Films, 1993. Basada de la novela de Laura Esquivel. 105min.

Esquivel, Laura. *Como agua para chocolate.* México D.F: Planeta, 1994. Print.

El banquete de boda. Dir. Ang Lee. Con Hsiung Lung y Manin See. Guión de Ang Lee, Neil Peng and James Schmus. Central Motion Pictures Corp. with Good Machine Production, 1993. 108 min.

Khaw, Winnie. "Review and Analysis of the Film *Eat Drink Man Woman.*" <http://www.eclectica.org/v16n4/khaw.html>. Oct. 2012.

Maslin, Janet. "Emotions So Strong You Can Taste Them." <http://www.nytimes.com/movie/review?res=9F0CE7DA 1438F934A25751C0A9659582 60> February 17, 1993

PART V

Sustenance & the Soul:
Representation via the Literary Arts

Introduction to Sustenance & the Soul: Representation via the Literary Arts

A. Writers & Writing/Fiction & Essay

This collection, sadly, does not include chapters on poetry in the context of food & drink, but the poems glorifying food in Pablo Neruda's Las *odas elementales/Elemental Odes,* e.g., *Oda a la alcachofa/Ode to the Artichoke* and those to *sal/Salt, tomate/Tomato and caldillo al congrilo/Eel Au Jus* would have been great candidates! Neruda paints eloquently with words; he is a master of the senses! I can absolutely "see" the armored warrior to which he likens the leaves of the artichoke, taste the briny salt throughout nature, savor both the tomato and the eel in its own juice. Rather like psalms of praise to the objects he exalts, perhaps the *Odas/Odes* can figure into the next collection this series, *Rites, Rituals & Religions,* to be published in 2023. How ironic that would be for a writer with the socioeconomic philosophy of Neruda to have his poems, intended to celebrate socialist/communist ideals of the everyday, featured in a collection of criticism with such a title, even though the tome will not be limited to denominational rites or rituals and certainly not to religions of the sort which might be expected in view of the geographic places highlighted! Of course, less-upbeat in the terms I use, but also highlighting food and much more in keeping Neruda's intent for his literature, his protest poem, *La United Fruit Co.,* a masterpiece of fruit images and metaphors—and other poems in other contexts—demonstrate Neruda's fascination with food & drink in the service of both his philosophy and his artistic production.

However, focusing on prose fiction, my study of how food & drink function as *Linguistic, Familial & Cultural Links: Memory, Identity & Comfort: The Short Stories & an Essay* for Rose Mary Salum's Lebanese/Mexican/U.S. immigration experiences, precedes and serves as a segue to her own, original, never-before-published essay, *Filminas,* which follows the chapter. Jorge Chavarro explicates similar relationships between functions of culture and food for Cuban identity in *Paradiso* by José Lezama Lima. These are the so-called "follow-up" identity chapters alluded to in Part II focused on food and drink and physical spaces, the kitchen and dining room.

Eduardo Cerdán's comparison of written works by Leonora Carrington and Adela Fernández expands scholarship per se since Carrington is much better known for her paintings and Fernández has been barely included in literary criticism thus far. As Cerdán notes in his study, "domestic space representation is configured as a disturbing element for the characters and the readers themselves in the stories of both. The kitchen plays a leading role in space construction and there are testimonies, both about Fernández and Carrington, that show their personal fondness for it." Were this study not emphasizing the literary representation of food preparation and presentation space and unsettling metamorphosis of both the kitchen and the food, this chapter would have been included in Part II which deals with actual food and physical space.

Harking back to the inclusion of the very many cultures (and the importance of their food in their identities) which make up the Latin American demographics, as in earlier chapters, Stephen Miller's chapter on Isabel Allende ties the various references to food and its cultural importance to various immigrant groups therein. I do feel constrained to mention (I added the parenthetical note in the text) that *Colonia Tovar* is a real place, established by German immigrants in 1843, "lost" in the Andes due to its geographic inaccessibility and the inhabitants' desire to maintain their separate identity until "rediscovered" in the early 20ᵗʰ century. Being personally very familiar with both Venezuela, at least pre-Chávez and Maduro, and Germany, I can attest to the then still-extant Bavarian-ness of its architecture, language, food and especially, the *Gemütlichkeit,* of Colonia Tovar, a time-capsule tourist attraction.

Particularly the last three chapters emphasize feminist critique, calling to mind the studies in the third book in this series, *S/HE: Sex & Gender in Hispanic Cultures.* The stereotypical association of kitchen, cooking and food with "acceptable" behaviors and responsibilities for women and their domestic and socio-economic history (apart from the "upgraded" ideas of "chef" and "cuisine" being associated with men) pops up as a motif through this collection but a bit in passing rather than as a major emphasis, as in these last three chapters.

16

Food Vocabulary & References as Linguistic, Familial & Cultural Links: Memory, Identity & Comfort— The Essays & Short Stories by Rose Mary Salum

Debra D. Andrist

By second, or certainly third, generation, the descendants of immigrants, no matter the country of origin or to which country they immigrate, are statistically both verbally- and writing-dominant, if not monolingual, in the dominant language of the country in which the immigrants establish residence, mostly due to language of instruction in the schools those offspring attend.[1]

For example, Mexican-origin writer, Rose Mary Salum, who now lives mostly in the United States since 1998, is no exception. Rose Mary is a second-generation Lebanese-Mexican whose great-grandparents immigrated to Tampico, Mexico with her grandmother and her siblings. Her father, however, strongly encouraged speaking in English throughout her childhood, though he spoke English, Spanish and Lebanese (Levantine Arabic) himself, Rose Mary herself is bilingual in Spanish and English, though she does characterize herself as Spanish-dominant and mostly writes/publishes in that language.[2] Content and motifs of her works, however, almost always are laced with references to Lebanon and Lebanese and most frequently to vocabulary about family, family cultural practices & attitudes, food and food preparation. As befitted a young woman of her background, she was educated in private Roman Catholic schools in Mexico until graduate school at University of St. Thomas/Houston. In spite of Rose

Mary's constant relationship with all four grandparents and parents up through adulthood, she speaks no Lebanese, save the words or phrases mostly related to food and its preparation. In fact, she visits Lebanon as a "foreign" tourist with her own adult children. As she says in the essay, *Filminas*,[3] which follows this chapter and tells the story of her own immigration to the U.S. and its aftermath,

> when I am in Lebanon . . . I have only been there twice but when I am there, I recognize everything. I recognize the food, the codes, the way its people communicate with each other. I can decipher body gestures. I know what the tone of the words conveys, even though I don't understand them because my grandparents and parents spoke Arabic for the sole purpose that we do not understand. The third generation loses the language, I read in an article that reflects on exiles and uprooting. (12–13)

Yet, even though third generation in terms of living in Mexico (and then the U.S.), with only the most rudimentary Lebanese language ability, Rose Mary's written works abound with the Lebanese vocabulary and references associated with food and food preparation. These words, phrases and actions corroborate cultural and personal identity, familial memory and, most importantly, serve as a psychological source of comfort in a confusing and increasingly topsy-turvy world.

Although she is talking about the power of food in terms of colonization and not in those of immigration, Linda Álvarez's observations reiterate the power of food in the terms I describe. I contend that the substitution of words relating to "immigration" where Álvarez uses "colonization" is utterly justified and supports the thesis of the function of food vocabulary and references in the case of immigrant writers, especially in the Lebanese content of the works of Rose Mary Salum.

> [Immigration] is a [psychologically, if not physically] violent process that fundamentally alters the ways of life of the [immigrants]. Food has always been a fundamental tool in the process of [immigration]. Through food, social and cultural norms are conveyed, and also violated . . . Yet, we must never forget that the practice of [immigration] has always been a contested matter as groups have negotiated spaces within this process . . . Understanding the history of food and eating practices in different contexts can help us understand that the practice of eating is inherently complex. Food choices are influenced and constrained by cultural values and are an important part of the construction and maintenance of social identity. In that sense, food

has never merely been about the simple act of pleasurable consumption—food is history, it is culturally transmitted, it is identity. Food is power.[4]

In Rose Mary's first collection of short stories from 2002, *Entre los espacios*,[5] two stories stand out in terms of the focus on food, first as a generalized leitmotif in the fictive *Entremés, entrada y despedida/Appetizer, Entrée and Goodbye!*, which centers around the eating disorder of the protagonist and in which the only and very few references to food itself are actually to Mexican items: *quesadilla . . . tacos . . . tostadita, doradita . . . botana . . . churritas* (62–63/44–45). Her later collection from 2016, *El agua que mece el silencio/The Water Which Rocks the Silence*, in which she sets stories in the conflicts in the Middle East, contains virtually no inclusion of either food, or references to it, in either Lebanese or Spanish.

Much more importantly for thesis of this study—and a story which might suggest autobiographical elements in terms of searching for identity—is *Las voces del agua/The Voices of the Water*. This second story traces the physical and psychological journey of *Naidín*/Nadine, the young Lebanese protagonist who "*había perdido su vida (15)*/had lost her life" (9), i.e., her identity, as symbolized by

> *una caja de maderas preciosas y trabajo damasquino [en la que] desde pequeña ella recopilaba eventos y presencias y los iba depositando [en ella] (15)*/a box made of precious woods inlaid with damascene [in which] from a young age, she had written summaries of events and company and stored them [there]". (9)

Not only food items but food preparation references appear from the first in this text, as *Naidín* initially tries to find the all-important repository of her being. Had she again, as on "la tarde anterior cuando su madre cocinaba, la habría dejado por descuido entre los pimientos rojos o las berenjenas (15)/the afternoon before, when her mother was cooking . . . carelessly left it among the red pimentos or the eggplants" (9)? All of these references underscore the roles of her parents and her grandmother in *Naidín*'s cultural identity formation and it is all intertwined with food. As a result of how "*las voces de sus padres cincelaban en su alma las tradiciones (16)*/her parents' voices chiseled traditions into her soul" (10), the young woman desperately seeks her own cultural identity in the dual world of the immigrated.

> *Decidió aprender las recetas de la abuela, los secretos de la miel de vainilla y la manera de preparar le mermelada de higo. También*

escuchó que la feminidad se encuentra en el seno de la dulzura y la prudencia (16)/she decided to learn her grandmother's recipes . . . the secrets of vanilla extract and the way to make fig marmalade. She had heard that femininity was to be found in the essence of sweetness and prudence. (10)

The descriptions and vocabulary go on to detail her home where

el ambiente donde la hospitalidad se expresaba a través de la confección de platillos suculentos . . . los olores de la cocina . . . ascendían y se deslizaban . . . hasta confundirse con el humo del 'arguile' que cada tarde se preparaba para el 'sajrille' . . . los 'belewes' y la' macrum' (16)/the atmosphere where hospitality was expressed by way of an extravagance of succulent dishes . . . the odors of the kitchen . . . heightened and dissipated . . . until they mixed with the smoke of the *arguile* that were prepared every afternoon for the *sajrille* [as well as] the *baklava* and the *macrum*". (10)

Paragraph after paragraph reiterates characteristically common ingredients in Lebanese food that *Naidín*'s grandmother utilizes, "*menta*/mint . . . *almendras*/almonds . . . *cebolla*/onion" (16–17 & 10–11), as *Naidín* and her grandmother "*se comunicaban a través del recetario* (17)/communicate through the recipe collection" (11), serving the Lebanese specialties like *kepe . . . humus betjine . . . falafel, kafta* (17) and more.

One night, *Naidín* and her grandmother meet in her room to talk about the meaning of life in the context of *Naidín*'s identity, where *Naidín* serves her grandmother a typical Lebanese *aperitivo*, "*un poco de arak sobre el que espoloreó algunos granos de anís* (18–19)/ a little *arak* over which she sprinkled some grains of anise" (12). Eventually, with her grandmother's understanding and blessing, *Naidín* goes on a perilous journey outside her home to track down the all-important box. She takes "*algunas frutas almíbaradas, lentejas y pistachos* (20)/some glazed fruit, lentils and pistachios" (14), eventually finding both herself in terms of her cultural identity—and the symbolic box—after stopping along the treacherous way fraught with challenges to her body and soul. But first, she "*evocó a su abuela, su olor a costumbre y su voz arrulladora. Recordó cómo amasaba el kepe enre las manos y cómo se lo daba a comer para convercerla de que era libanesa y no árabe* (22)/she recalled her grandmother, her customary smell and her lulling voice, remembered how the older woman kneaded the *kepe* between her hands, and how she gave it to [*Naidín*] to eat to prove to her that she was Lebanese and not Arab" (16). *Naidín* then realizes that she can/must go home and does just that!

Rose Mary's artful, but necessary, inclusion of cultural references and, especially, to food, in this short story functions to support the title of this article, *Food Vocabulary & References as Linguistic, Familial & Cultural Links*, leading to *Memory, Identity & Comfort*, particularly since there are autobiographical elements related to identity, not to mention the "happy ending."

However, the essay, *Filminas*, printed after this chapter in this collection, while utilizing food and food references as linguistic, familial and cultural links, is far less comforting as memory and identity are far more problematic aspects of the situation. These constant familial, cultural & linguistic references to Lebanese food in the essay trace the heart-wrenching (for both author and reader) true story of Rose Mary's own, albeit forced, unintended and mixed-feeling immigration to the United States from the Mexico to which her great-grandparents immigrated long ago with all the hopes & trappings of an American Dream (remembering that the U.S. is but one of the countries in the Americas). In this episodic essay, Rose Mary recalls

> my maternal grandma, Lorís, tells us stories all the time. She tells us about her father's departure for Mexico. How she, her sisters and her mother had to wait for him in Lebanon until they received the go-ahead to leave; not a moment before they had obtained the coveted fortune that this new promised land offered them. (3)

And food, too,

> My grandma remembers the boarding school and the principal in charge; how she gave up all the food that was donated to them. The *kibbeh* trays that my great-grandmother prepared for her children were distributed amongst all the girls at the school. The principal would die a few years after her belly swelled like a ball from starvation. Grannie Hanne takes the walnuts out into the yard. She wants them dry to make chicken and rice. But I'm hungry and I sneak out. I casually walk from one side of the patio to the other and every turn, I steal some; I'm sure no one will notice. After a few hours, my grannie scolds me. If I wanted nuts, I should have asked for them, she tells me. I can't understand how she finds me out. The image remains vivid in my memory, accompanied the word "betrayal," although an internal voice forgives some of the weight and adds the word disobedience. Still, something inside me remains uneasy. When I repeat the exercise,

"betrayal" returns. I always deeply adored my grannie; My grandma
I learned to love and treasure through her stories. (3–4)

Betrayal is a key leitmotif of Rose Mary's accompanying musings
about immigration & politics, though not of either culture, not of her
family, but certainly of the promises that immigration to either "new"
country was supposed to have kept!

The summers of my childhood are spent in Tampico; my grandparents arrived there when they left Lebanon. There are my uncles, my
cousins; my maternal family. Tampico is humid. My mother leaves us
in our underwear and a T-shirt. This is her way of saving us from the
heat. My sister prefers to be dressed. Her sense of her shame cannot
let her tolerate this. She cries, but my mother ignores her. I attempt to
turn on the fans at full speed, but my grandmother forbids it; she says
they can break down. In response, I throw a tantrum and tear off a
piece of her curtains with my teeth. I can still feel the pull of the fabric
on my teeth to this day. My grandmother doesn't love me nor I her.
She is unreasonable, her requests are absurd. My father calls us on
Sundays and I cling to the phone like it's the last foothold in a sink-
hole. The city's heat and ideology are suffocating. At noon, everyone
stops their activities to take a nap; even the service girl does. I sit in
the living room, rebelliously turn on the fan at full speed and read the
newspaper. In Tampico, they only report yellow news: rapes, murders
and crimes of passion. Now, they call them femicides. I wait patiently
for my mother to wake up because it is only in the afternoons that the
possibility of playing with my cousins arises. On Sundays, we go to
the beach. It is the best day in the world when we are in the port,
which welcomed the English at the beginning of the twentieth century
who came to expropriate oil. Back then, Tampico was the most important port in Latin America. Now, even Houstonians can't find it on a
map. Despite the two being sister cities. Despite looking at the same
gulf. Despite its closeness. My aunts make grape leaves, my mother
tabouleh and *hummus* with *tahini*. The beach is not the beach without
Lebanese food. The tent that my uncles set up week after week is red
and green; the shade it casts is heavenly. The surf is rough and the
sound of the waves envelops us in a kind of spell. We stay until sunset
and by then, most people are gone. Upon our return, we wash the
car and rinse the saline crust that has built up on our skin with
the thick jet of water from my grandmother's glaucous hose. My
brothers, my cousins and I laugh as we brush the sand off ourselves.
The night arrives imperceptibly. My grandmother dines on black
olives with Arabic bread, as she has done every night of her life.

The darkness lulls us with the sound of crickets. The next day it returns us to hell.

Finding the culture and traditions of Lebanon "out of context" begat betrayal of feelings and self-determination which the "new" country (Mexico) might promise to her grandmother, even before the socio-political betrayals by both Mexico and the U.S. related to Rose Mary's own immigration from one to the other.

[After arrival in the new country] my grandmother meets Emilio Portes Gil. They play chess every time he visits Tampico, and he always asks my grandmother for his favorite dish: *tahini* with parsley. My grandmother is still young, but when she reaches adulthood, she is introduced to Juan Nemer, her future husband. She is attracted to another young man, but great-grandfather insists that Juan Nemer must be her fiancé.

Yet, perhaps there is hope amid all the political and philosophical mayhem, via the newest generation, via focus on plurality of languages, cultures, traditions and the all-important, food and food preparation, in order to transcend what earlier generations have endured and establish a multi-identity of diversity in harmony!

[My granddaughter is] Samara Rose. She is an American by birth, even if she does not fully belong to this country. I speak to her in Spanish and observe that she begins to understand some words. She is a restless but serene baby. When I see her, she extends her arms to me and an involuntary complicity is generated between us. She awkwardly points out what she needs. I guess at her wishes and she has no choice but to settle for what I am able to offer her. I want her to know that she carries Lebanese, English and Mexican blood. I want her to learn to cook the dishes of those countries. I want her to understand that there is a past, and within it, her grandparents and her great-grandparents. (19)

Notes

1   Numerous sources, a few of which are listed in the Bibliography of this essay, support this generalization.
2   Her publications and other accomplishments are detailed on the web at Rose Mary Salum—Writer & Editor.
3   An as-yet otherwise published essay in either Spanish or English, Rose Mary's own translation of her essay follows this chapter in this

collection. Rose Mary & I discussed at some length the best translation for her title, *Filminas,* literally a *filmstrip* in English. She suggested *slides;* I initially countered with *snapshots* to give the ideas of the episodic nature of the essay, then *moving picture frames* to get the idea of a continuing saga but that felt unwieldly. *Cinéma verité,* described by Wikipedia as "a style of documentary filmmaking, invented by Edgar Morin and Jean Rouch, inspired by Dziga Vertov's theory about Kino-Pravda combines improvisation with the use of the camera to unveil truth or highlight subjects hidden behind crude reality" actually came the closest to the concept she intended but requires a double French translation (*true cinema*) and film vernacular footnote.

4   Álvarez, Linda. "Colonization, Food and the Practice of Eating." *Food Empowerment Project.* Colonization, Food, and the Practice of Eating— Food Empowerment Project (foodispower.org).

5   As I have explained elsewhere in writing and verbally, as translator, I overtly chose to rename the translated tome, *Spaces In-Between,* rather than the literal, *In-Between the Spaces,* for several reasons related to the duality of the word, *entre,* in Spanish, which is variously translated to English as *between* or *among.* Likewise with the title of the story about an eating disorder, I chose *Goodbye!* rather than *farewell* or a similar translation of *despedida* to emphasize the finality (death) in many of these cases. Since my philosophy of translation is informed by the concept of messages, not words per se, as well as the sometimes-controversial view of some translators that a translation is something new in itself. Thus, I felt these differences were important points to make. I'm not sure that Rose Mary has ever forgiven me, however. Furthermore, in this essay, I will not attempt to translate the names or content of foodstuffs and dishes from Lebanese Arabic, as the references suffice for the presence of said vocabulary—the actual description is somewhat superfluous.

Bibliography

Álvarez, Linda. "Colonization, Food and the Practice of Eating." *Food Empowerment Project.* Colonization, Food, and the Practice of Eating— Food Empowerment Project (foodispower.org)

Isphording, Ingo E. "What Drives Language Proficiency of Immigrants?" Germany: *IZA World of Labor.* Aug. 2015.

McWhorter, John. "How Immigration Changes Language." *The Atlantic.* Dec. 14, 2015. Multiethnolects: How Immigrants Invent New Ways of Speaking a Language—The Atlantic.

Salum, Rose Mary. *El agua que mece el silencio.* Madrid: Vaso Roto Ediciones, 2016.

——. *Entre los Espacios.* México, D.F.: Editorial Tierra Firme, 2002.

——. *Spaces In-Between.* Debra D. Andrist, translator. Houston: Copper Hands, 2005.

——. Rose Mary Salum—Writer & Editor. Web.

Toppelberg, Claudio O. and Collins, Brian A. "Language, Culture & Adaptation in Children." Language, Culture, and Adaptation in Immigrant Children (harvard.edu).

17

Filminas: An Essay

ROSE MARY SALUM

It is Friday, October 2nd, 1998. I am about to take a shower when I hear my husband answering the phone. I can hear that he's nervous; his voice sounds disturbed. This immediately sets off something in my gut; an explosion that shoots tiny needles into my body. Something is wrong. It's ten o'clock and my children are already at school; we left home early like every other day, listening to our usual classical music. My husband's voice drifts further and further away . . . just before it disappears, he hangs up. He approaches me and, with eyes open wide, he tells me that our thirteen-year-old nephew has been kidnapped. He is the same age as our son. He has the same last name.

My husband carries on in a state that is becoming contagious. He tells me that he just spoke with his father and that we should leave the country. The very notion injects a cloud of white air into my head that paralyzes my brain. I am intoxicated by the adrenaline. All I can manage is the realization that what I have conceived as my future, what I created and nurtured with devotion since my childhood, has been cut into pieces. What follows is to pack and to wait for the afternoon to pick up my children from school and head to the airport. My rebellious and analytical nature disappears as all my future projects are being mutilated.

The situation in Mexico is overwhelming. A man rises in fame, nicknamed the "ear cutter," who has earned his moniker by kidnapping people and dismembering them. Criminality in Mexico City reaches unprecedented figures. Years later, López Obrador[1] would come to power, rising in prominence by initially making fun of people who march the streets dressed in white, protesting the violence. "It is a march of nitwits," he says, laughing at what he now calls the upper class, bourgeois or "fifís" now that he's been elected president of the Mexican Republic. Still, all social strata are affected by this wave of crime; all of Mexico is represented in this demonstration, regardless of the government's myopia. The ransoms that are paid for family members range from five hundred pesos to millions of dollars. The situation is appalling. What is true is that only a few people with significant means have access to private security. The government is unable to guarantee our citizens' lives, a primary guarantee of the Rousseau's Social Contract.[2]

My children leave school and are surprised to see us. There were certainly no plans for the day that included moving out of the country, and they tell us as much, distraught. The way to the airport is a trail of tears and anxiety. The pain of my children clings to my skin like a chewy paste; it's impossible to take it off. At ten in the morning, I live in Mexico; at eight at night, in the United States. One can't begin to contemplate sleep . . . This is a nightmare. The question is how does one open one's eyes to get out of it?

I am sitting in my childhood classroom. The sun has painted diagonal lines along my classmates' desks. One side looks shaded, the other bright. We seem attentive in spite of the teacher's drowsy, monotonous voice. He tells us about pre-Hispanic cultures, about our common past, about our origins. There is something about it that I do not recognize; it is an artifice imposed on me, as it does not fit with the stories that I have been told at home about my past. Something is dislocated. In the void of this detachment, my parents and grandparents' versions of our origins are superimposed on each other. They tell us about the Phoenicians, the First World War, the famine, the ships leaving Beirut bound for America, their ultimate decision to stay in Mexico, the stops in Cuba, Tampico, Veracruz and other ports, the need to assimilate so as not to be called Turks, the bewilderment inflicted by someone else's language. The teacher tries to call our attention but I'm not interested in his stories. They don't sound real, nor do mine.

I am fascinated by my grannie's crooked finger. Her name is Hanne; my father's mother. She is an educated woman and was punished for it. She knows five languages: Arabic, French, Spanish, Italian and English. My curly hair emulates hers, my chubby legs take after her genetics. I am proud to look like such a woman. Over the years, I understand why. In contrast, my maternal grandma, Lorís, tells us stories all the time. She tells us about her father's departure for Mexico. How she, her sisters and her mother had to wait for him in Lebanon until they received the go-ahead to leave; not a moment before they had obtained the coveted fortune that this new promised land offered them. My grandma remembers the boarding school and the principal in charge; how she gave up all the food that was donated to them. The *kibbeh* trays that my great-grandmother prepared for her children were distributed amongst all the girls at the school. The principal would die a few years after her belly swelled like a ball from starvation. Grannie Hanne takes the walnuts out into the yard. She wants them dry to make chicken and rice. But I'm hungry and I sneak out. I casually walk from one side of the patio to the other and every turn, I steal some; I'm sure no one will notice. After a few hours, my grannie scolds me. If I wanted nuts, I should have asked for them, she tells me. I can't understand how she finds me out. The image remains vivid in my memory, accompanied the word "betrayal," although an internal voice forgives some of the weight and adds the word disobedience. Still, something inside me remains uneasy. When I repeat the exercise, "betrayal" returns. I always deeply adored my grannie; My grandma I learned to love and treasure through her stories.

The first weekend in the United States and all I can feel is a dark mass inside my chest. I was only just an insect that was walking on the cement streets of Mexico and a swift wind has blown me onto the "gringo" sidewalk. Such is human vulnerability. The degree of control that I can exercise in my life is zero. The United States has wide streets but lacks a measure of chaos. Its order irritates my senses. Everything looks like plastic; it *is* plastic. Women speak in high tones, their voices emulating parrots. It is their way of pleasing everyone around them. Men repeatedly wish us a good day. The sounds hurt my eardrums; the light, my corneas. Everything feels like a huge vacuum, a bubble without oxygen. The space cannot contain anything; not even air to float inside it.

I worry about my children. In the United States, they are no longer someone's children, cousins, or grandchildren. They will be perceived as "wetbacks." If we are to endure this country, it will be in the legal way; the idea of remaining undocumented is inconceivable. Damned be this moment when the country that once welcomed my grandparents now forsakes me. It no longer cherishes the most precious thing there is: life. Mexico has betrayed me, as it has betrayed the hundreds and thousands of others who have disappeared, their families, who mourn the absence of their loved ones every day, and the dead, about whom I am not sure are resting in their graves. Presidents allow themselves to be bribed by organized crime; corruption is an essential part of the Republic. Whoever complains about insecurity gets ridiculed by their peers and leaders alike. They are silver-spooned people, they say, without acknowledging that violence does not understand class nor origin. I come to realize that I will not be able to finish my degree; the one I started late in life given "my traditions." Or rather, the traditions of my grandparents, who were people raised in the country. More specifically, a misunderstanding of what it means to be a decent person: confinement as a symbol of modesty, of decorum. After so many years under the tutelage of my parents, trapped by my status as a decent young lady born to Lebanese immigrants in Mexico, I had reclaimed the right to education for myself, stealing time for my studies. And yet all that was about to vanish.

Sometimes I walk home. The school bus leaves daily at three in the afternoon. When my class schedule allows me to leave earlier instead of staying in the schoolyard to talk, I walk home. I'm fifteen, and I walk along the sidewalks of *Amores* Street, backpack on my shoulder, white tennis shoes, thigh-high socks hugging my calves, finally free to think. Here is a kind of freedom that I love; it has made me addicted to those walks. In that space, I own myself. I am not the daughter of a conservative family nor the student at a nun's school. Nobody there forces me to do anything I don't want to. I'm just me; a young woman who walks, lost in thought, enjoying my surroundings and every thought that comes unexpectedly, my speed, my rhythm, where I'm going . . . It would be impossible to have that at home or at school; impossible to share my concerns with the family. All I ever get is a resounding "no." I can't understand this many negatives. Over the years, I attribute it to a lack of resources but then I understand that fear lies at the bottom of making those decisions: no, because this and that could happen. No, because you are a good family girl. No, because we cannot calculate the consequences of a decision of that magnitude. No, because after that, we will not be able to control you. No, because I don't want to . . . As if studying with the nuns of San Antonio could be threatening to anyone or anything. As if the hymen that I have never seen and cannot even be sure I have is what gives me value. As if reading were synonymous with prostitution. As if thinking were leprosy. When I walk home alone, none of those thoughts crush me.

I don't feel free in the United States. That idea is a mere artifice, it's a flag that the country waves to convince its inhabitants to give up 30% of their earnings in taxes and sacrifice their privacy, watching them at all times. It is true that their bridges lighten traffic, that the streets are clean, that there is a system of laws. But there is an omnipotent eye that sees everything once you are connected to the internet. And against the will of the powerful, their interests and subjectivity, there is no defense.

Each of us has a different version of October 2nd. My children remember it perfectly. At least, that's what they assure me. My memories are similar to theirs. My husband's disagree diametrically. None of our memoirs pays homage to 1968's, however. Personal tragedy has obliterated our relationship to the national and international history. The memory of the three hundred dead in the Plaza de Tlatelolco overlaps with the loss of our home. My cousins are part of that official figure. And though I never met them, I know about them from the stories they tell at home. My aunt, whose face I have forgotten, welcomed the students into her room. She fed their desires for justice, my grandfather says at some of the Sunday gatherings. If they died, it was because she stoked the fires at student meetings, says one of my uncles, the blame is hers. They had communist ideas and did not know their parents, says another of my uncles. They got it into their heads that the parents were a mere biological accident and they believed it, my dad tells me as we walk to the *Hacienda* club, a club that is subsidized by the Mexican government and where my father has been the tennis league champion for years. They disappeared and we never heard from them again, he tells me. There is a belief that the oldest survived, but no one knows for sure. *Fued* and his wife never saw them again, despite having paid detectives and bribed contacts within the power strata. What if they were seeking justice? I wonder. But I must believe otherwise and try to erase the sentiment that just crossed my mind. What is certain is that my family has their share of absent members and they are willing to say a number of things to each other, as long as no one disappears again. Although I no longer live in my country, the disappearance of two strangers who carry my blood connects me to the national tragedy, yet it makes me feel nothing. Not even pain for them. Now the missing have surpassed the most unthinkable figures. Communists or not, "fifís" or proletarians, rich or poor, people are taken out of circulation against everyone's will. Mexico is a swamp that swallows its people, and we are still in a state of denial. There's no place like home.

I am sitting in a cafe with some friends and we're enveloped in the patio's bustle. People are animated. From the balcony, you can see some orange clouds floating in a peaceful, light blue sea. It is a country of immigrants, they tell me, it is a very powerful country, they tell me, the laws apply to everyone equally, they tell me. A gap opens between ideas and reality. The first American immigration law was conceived in 1792 and limits citizenship to white and free people. The ideals to which one aspires in the country are not fraternity and equality but life and happiness. Although only for whites. Benjamin Franklin said it well at the time of him: neither blacks nor browns are welcome in the country. Only Europeans. Hence, the Statue of Liberty faces East. And since then, only part of the gap has narrowed.

The summers of my childhood are spent in Tampico; my grandparents arrived there when they left Lebanon. There are my uncles, my cousins; my maternal family. Tampico is humid. My mother leaves us in our underwear and a T-shirt. This is her way of saving us from the heat. My sister prefers to be dressed. Her sense of her shame cannot let her tolerate this. She cries, but my mother ignores her. I attempt to turn on the fans at full speed, but my grandmother forbids it; she says they can break down. In response, I throw a tantrum and tear off a piece of her curtains with my teeth. I can still feel the pull of the fabric on my teeth to this day. My grandmother doesn't love me nor I her. She is unreasonable, her requests are absurd. My father calls us on Sundays and I cling to the phone like it's the last foothold in a sink-hole. The city's heat and ideology are suffocating. At noon, everyone stops their activities to take a nap; even the service girl does. I sit in the living room, rebelliously turn on the fan at full speed and read the newspaper. In Tampico, they only report yellow news: rapes, murders and crimes of passion. Now, they call them femicides. I wait patiently for my mother to wake up because it is only in the afternoons that the possibility of playing with my cousins arises. On Sundays, we go to the beach. It is the best day in the world when we are in the port, which welcomed the English at the beginning of the twentieth century who came to expropriate oil. Back then, Tampico was the most important port in Latin America. Now, even Houstonians can't find it on a map. Despite the two being sister cities. Despite looking at the same gulf. Despite its closeness. My aunts make grape leaves, my mother tabouleh and hummus with tahini. The beach is not the beach without Lebanese food. The tent that my uncles set up week after week is red and green; the shade it casts is heavenly. The surf is rough and the sound of the waves envelops us in a kind of spell. We stay until sunset, and by then most people are gone. Upon our return, we wash the car and rinse the saline crust that has built on our skin with the thick jet from my grandmother's glaucous hose. My brothers, my cousins and I laugh as we brush the sand off ourselves. The night arrives imperceptibly. My grandmother dines on black olives with Arabic bread, as she has done every night of her life. The darkness lulls us with the sound of crickets. The next day it returns us to hell.

I remember it like it was yesterday. We all arise to a shared night-mare. On January 19, we live within a democracy that minds its institutions. On January 20, the president of the most powerful country in the world dedicates himself body and soul to erode them through Twitter. The FBI is made up of a bunch of criminals; the media of liars; Muller's investigation, a witch hunt. The power strata protects itself. It regenerates himself and adapts to its own circumstances. The country loses credibility day by day, and its moral authority in the world becomes laughable. The truth is gone, and it is hard to conceive that anyone else could share it with you. The country is a tennis court split in two by a net where the ball, though it comes and goes, fails to topple the division. The white line that delimits the country divides families seeking asylum. Our sense of unity is a thing of the past, it belongs to the history books that will never be read because it is being written on Instagram. Especially now that our thinking is fragmented every day, thanks to social networks. They now dictate our values, what's cool, which only fuels our collective narcissism. In the meantime, we are watched and censored. The silence that surrounds this situation scandalizes me and I don't even know how to begin to denounce it. My words rot in a sea of indifference. The first chapter of *Black Mirror,* that series so distressing because of its accuracy, opens with an angry man. His anger is part of the performance that those in charge of creating content for networks offer, receiving in return an eye that sees everything. The air brings new winds, and my anger serves only to fuel the collective entertainment.

The street where I grew up is named after Pythagoras. Number 20, Pythagoras St. The street where I live in the United States is called West Oak. In my mind, Pythagoras is the quintessential mathematician; oak trees don't interest me. I know that in Jungian language, they have important connotations: the tree as a source of life, as the archetypal figure that usually inhabits the dream world or the symbol that fascinates so many people. The tree as a representation of the cyclical, as the channel that communicates the three levels of the cosmos; the underground, where Persephone ingests the pomegranate seeds, the trunk on the surface of the earth that the Phoenicians use as channels to promote trade, and the leaves that sow ideas in the sky. My stay in this country has forgotten the symbols, it only brings work. The US lives to work. This is how *its* system is designed. Everything is achieved when day passes from nine to five; the rest does not count. This is the only way to get health insurance, friendships, loans. I remember the house number from Pythagoras vividly. I can still repeat my home's phone number from memory because, back then, you kept the information inside yourself. Pythagoras' floors are black and have white polka dots scattered throughout. It is those white spots that awaken my imagination. In some blocks, you can see sea foam, in others, a lost girl. A silver line separates the dark tiles. When I am up-to-the-brim with boredom, I follow it with my feet, playing rooster, hen. On Pythagoras, my mother welcomes us with surprises: she makes strawberries with cream or bananas with caramel. She sometimes cooks beef and on those days, I hide it under the rice or throw it on the ground. The meat has a serious, dark flavor. It tastes like an old man, I think. My father hides his candy under the seat of his Dodge truck. My brothers and I know this and he knows that we know, because we often steal them. The Dodge truck is like his office. When we accompany him, he rewards us with a visit to the Twinky Wonder factory that is located on the other side of the forge where my father and my uncle work. He buys Twinkies for us and we devour them, even though we like the Ho-Hos, chocolate cakes, cream and jam made in Mexico more. Inside the plant, there are two ovens that melt the metals as if they were chocolate. There, my father became an alchemist; everything transforms. His company: *Recuperadora Metalúrgica*. Over the years, the factory disappears, like so many other companies started by Mexicans. Only industries of foreign origin have survived. On Pythagoras, the confusion begins: am I Mexican or am I Lebanese? These doubts are deepened on West Oak; am I Lebanese, Mexican or American? On that street, I learn that it does not matter to others; they have already classified people under the criteria of color and race. My questions, my search for identity, run up against the pre-established catalog; my internal problems are obsolete in the eyes of my environment. The color of my skin, my features, my accent differ from the mean and end up determining the rest of my stay in exile. In the first months after our arrival, we see a documentary that talks about races. The Lebanese are the only ethnic group in the Middle East that considers itself white. After 9/11, we are all terrorists. A customs officer stops me at the airport. Where are your surnames from? he asks me. From Mexico, I lie, relying on my Mexican passport. That's not true, he answers angrily. I remain silent. Where are your parents from, the customs officer asks again. From Mexico, I reply. And your grandparents and great-grandparents? From Mexico, I repeat. The officer loses his patience and drops his hand on the pistol hanging from his belt. My throat swells like a melon and I hold my tears. The man storms out of his office to bring in someone else. I peek in to see if my kids are okay in the waiting room. They are not moving, they are glued to each other and their eyes have doubled in size. The officers return with a string of questions, but are hit by a blank screen. Nerves have taken possession of me and I am unable to remember anything. The Oak of the West does not do justice to its symbolism. It does not connect any world. Pythagoras only offers longing, nostalgia, and now, problems.

It has been 20 years. Twenty laps around the sun on this globe. Twenty years of long discomfort before being able to settle. Twenty ways of seeing the world, twenty steps to get where we are. This time has been important to observe the evolution of the country. In this time, I have been able to witness its movements and reach one or two conclusions about the character of the nation that is now called home. I follow the line of life that beats in its people, observe its ups and downs in its recent divisive years. I see two tectonic plates in the process of separation, two groups attacking each other incessantly, two ideologies clashing. I see a country divided both economically and ideologically. The division arises from its lodges. It is born from perceptions, from beliefs so misplaced that reality has been affected. Up until 2017, what I perceived as true gave me a feeling of stability, it was a playground where common facts are shared. The discourse was relatively unified and we all agreed that, within that playground, the color blue is, incredible as it may seem now, blue. We know that if the yard fills up at certain times of the day, we can refer to it as a full yard. When it is empty, we can verify it without much effort. But those times are in the past. It happens one day and from that moment on, we cannot agree on the information that is offered to us on a daily basis, and all because someone changed the dynamic and decided that although the patio is half empty, we are going to say that it is full. Record-breakingly full. Period.

Why insist on one's origins? Why the need to stand in the land of the ancestors and from there make our judgments? Every time I address these questions in my mind, I come to a silent wall. There is a degree of emotionality that blinds me. It is the same blindness that I acquire when I am in Lebanon. I have only been there twice but when I am there, I recognize everything. I recognize the food, the codes, the way its people communicate with each other. I can decipher body gestures. I know what the tone of the words convey, even though I don't understand them because my grandparents and parents spoke Arabic for the sole purpose that we not understand. The third generation loses the language, I read in an article that reflects on exiles and uprooting. I realize that I am the third generation to grow up in the "new" country, and I am already part of the statistics. I only have the residue of sounds and words. I protest. His intention when he arrived in America was to prevent us from being discriminated against, my father explains, laughing at my grandparents. His reasoning tries to reassure me. And it does, until I move to the United States and I am forced to talk to someone from Lebanon in English because I have lost the language, until I become the subject of a certain contempt, because I was not born in Lebanon, until I find myself avoiding questions that inquire about my race in official questionnaires. When I am in Beirut and they speak to me in Arabic, fully expecting an answer in kind, something about me mourns the loss. I suffer from a generational longing. I force myself to shut it up. There is nothing left to do but deal with that which has never been mine. I am not going back to Arabic, not when I have a genetic clumsiness when it comes to languages. The postmodernists argue that all truths are partial, that all ways of representing a truth are legitimate. All speech must be heard; from the one where we're informed eggs and beans were had for breakfast, accompanied by a selfie and the eloquent phrase "yummmm," to the one where we're told the world was created by UFOs. There are entire communities that get their news from social media. Not only in Mexico or the United States, but throughout the world. The need to capture the attention of others at the cost of privacy, of the most basic intimacy, has disrupted social codes and the way people interact. In short, it's cost us our mental health.

El destierro trae consigo la desmemoria. Es una desmemoria impuesta. Sartre dice que la realidad existe gracias a la mirada del Otro. Pero si esa mirada nace de la ignorancia y hay que portarla con camisa de fuerza, la realidad se desvirtúa. En Estados Unidos soy una Hispanic. Así, en inglés. He buscado todo tipo de etimologías para darle vuelta a una etiqueta que se me antoja peyorativa, pero vuelvo al mismo lugar: Hispanic. ¿Saben los estadounidenses exactamente a qué se refieren con ese término o sólo repiten como nosotros repetimos tantas palabras desconociendo su origen, las razones por las que esas expresiones han proliferado perpetuando el dolor entre nosotros? ¿Saben de la escisión que han causado en la sociedad? ¿Son conscientes de arrancar de un tirón la identidad de lo que conforma la esencia del país, es decir, del inmigrante? Las respuestas pierden importancia siempre y cuando esos grupos puedan ser manejados en términos del mercado y el grado de su consumo sea satisfactorio para la economía. No importa si mi presencia puede ofrecer algo bueno al país. Aquí nada importa. Sólo el color.

La inseguridad en México va en aumento. Los asesinatos, los femi-nicidios, los desaparecidos siguen nutriendo las cifras de forma alarmante. La violencia no cesa. Al final de esta década se han regis-trado 8.493 homicidios, 9.6% más que el año anterior, según datos del Sistema Nacional de Seguridad Pública. Los políticos nos reiteran que todo va a cambiar. Yo me pregunto en dónde se localiza ese futuro especulativo. Las soluciones propuestas por el nuevo gobierno no funcionan. Seguimos matándonos entre nosotros. Dañándonos. Desapareciendo a los demás. No importa el gobernante en turno. Nosotros a matarnos que al n y al cabo llevamos el México bronco en cada uno. Y eso hay que presumirlo.

Exile brings with it forgetfulness. It is an imposed forgetfulness. Sartre says that reality exists in the gaze of the Other. But if that look is born out of ignorance and you have to wear it with a straitjacket, reality is distorted. In the United States, I am Hispanic. I have looked for all kinds of etymologies to turn a label that strikes me as pejora-tive, but I return to the same place: Hispanic. Do Americans know exactly what they mean by that term? Or are they just repeating it, as we repeat so many words, ignoring their origin or the reasons why these expressions have proliferated, perpetuating the pain among us? Do they know about the split that you have caused in society? Are they aware they are tearing off the essence of this country's identity; that is, of the immigrant? The answers don't matter as long as these groups can be managed neatly in market terms, and their consumption is satisfactory for the standards of the economy. It does not matter if my presence can offer something good to the country. Here, nothing matters, only your color and bank account.

Insecurity in Mexico is on the rise; murders, femicides and disappearances continue to inflate the figures in an alarming way. The violence does not stop. At the end of this decade, 8,493 homicides have been registered, 9.6% more than the previous year, according to data from the National Public Security System. Politicians continually promise that everything is going to change. I wonder where these promises are located. The solutions proposed by the new government do not work; we keep killing each other, damaging each other, disappearing each other. It does not matter who happens to be in charge, we are going to kill ourselves off because, at the end of the day, we are all proud to carry the "wild Mexico" inside, as if it were something to show off.

Now, I realize why the lies baffle me. When I listen to them, my first impulse is to go to a psychologist to cure this madness and find my way back to a state of inner silence impervious to what happens outside. It is not borne out of fear meeting someone who might try to convince me that, in fact, the patios I observe are full, whether I like it or not. But I have given up the search because no doctor is qualified to correct the political problems of the world. Would that I could turn my face towards some superior and beg him to return the waters to their course; ask for severe punishment for those who lie, who try to convince me of the non-existent, of what common sense imposes on me and they deny. These types of situations tend to silence me, to paralyze my mind as a deer when in danger. Like Eduardo Nicol,[3] I think that anguish occurs when thoughts are lost in a formless void without outlines or nests; something stable to hold on to. What can be said when we no longer share the same reality? To whom does one extend the bond of dialogue and receive congruent answers in return? My paralysis is not normal; seemingly everyone has something to say about this situation on social networks, and my silence only makes me invisible. I go back to my desperate thoughts. Since when does lying keep me awake? A series of memories are filtering in my memory: my personal work on that subject, my undergraduate thesis on Socrates vs. the sophists, and my master's thesis on truth in alchemy; my comments on truthfulness in politics. Such an obsession with the subject will have to be addressed.

Today, reality adapts to one's own visions, as do the algorithms of social networks and the excellent work with which the internet manages to adjust everyday life, expectations and ideology of the average person. The facts, the verifiable truth, is replaced by what is perceived. The ability to communicate is lost. Or better yet, the internet does not reflect reality, on the contrary, it bends it until it presents it as one more expression of its infinite chatter. Freedom is then a noun that only inhabits the universe of utopias.

My great grandfather is the first Hudson car supplier in Tampico. Most of them are rented out to the English who came to the port in the early twentieth century to extract oil from the Gulf. They pay with gold coins that my great-grandfather deposits in sacks of rice. When the Mexican Revolution begins, my great-grandfather does not leave the city despite the fact that the United States sends a ship to rescue those who decide to save themselves. His interests are there, and he does not intend to abandon them, having lived through poverty and famine in Lebanon. Soon enough the Spanish arrive, bringing European bakery in their wake. The city promises changes. After several years, my grandmother meets Emilio Portes Gil. They play chess every time he visits Tampico, and always asks my grandmother for his favorite dish: *tahini* with parsley. My grandmother is still young, but when she reaches adulthood, she is introduced to Juan Nemer, her future husband. She is attracted to another young man, but great-grandfather insists that Juan Nemer must be her fiancé. Upon the death of my great-grandfather, the only male inherits his fortune, as dictated by the customs of the Middle East. Life in Mexico is just circumstantial; its laws are not to be obeyed. Gender equality is not even a coherent thought in their world. Whatever use would that be?

The internet as the laboratory of falsehood is successful to the extent that it encourages and protects anonymity. The Platonic approach to human justice from invisibility, which I had questioned in my early years, has now been more than resolved. The contempt for the truth, the fraud in ignoring it, the exaltation of emotions over reason and the arbitrary use of language become an alienation that makes dialogue impossible. The displacement of reason by emotions corrupts language. It gives way to a new and more radical way of irrational thinking that no longer draws its content from refined thought, or from the rigor of any tradition. As the muses tell Hesiod, we now refine the way to say false things that sound like truth. And in English.

I wonder if the future will bring some sort of return to truth? Computers and artificial intelligence are laying fertile ground for such a thought. The digital world is Manichean and doesn't allow for any of our subjectivity. Then again, it sometimes seems like our own reason's wishful thinking betraying its most intimate and obsessive feelings.

October 2, 2018. It is Tuesday, and I have to pick up my grand-daughter, Samara Rose. She is an American by birth, even if she does not fully belong to this country. I speak to her in Spanish and observe that she begins to understand some words. She is a restless but serene baby. When I see her, she extends her arms to me and an involuntary complicity is generated between us. She awkwardly points out what she needs. I guess at her wishes and she has no choice but to settle for what I am able to offer her. I want her to know that she carries Lebanese, English and Mexican blood. I want her to learn to cook the dishes of those countries. I want her to understand that there is a past, and within it, her grandparents and her great-grandparents. But she only lives in the moment. Nothing mortifies her, neither identity nor origin. She only wants milk when she is hungry and for me to take her to see the fountains that adorn the apartment complex where she lives when I visit her. She has renewed my ways of loving, as well as the need to live without intellectual or physical artifice. Although there is an important possibility that in her future she will not have to deal with the devastating effects of femicide in Mexico, she may have to face the veiled violence, abuse and mistreatment that lie latent within US society. Or maybe she'll be a product of her own deception. But we don't know that yet. I would like to think that everything is going to change in both countries in the next twenty years but there are no guar-antees. Nothing that happens around my girl, however, complicates her life. Everything is as simple as a toy on the floor or her stuffed doll that her mother has named Tuki. The rest is irrelevant. She instructs and loves me. For now, that's all that matters.

Notes

Unpublished until now, this essay is Rose Mary's own translation from Spanish or English. She & I discussed at some length the best transla-tion for her title, *Filminas*, literally a *filmstrip* in English. She suggested *slides*; I initially countered with *snapshots* to give the ideas of the episodic nature of the essay, then *moving picture frames* to get the idea of a continuing saga but that felt unwieldly. *Cinéma verité*, described by Wikipedia as "a style of documentary filmmaking, invented by Edgar Morin and Jean Rouch, inspired by Dziga Vertov's theory about Kino-Pravda. It combines improvisation with the use of the camera to unveil truth or highlight subjects hidden behind crude reality" actually came the closest to the concept she intended but requires a double French translation (*true cinema*) and film vernacular footnote.

1   Andrés Manuel López Obrador, three-time but non-concurrent president of Mexico, including at the time of publication of *Sustenance for the Body & Soul.*

2   *The Social Contract* by Jean-Jacques Rousseau is a 1762 book in which Rousseau theorized about the best way to establish a political community in the face of the problems of commercial society, which he had already identified in his *Discourse on Inequality.*

3   "Nicol was one of a group of Spanish philosophers exiled after the fall of Republican Spain who went to Mexico . . . In his book of 1961, Nicol identified a paradox in José Vasconcelos's concept of the 'cosmic race' by noting that *indigenismo* and negritude are racial concepts put forth as worthy of special attention at the same time as Vasconcelos holds the ideal of purging racial consciousness from society." Nicol, Eduardo. "Mexican Metaphysician." *World Biographical Encyclopedia.* prabook.com. Web.

18

Real Recipes and Willed Eroticism in Isabel Allende's *Afrodita*

STEPHEN MILLER

Around the turn of the 21st century, Isabel Allende's literary reputation began to be discussed a lot in an unflattering way: not, to be sure, in terms of being a bestselling author but rather as related to the criteria of the high-culture literary establishment. The matter was highlighted in Allende's August 31, 2003 interview with Leila Guerriero in the *La Nación* of Buenos Aires, the acknowledged newspaper of record for Argentina, and with Buenos Aires itself being one of the two or three Latin American capitals which have a long and strong claim on cultural leadership and prestige in the entire Spanish-speaking world. Moreover, *La Nación* has been continuously published since the last third of the nineteenth century. During those 150 years, columns by prestigious literary writers from both sides of the Atlantic, articles about and interviews of them have continuously appeared in the pages of *La Nación*. What appears in those pages has counted and counts in a very special way, just as have in the past and do in the present, comparable writings in the pages of the *New York Times* or, crossing the Atlantic, leading periodicals in the United Kingdom and Spain. In the case of the most prestigious writers—and Allende is one of them under any circumstances—translations, interviews and reviews of their works are at the center of today's cosmopolitan literary world produced by globalization's patterns of travel and migration among the countries today that were once part of the former Spanish and British empires.

To understand more precisely Allende's literary reputation, a close examination of certain parts of the Guerreiro interview in *La Nación* is useful. In response to Guerreiro's question, "How do you react to the opinions of those who claim your writing is lightweight and pretentious?"[1] Allende stated she did not care and gave pointedly and self-interestedly the historical context of that kind of criticism from her viewpoint: "When the possibility arose in 2002 that I could be awarded the Chilean National Literary Prize for that year, horrible things were said" and "The people who said them were failed writers, who did not sell even one book."[2] Then Guerreiro insisted. She inquired about a specific criticism of Allende and Mexican writer, Ángeles Mastretta's, writing by the Chilean-born, high-literature prestigious, and much-traveled Roberto Bolaño, who died at age fifty in Barcelona about a month-and-a-half before the Guerreiro–Allende interview. With his customary acerbity and arrogance, Bolaño had contrasted himself with Mastretta and Allende in an issue of the Mexican edition of *Playboy*: "not even in my worst drunks have I lost a certain minimum lucidity, a sense of prosody and rhythm, a rejection of plagiarism and mediocrity."

Now the sometimes opprobrium between one generation of authors and another, between financially successful ones and those who are not in the same generation is age-old, and a critic so prestigious as the late Harold Bloom in the *Anxiety of Influence* studied in perhaps the most scientific of terms aspects of that rivalry. But even without following Bloom in all the details of his analysis, there can be no doubt that there is nothing unusual about a great contention among writers and artists of all sorts because they are all seeking—even posthumously—their place in the "artistic sun" and their piece of the "artistic pie."

This stated, I believe it could be documented in a more research-oriented article that several earlier books by Allende are simply part of the contemporary canon of high-culture Spanish-language literature: her great breakthrough and best-selling novel, *The House of the Spirits* (*La casa de los espíritus*), first published in Spanish in 1982, *Eva Luna* (1987), *The Stories of Eva Luna* (1989) and the non-fiction memoir *Paula* (1994), are at least four titles which mark their author as a world literary presence of the first rank. Yet, as still seems to happen, female more than male authors must conform or live up to a largely unwritten, not-universally-accepted set of socio-literary expectations which reflect centuries and even millenia of criteria for works to enter into the canon. This is not the place to engage that discussion but rather only to address it briefly before considering Allende's treatment of food in her early work.

My reading of *The House of the Spirits*, in this regard, is that unlike some of Ibero-America's younger literary "Turks." Allende in her break-through novel openly, graciously and wholeheartedly acknowledges and engages the García Márquez of his own breakthrough novel of the previous generation, *One Hundred Years of Solitude* (1967).

But Allende's rural, semi-rural and urban Chile is very different from the trackless wilds and, on balance, the abiding isolation of García Márquez's Macondo and its environs. Moreover, not only in place, but by reaching to the early 1970s of General Augusto Pinochet's Chile, Allende comes to focus sharply on the primary event of Chile and Latin America's then contemporary history: the American CIA assisted coup of September 11, 1973, which resulted both in the death of President Salvador Allende and its immediate aftermath of persecution—experienced first-hand by the real-life Isabel Allende as well as the future, twice-elected Chilean president, Michelle Bachelet (b. 1951)—death and Pinochet's dictatorship (1973–1990). The earlier supernatural events of *The House of the Spirits*, like those of all *One Hundred Years of Solitude*, are simply "muscled out" of social, historical and political protagonism in Allende by the Chilean equivalent of "blood and steel," with no backward look, no space nor time for the earlier, more geographically distant realities and supernatural events which fully center *One Hundred Years of Solitude*. The second half of *The House of the Spirits* is closer to the similarly contemporary, coup-dominated realities of the kind which the Peruvian Mario Vargas Llosa (b. 1936)—half-way in age between García Márquez and Allende— presents later in his own blood-and-steel, historically oriented, urban novels: the year 2000's *The Feast of the Goat* set in Trujillo's Dominican Republic of the early 1960s and 2019's *Fierce Times* which novelizes the history of 1950s' CIA-interrupted Guatemala.

Allende's second major novel, *Eva Luna*, has elements of the urban and semi-rural picaresque, but for our purposes, is most significant for setting up the rest of Allende's work. By the time in the novel from which the following quote comes, the namesake protagonist—and alter ego in this regard of Allende herself—has discovered her gifts for storytelling. She could be the creator of "her own world," which would be "populated by living characters where I declared the norms and changed them at my whim. Upon me depended the existence of everything that was born, died or happened in the sands wherein my stories germinated."[3] And perhaps it is her next book, *The Stories of Eva Luna*, where she gives the freest rein—to that point in her work— to that philosophy of authorial control and inventiveness. In twenty-three different stories, Allende has her creation, Eva Luna, experiment with realism, humor, graphic sexuality and, to abbreviate, full-blown magical realism in the lives of a wide variety of social and gendered situations. Strictly speaking, the stories are independent creations and the reader experiences Allende through her fictive creation, Eva Luna, as she decides who and what, why and to what purpose her stories will be told. Importantly, as with any author more or less influenced by or involved with magical realist creation, Allende tends to declare her freedom, in theory and practice, from the constraints of possibility and probability when understood in the traditional mimetic terms of how people live and have lived over generations and, in fact, millenia. The most important limit on her fiction, then, is not external to it, but organic to the kinds of characters and situations she invents and—bottom line—to her ability to interest readers in "her own world . . . populated by living characters where [she] declared the norms and changed them at [her] whim." Simultaneously, Allende in her fiction and her own life, both embraces traditional heterosexual romance between two partners, and freer, not-necessarily "until-death-do-we-part" relationships.

Part of this liberty flows from the non-specific tropical setting shared by both the *Eva Luna* novel and book of stories: the environs of a place like the Caracas of Allende's post-Pinochet-coup exile in Venezuela. In *The House of the Spirits*, a multi-generational retelling in essence of what led up to and then followed the anti-Salvador-Allende coup of 9/11/1973, neither Chile nor Allende (typically, "the Candidate"[4]) are ever specifically mentioned, just as the Nobel-Prize poet Neruda ("the Poet") never is. But everything in the second half of the book focuses on the social, political and economic precursors to the coup and its comparatively immediate consequences for the matriarchal line of the female protagonists (the descendants of Clara del Valle), which, even in estrangement, are financed by the riches of Clara's once-brutal, always conservative and self-made husband, the patriarch, Esteban Trueba. His and theirs is an unmistakable Chilean story of that society's upper classes. Eva Luna, on the other hand, is the early-orphaned, mestiza offspring of unmarried parents whose eponymous novel and volume of short stories has her moving in the poor, semi-permanently revolutionary countries of Latin America's *tierras calientes*, and, because of the references to petroleum riches, specifically Venezuela.[5]

For our purposes, most significant is that the primary physical setting for *Eva Luna* is a curious, anachronic Germanic enclave—*Colonia Tovar*/the Colony—in the mountains above Caracas (which actually exists in the cultural, and now touristic, context Allende mentions). In that peaceful, Alpine-like space of weekend tourism of good eating, music and dancing, co-protagonist Rolf Carlé's distant relative, "Uncle" Rupert, his wife, Burgel, and their two daughters run an inn at the center of life there. And strictly to the point of this essay: "Food had a fundamental importance for them;" "their lives revolved around the kitchen and the ceremonies to sit down at table."[6] Rolf's thinness contrasts with his relatives' plumpness. But "Aunt" Burgel has a special skill. She "had created an aphrodisiac plate which attracted tourists and maintained her husband always in flames," and she took pride in her work: "look at him, he looks like a tractor."[7] Then follows over nearly a complete page the recipe for this dish and the complicated manner, even rituals, of its preparation. With time, the healthy Rolf and his cousins, right under the noses of their parents and his uncle and aunt, come to form a sexual threesome fueled on one hand by the youthful vigor of the three and on the other by Aunt Burgel's aphrodisiac preparations. But this happy situation is interrupted by Aravena, a newspaperman of great standing who also was the inn's most important client. At Rolf's twenty years of age, Aravena introduces him to what will become his life work as a photojournalist. This means he must leave the Colony, to the great disappointment of his German family, and begin his life in the capital city. However, by the last chapter of the novel, perhaps fifteen years later, both Rolf and Eva Luna have enjoyed professional success. He because of his work in the field with the revolutionary forces and she in the capital as a successful writer of *telenovelas*. Yet, because of their work and contacts made during the generally successful but not completely resolved revolution, it is safest during that time of transition for them to absent themselves from the political center and lay low in the Colony. By then, Rolf's cousins remain unmarried but happy and active in their parents' inn and, along with their parents, welcome Rolf and Eva as a deeply enamored couple for whom Aunt Burgel prepares one of her "aphrodisiac plates."[8]

The twenty-three narrations which are *The Stories of Eva Luna* have a two-page fictionalized prologue which, in its turn, follows an epigraph taken from the *Arabian Nights*. It is the short section in which Sheherazade, a daughter of the king's vizier, is first mentioned in the context of the king's having exhausted, after three years, his kingdom's supply of virgins. But the framing story of those two pages is different from that of the classic Middle Eastern folktale collection. Here the prologue is by Rolf Carlé and, without any real transition, takes up where *Eva Luna* ends, i.e., with Eva and Rolf in bed together. But now for these two pages, it is Rolf who takes over from Eva as the first-person narrator. He simply requests of her to "Tell me a story," and to her unblinking inquiry as to what kind, he responds: "Tell me a story that you haven't told to anyone else."[9]

In five of the stories, Eva herself has some degree of protagonism but for our purposes, the most important story, "The Little Heidelberg," is set in the inn of Rolf's uncle and aunt, which they continue to run. But there is no reference to Rolf nor to Eva, and only one in passing to the two daughters/cousins who now are women and, it seems, unmarried. Also, the clientele seems to have evolved. It is now older and composed of refugees from a WW II-down-beaten Europe; their only desire is to be left in peace while enjoying the food, music, dancing and hospitality—the *Gemütlichkeit,* it could be said—of the inn. In the mere six pages of the story, there are four references to Aunt Burgel's aphrodisiac plates.[10] Of the greatest interest for this study is that it is only in this one story of the twenty-three in the collection where the aphrodisiac dimension occurs. That combines with the only story in the collection with a full-blown magical realist dimension.

There is something extremely voluntaristic about magical realism, given that it (1) does not conform with any common or normal sense of what is possible and probable in human affairs; and (2) it shuns the most usual—the mimetic—mode of literary art which Aristotle's' *Poetics* (c. 335 BC) memoralizes while retaining its status as its fundamental theoretical document. From this millennial perspective in the Judeo-Greek-Christian tradition, what we call magical realism is really but a name for author-created, audience-experienced, and in the most literarily successful instances, audience-endorsed, supernatural occurrences, even while contrasting with, and truly contradicting, the natural order of things possible and probable in human society. Such occurrences are miracles in divine histories or *Deus ex Machina* events in literature. They need no explanation because, for whatever reasons, some sufficiently large or influential group of people or readers is disposed to accept them as verisimilar—albeit contradictory to real life experience today, yesterday and as far as is known, forever. Hence, the superheroes of the *DC Comics* world beginning in the 1930s America and later the *Marvel Comics* world which rose in the 1960s combine to support and enforce each other mutually among those disposed to "suspend their disbelief" in religious and fictional spheres which are alternative to everyday life in the real world during millenia. There are, though, no real words where the truly dead rise or can be risen from the dead, nor the unaided human being who can fly or exhibit x-ray vision or demonstrate supernatural or miraculous powers. Rather it seems that the supernatural powers of comic book heroes are simply the secularization, amplification and exaggeration of the miraculous powers and actions which, as recorded first in the *Old* and *New Testaments* of the *Bible* and then renewed over the centuries through the Christian saints, of Christianity, are fundamental, among believers, to a religious view of the world. That is, to a worldview where the omnipotent, supernatural divinity, directly or through its agents, intervenes in human affairs by controverting the natural order according to its whim or desire. Perhaps it is for that reason that magical realism, so indelibly associated with the likes of García Márquez and Isabel

Allende, can really be considered as the secularization of Hispanic culture's acceptance of, and dependence upon, the fact and providential occurrence of supernatural interventions in natural human affairs. No matter that such authors may be religious sceptics or outright atheists, they were brought up in a world that makes them culturally Roman Catholic. That means they—and much of their readership—have been culturally formed to accept, even expect, that the religious histories of divine, supernatural interventions into humankind's natural order—the normal inventory of the probable and the possible—can recur according to mysterious reasons not accessible to human understanding. Allende's story, "The Little Heidelberg," is a case in point.

It is noteworthy that the seventy-year-old protagonist, The Captain, perhaps Finnish in origin, has over forty years shown no interest in Burgel's aphrodisiac plates nor demonstrated any behaviors but those associated with the totally gray everyday life of a solitary expatriate who gets along with everyone because he pays for what he consumes, causes no trouble, neither socializing nor speaking in any language with anyone. Then one day, by chance, two young Scandinavian tourists arrive at the inn and soon, due to their drink-aided loud voices, The Captain understands what they are saying, goes to their table and with some effort, speaks with them in their tongue. As a result of a conversation in broken English and the Scandanavian tongue, Uncle Rupert is prevailed upon to translate into Spanish from his and the young Scandinavians' poor English The Captain's request to another long-time patron, the eighty-year-old, frail but carefully turned-out Spanish-speaking Niña Eloísa whom, it turns out, The Captain has admired for forty years. "Niña Eloísa," Rupert states, "The Captain asks if you want to marry him."[11] When the woman reconciles with The Captain's unexpected, but welcomed request, the couple begin to dance waltzes. As they dance harmoniously on into the night, The Captain feels her hand becoming lighter and her presence more incorporeal. Then the unexplained, but all the same powerful, supernatural moment of magical realism: Niña Eloisa goes from being flesh and blood to "becoming lace, foam, fog until imperceptible, she disappears completely and [The Captain] is left turning and turning dance steps with hands and arms empty."[12] The supernatural—miraculous or magical according to the reader's background and preference—transformation is now complete, accepted by all in the dance hall. A middle-aged Mexican flamenco dancer resolves the story. She gets up from her table from which she saw the dance and Niña Eloísa evaporate, goes to The Captain still on the dance floor and, taking his trembling hands in hers, dances with him. The story ends. The real-world probabilities and possibilities are not altered for either the characters or for the readers. Simply, for a brief moment, a sentimental, pleasant alternative reality is created. And perhaps some of Allende's critics could accuse her of merely giving a magical realist twist in her 1989 short story to the carefully realistic portrayal of how, after many decades, Florentino's love for Fermina Daza was finally reciprocated by her four years earlier in García Márquez' long novel, *Love in the Time of Cholera*. But the main point here is how, through pure voluntarism on one hand and literary skill on the other, Allende makes The Captain and Niña Eloísa real enough to evoke interest, concern and finally, as with the flamenco dancer as stand-in for the reader, active compassion for their fates. But the whole experience is invented, not a reflection or transcription or version of real life.

With this last point in mind, Allende's reasoning for writing and subsequently publishing *Afrodita: cuentos, recetas y otros afrodisíacos* eight years after *The Stories of Eva Luna* is striking. In her *"Introducción y rondo capriccioso"* to the book, she acknowledges that cooking and sex manuals abound and that, in the end, few purchasers of such volumes actually take them into account when cooking or having sex. Hence, with complete honesty, she rhetorically asks: "Why then this book?" and she responds: "Because the idea of finding out about aphrodisiacs strikes me as amusing and I hope to you [reader] it also does."[13] Then she states that "In these pages, I try to get close to the truth but that is not always possible. What, for example, can be said about parsley? Sometimes, it is necessary to invent."

Six years later in *My Invented Country: A Memoir,* Allende discusses the religiosity of Chileans but asserts that "in practice, there is much more fetishism and superstition than mystical inquietude or theological learning."[14] Then, she proceeds to give an inventory of practices which support this assertion, including family anecdotes, especially concerning attributes of a grandmother, that are pure magical realism but which she, because of her age, does not know if she witnessed or simply heard told so many times that they became real for her. As a result, she admits that such experiences have abounded in her life and that "many of my life's events and anecdotes come across as having been lived" but that, when it comes to "putting them in writing and subjecting them to logic, they seem improbable." But not to worry: "What difference does it make if they really happened or if I imagined them? In any case, life is a dream."[15]

I came to this article on Isabel Allende a full generation after researching and writing a literary encyclopedia entry titled "Pardo Bazán, Emilia (1852–1921): Reception of Her by Male Colleagues."

And truth be told, I began and complete this essay feeling some of the same resentment toward the criticism and treatment of Allende that I documented was endured by the tireless Pardo Bazán in her day. This feeling, if anything, is deepened by the recent novel by Carlos Mayoral, a young Spanish novelist, titled "A National Episode," in which a subplot is the wonderfully-rendered romantic relationship between two of Spain's principal novelists since the death of Cervantes in 1616: Benito Pérez Galdós (1843–1920) and the Countess Emilia Pardo Bazán.[16] Like the now three-times married and sexually-adventurous Allende, Pardo Bazán lived a fully-corporeal life while becoming an author whose times cannot be understood without reference to her life and work.

This said, it also may not be surprising that the best study of the complex role of food in Allende is by a woman: Durango Pacheco's 2009 MA thesis titled "Woman, Food and Body." Most convenient for our purposes, she focuses on two of the same works by Allende as in this present study, *The Stories of Eva Luna* and *Aphrodite*, albeit from a more feminist viewpoint or exploration than adopted here, and which frees us from pursuing that most basic dimension to the books and their theme of food, woman and her body. Our central interest has been how Allende steadily claimed her right to remake or recast reality in her own terms. And what are those terms? Not mimetic reproductions nor reports nor recipes nor formulas, but rather Allende's considered vision of life, things and relationships. And most definitely, of the books we have explored, the relation between Eva Luna and Rolf Carlé is the most exhaustive. The novel, *Eva Luna,* traces their respective troubled early lives and the forces which make finding each other the realization of all that had been missing in them. Rolf's two-page prologue to *The Stories of Eva Luna* is the equivalent, in Allende's world, to an "and they lived happily ever after" ending of the fictions, beginning of their lives together. However, there is one dimension left to be indicated here that flows from the *New York Times* review of the 1995 translation to English of *Paula*, Allende's memoir of the irreversible genetic disease which caused her daughter to go into coma and then die at age twenty-nine, less than a year after they learned what would be her fate.

In that review, the multi-lingual, multi-cultural novelist, Suzanne Ruta, demonstrates an impressive knowledge of and familiarity with the entire corpus of Allende's life and work to that date. Hence, when she declares *Paula* to be the author's masterwork, until then, it is a noteworthy claim. For *Paula* reveals the voluntaristic idealist, magical-thinking Allende confronted by a reality she simply cannot contemplate as a dream or turn into a wonderful story. Allende will,

of course, continue in literature and life to reaffirm a joyous exploration of her and her fellow women and men's needs, desires and
possibilities. But the real limits, the real dampers, life imposes on us
all are now always hovering in the shadows of Allende's joy, as well
as that of even her most voluntaristic, life-affirming readers. There was
no saving grace, no authorial intervention in Paula's demise that could
make it anything but what it was: the senseless end of her still-young
life and a most horribly sad before-and-after in her mother's life and,
differently, in that of her most heedful readers. At such moments,
mostly it is pleasant to think of the younger Rolf and his two cousins,
fueled by Burgel's aphrodisiacs, fully enjoying their youth and
health.

Notes

1 The rendering into English from the original Spanish is my translation.
For the sake of offering an easily-read essay, I leave for these notes even
fuller quotes in Spanish from the relevant section of the interview:
"-¿Qué te producen las opiniones de quienes señalan que escribís cosas
livianas, cursis?
-No me importa. Cuando surgió la posibilidad de que me dieran el Premio
Nacional de Literatura en Chile en 2002, se dijeron cosas horrendas.
Surgió una oleada de odio, de envidia. Se dijeron cosas espantosas. La
gente que las dijo fueron otros escritores fracasados, que no venden ni un
solo libro. Pero no me dolió nada.
-En una de las últimas entrevistas que dio el escritor Roberto Bolaño
(N. de la R.: una de las voces más respetadas de la literatura chilena
actual, fallecido en julio último a los 50 años) . . .
-Sí, se murió.
-Sí, en una entrevista de *Playboy* de México, la periodista le pregunta
acerca de tus libros y los de Ángeles Mastretta, y él contesta que "ni en
mis peores borracheras he perdido cierta lucidez mínima, un sentido de
la prosodia y del ritmo, un rechazo ante el plagio y la mediocridad".
-Me tenía un odio parido. Fue uno de los que dijo las peores cosas.
-¿Leíste sus libros, te produce algún respeto lo que hacía?
-No, ninguno.
-No leíste nada.
-Eché una mirada a un par de libros y me aburrió espantosamente."
2 Allende, in fact, did not receive that award in 2002. She had to wait for
it until 2010 (five years after induction into the United States' American
Academy of Letters, which was followed by the award to her by then
President Obama of the 2014 Presidential Medal of Freedom). For over
fifty years, the ambient, *The New Yorker*-like meanness and snobbery of
too much of the literary and artistic worlds, sometimes conflated with
that of politics—long before our present time of political correctness and
"cancel culture"—has impressed most negatively. The reader will decide

how to receive/evaluate Allende's "tit-for-tat" response to those criticisms of her.

3   Again, I give my translations from the Spanish to English to keep a mono-lingual text for the body of this essay, be it citing titles or textual materials. The Spanish original reads: "Me consolaba la idea de que yo podía . . . crear . . . un mundo propio, poblado de personajes vivos. [...] De mí dependía la existencia de todo lo que nacía, moría o acontecía en las arenas inmóviles donde germinaban mis cuentos" (*Eva Luna* 177).

4   Recall that Salvador Allende was a perennial candidate for the Chilean presidency for the eighteen years between 1952 and his fateful win in 1970 with a mere plurality vote win of 36.2% of the vote as compared to that of his nearest rival, Jorge Alessandri, who obtained 34.9% of the vote.

5   *Eva Luna*: 14, 72, 118, 134, 169, 172, 195, 204, 222.

6   As above the translation from the Spanish is mine; the Spanish reads: "La comida revestía una importancia fundamental para ellos, sus vidas giraban en torno a los afanes de la cocina y la ceremonia de sentarse a la mesa" (*Eva Luna* 90).

7   *Eva Luna* 90: "mírenlo, parece un tractor."

8   *Eva Luna* 285: "comenzaba a picar y sazonar los ingredients del guiso afrodisíaco."

9   *Cuentos de Eva Luna* 12: "Cuéntame un cuento . . . ¿Cómo lo quieres? . . . Cuéntame un cuento que no le hayas contado a nadie."

10 The Spanish text of "El pequeño Heidelberg" occupies pp. 131–137 of *Cuentos de Eva Luna*; the references to Aunt Burguel's aphrodisiac preparations are on pp. 131, 132, 133, 135.

11 *Cuentos de Eva Luna* 136: "Niña Eloísa, pregunta El Capitán si quiere casarse con él."

12 *Cuentos de Eva Luna* 137: "iba tornándose de encaje, de espuma, de niebla, hasta hacerse imperceptible y por ultimo desaparecer del todo y [El Capitán] se encontró girando y girando con los brazos vacíos."

13 I follow here the same practice of giving my extended Spanish to English translations in the body of the essay, and reserve for these notes the orig-inal Spanish: "¿Por qué entonces este libro? Porque la idea de averigüar sobre afrodisíacos me parece divertida y espero para usted también lo sea. En estas páginas intento aproximarme a la verdad, pero no siempre es posible. ¿Qué se puede decir, por ejemplo, del perejil? A veces hay que inventar . . . " (*Afrodita* 11).

14 *Mi país inventado* 77: "Los chilenos son religiosos, aunque su práctica tiene mucho más de fetichismo y superstición que de inquietud mística o conocimiento teológico."

15 *Mi país inventado* 87: "Esto me ocurre con muchos eventos y anécdotas de mi existencia, que me parece haber vivido, pero que al ponerlos por escrito y confrontarlos con la lógica, resultan algo improbables, pero el problema no me inquieta. ¿Qué importa si en realidad sucedieron o si los he imaginado? De todos modos, la vida es sueño."

16 For gendered reasons, is it surprising that Pardo Bazán who, following

separation from her husband, lived by her pen, Did become the author of a cook book: "Old Spanish Recipes" (*La cocina española antigua*), first published in 1913? In turn, that book became the starting point for a more famous cookbook: the frequently re-edited, two-volume "Culinary Encylopedia" (*Enciclopedia culinaria*) by another noblewoman: the Marchioness of Parabere.

Bibliography

Allende, Isabel. *Afrodita: cuentos, recetas y otros afrodisíacos*. Illustrated by Robert Shekter, recipes by Panchita Llona. NY: Rayo/Harper-Collins, 1998.

——. *L a casa de los espíritus*. NY: Rayo/Harper-Collins, 1995.

——. *Eva Luna*. NY: Harper-Collins, 1995.

——. *Mi país inventado. Un paseo nostálgico por Chile*. NY: Rayo/Harper-Collins, 2004.

——. *Paula*. Barcelona: Plaza & Janes, 1994.

Bloom, Harold. *The Anxiety of Influence. A Theory of Poetry*. 2nd ed. NY: Oxford UP, 1997.

Durango Pacheco, Nohemy Cecilia. *Mujer, comida y cuerpo*. Magíster Tesina [145 pp.] Bogotá, Colombia: Pontífica Universidad Javeriana, January, 2009. https://repository.javeriana.edu.co/bitstream/handle/10554/461/tesis54(2).pdf?sequence=5. Accessed 17 March 2021.

Guerriero, Leila. "Isabel Allende: la latina más vendida." https://www.lanacion.com.ar/lifestyle/isabel-allende-la-latina-mas-vendida-nid522537/. Accessed 22 April 2021.

Mayoral, Carlos. *Un episodio nacional*. Barcelona: Espasa/Planeta, 2019.

Miller, Stephen. "Pardo Bazán, Emilia (1852–1921): Reception of Her by Male Colleagues." *The Feminist Encyclopedia of Spanish Literature*, Vol. N-Z, ed. Janet Pérez and Maureen Ihrie, Westport, CT: Greenwood Press, 2002, 459–62.

Ruta, Suzanne. "The Long Goodbye." https://www.nytimes.com/1995/05/21/books/the-long-goodbye.html. Accessed 24 April 2021.

19

Cultural & Culinary Symbiosis: The Art of Describing Cuban Identity in José Lezama Lima's *Paradiso*

Jorge Chavarro

First of all, a labyrinthine narrative that eschews the usual narrative schemes, *Paradiso,* the novel by José Lezama Lima (1910–76), elucidates elements of Cuban identity. The novel appears in 1966, a year before the explosion that accompanied the first edition of Gabriel García Márquez's blockbuster novel, *Cien años de soledad.* The overwhelming success of the *Cien Años*[1] was based on the spell of an uncomplicated narrative, available to all despite its historical and geographical symbolic modes, each reader being able to make the stories of the saga of the *Buendía* family his/her own. *Paradiso,* too, is etched in what came to be called the Latin American Boom, the phenomena of Magical Realism (RM) and the Real Wonderful American (LRMA), which gave preponderant places to the novelistics of Guatemalan Miguel Ángel Asturias (1899–1974), the 1967 Nobel Laureate; Alejo Carpentier (1904–80), though born in Switzerland, self-identified as Cuban; and Juan Rulfo of Mexico (1917–86) (Chiampi 1991).

However, *Paradiso* could benefit neither from the paraphernalia surrounding the Boom (due to the policy of continental isolation to which Cuba was subjected or from acceptance by the public as the island and Latin America critics generally adhered more to rejection by the Cuban regime) nor from the favorable literary criticism. The non-confluent approaches of both novels made the difference. Immediate enthusiastic recognition came from well-known and esteemed Latin American writers like Octavio Paz of Mexico (1914–98), 1990 Nobel Laureate, Julio Cortázar (1914–84) & Carlos

Monsiváis (1939–2010) of Argentina, Mario Vargas Llosa (1936–, 2010 Novel Laureate) of Peru and Emir Rodríguez Monegal of Uruguay (1921–85), among others. They highlighted elements of Lezana's novel such as the architecture of a language in continuous metamorphosis, which reaches the untouchable point between the creation and destruction of language and is the heart of language, according to Paz. *Paradiso* is a ceremony that preexists all literary reading and is the first vision of the poem and philosophy, says Cortázar. Monsiváis explains that everything in *Paradiso* is reconquest, childhood, first joy, astonishment at first knowledge, a platonic dialogue about being, orthodox and heterodox sex, consciousness, fabulation and myth (all in Chiampi 1991).

This is how *"Paradiso"* begins, as a journey from hand-to-hand among readers who determine the next readers to take over the part of the discourse that they feel corresponds to them, in addition, of course, to the difficult integral readings. *Paradiso* is, well, contemplating history, in precise terms, the story of the initiation of a child who grows up in Havana, and discovers his destiny as a poet. Lezama tells us about the whole childhood environment of José Cemí, his alter ego; the internment of adolescence in denser and suffocating sub-plots which will be due to a first estrangement that makes the experience awake our senses.

The surname *Cemí* sounds strange and has given rise to various interpretations of its significance, some of them citing the hair as the possible allusion to Jesus Christ, others, perhaps more reasonably, attribute it to onomastic anagrammaticization[2] by/of the author. But, in my opinion, the most convincing explanation is that given by Juan José Arrom (1975) in his essay on the novelistic world of José Lezama Lima: in *Taino* mythology, *cemí* is the word that symbolizes the gods and their images.

In this way, the author is mythologized at the expense of his protagonist, who we denounce as his alter ego, and who gives meaning to the title *Paradiso*, soaking it with the spirit of the last thirty-three songs of *The Divine Comedy*, so the *Paradiso* of Lezama is an island, that of Cuba, the paradise of the *Taínos*. Lezama, in constructing the poetic image of the *Taino* paradise, continues the tradition of the chroniclers of discovery, Colón/Columbus in the first place, who overflow in imaginative narration about the newly discovered Eden of the Americas.

But Lezama is also the transgressor accused of pornography for his "baroque, Cuban and homosexual" novel (Sarduy 1987), exuberant from the power of "the erotic metaphor" (Goytisolo 1992), all achieved with profusion in the treatment of homosexuality. Cemí does not propose homosexuality as a different sexuality but as those with "a fixation on the normal development of sexuality . . . an unhappy resolution of the Oedipus complex . . . an Oedipus before revelation and repentance," which leads them to prefer maternal darkness. Night, darkness and hell are identified with the maternal figure, the son identified with the mother and refusing to separate from the maternal body (Cruz-Malave 1991). When Lezama was asked about the supposedly pornographic character of his novel, he alluded to the beauty of the human being and claimed not to separate the aberration from the sensual, the loving feeling or the intellect. Cuban institutional criticism of the novel led to the fact that shortly after it had been incorporated on the shelves of public libraries, some pages of the eighth chapter disappeared from the volumes of the first edition.

About the biographical work that the author assumes in the novel, most of Lezama's scholars refer to "*Paradiso*" as a diptych in which the first seven chapters are directed to the rescue of the lost family paradise, the sanctification of a Creole golden age that gives way to initiation into poetry. The second part of this diptych, which uses the eighth chapter as the hinge of the diptych, refers to the true contact of José Cemí with the outside world. The work is understood as a family story whose axis is the home, which persists as a place of reference or solid ground for the explorations of José Cemí in the second part. However, it is not the nostalgia of childhood or lost time that guides the author but the space to build the present with writing and make it immortal. That is why he has no time, as he is reborn every time someone approaches him; the recreation of that lost paradise is the true possibility of a "utopia of hope" (Ainsa 1983).

The utopias in which philosophers and poets claim a lost paradise or golden age, hoping for a better future for the world, do not correspond to the observation of man from the ambiguity of his realities, they place him between the excited wait and the awareness of irremediable loss, all because paradise is not a static image compatible with the fabric of nostalgia. For Cemí, the ease of reconstruction of paradise is possible because its home is on an island, Cuba, and utopias have been imagined absolutely in islands, the sea that surrounds them also protects them and makes possible the happiness in them that allows projecting the singular and inscribing it in the universal (Ainsa 1983).

It is a closed world which favors the absence of tension with the outside world for the world of José Cemí, the concentric structure of the same, family, servitude, friends, is traveled smoothly. Each circle guarantees the stability of the next, which guarantees a return to the central element of support because the image of greater strength is the mother. The excellent relationship of José with his mother guarantees the cohesion of the structure. Upon the death of José Eugenio Cemí, Rialta, who at the time is a woman of only thirty years, turns to her affection for her orphaned son. It is all that allows us to say that the true heads of that home are the women, centered in the house but energetic; in addition, the men, apparently strong, die young. José María Cemí dies shortly after marrying, José Eugenio at thirty-three years old, Don Andrés Olaya at forty-four, uncles, Luis and Alberto, also die young. Andresito dies in childhood. That is why women must ensure family stability. Rialta, upon marrying at the age of twenty, becomes the third generation of mothers in the novel. She determines the life of her son so completely that it makes the author claim it as a conspiracy against death—and guarantee of happiness—because, without the maternal presence, every shadow of death is a serious threat. When Rialta's life is in danger, Cemí discovers, as his uncle Alberto had done, that the security of feeling young is linked to a mother's life because, in reality, the humiliation of a man begins on the day of his mother's death. Lezama conjures death and makes the triumph of that life apparent when, once Rialta is operated on, he describes "the fibroid removed in great detail" (Ainsa 1983).

Of the central themes of the present essay, the aspects of family biography that continue to seek a paradise lost are already exposed; that of the Cuban identity, we now recognize is built on the abundance and exuberance of the landscape and food. The one that precedes in *Paradiso* is the first approach to sexuality. However, the two themes, food and sexuality, merge in the construction of the image. The image is not only Cuban but, in general, the Latin American image that Ingenschay (2007) portrays as the erotic and libidinal excesses that constitute the Baroque tradition of Latin America and the irrational subjectivity of that subject (taken from the speech of Sarduy), who seeks scenarios of wastefulness and opulence in "art, luxury, mourning, non-reproductive sexuality and gluttony."

Having established that the Cuban identity is characterized in the novel as in reality, through the landscape and food, with the description of the preparation process and the banquet itself as a social event, allows the reader to perceive the relationship between food and poetry in the narrative, the transformation experienced by food is transferred to the word. That is why the appearance of the mulatto chef, Juan Izquierdo, who dominates the style of eating in five countries, announces the arrival of the contributions that the creole-ism will receive from a first vestige of modernity. The event occurs after the asthmatic attack of José Cemí. The presence of the ladies of the house causes the perception of the risk of displacement of the chef's skill upon Rialta and her mother, Doña Augusta. The latter is brilliant in the concoction of sweets, especially the *natilla*/custard, with a touch of pudding. The house surrenders at her feet to facilitate her culinary office; she was a queen with the whole house, "the court" arranged for her to do her will. Lezama describes exuberance, not only due to grandma's art, but of family gluttony. This defines the voracity of this bourgeois family, aware of its roots and creole social layer, proud of being so and more, and differentiates it from its presence in the bosom of the military. That is why, because of the concept of tradition, Juan Izquierdo and his conceptions of an internationalized cuisine do not fit into the complex structure of the family and that is why he must leave, since he perceives the lack of recognition by his masters (Ingenschay 2007).

But Izquierdo returns and then exposes how, after the wars of independence, Cuban cuisine also begins to emancipate itself from the colonial model, which, in turn, recognizes it as not dominating in all its particularities. When he prepares the *ombombó*,[3] a typical Creole dish par excellence, Rialta enters the kitchen and criticizes him for having mixed two types of shrimp. Here comes into play the element of social superiority of women, built on a kitchen without vanities (that is the discourse that is then denied by emphasizing the recipes of the family book), a kitchen of their own, Cuban and Creole. The colonel's father, of Basque origin, recalls at family gatherings the debates about supremacy between Spanish and Cuban fruits, which for the new generation is meaningless and falls on deaf ears. Juan Izquierdo returns to the ineptitude of his successors at the end of the first chapter to serve the family (Ingenschay 2007).

In *Paradiso*, the function of the feast is to demonstrate how the life of the "American lord" takes place in an everyday baroque-ism, resulting from its strictly Creole character that corresponds to linguistic exuberances. In food descriptions, the narrative often assumes an explicitly erotic dimension, as in the scene in which the colonel opens the melon and takes out *la mogolla*[4] before slapping Juan Izquierdo (Ingenschay 2007).

Cuba cannot be imagined apart from association with tobacco and sugar, both constituting the national heritage, and in the novel, established in the coat of arms of the paternal family, its metaphor and the family entrenchment in Cuban cultures. The two characterize the family due to the peculiarities of their crops. Sugar is preponderant and its expansion represents the fortune, as well as the vigorous symbol of the grandfather who claims his Basque ancestry. Sugar is autonomous and Lezama, by associating it with the grandfather, gives it a connotation of continuity, alive in the long cycle of its production.

It represents the strength that the narrator sees in the paternal family because, although the plant grows easily, the final product requires a sophisticated path of transformation.

The grandmother's family is represented by the subtlety and calmness of tobacco and its artisanal production, which is related in a poetic way: a tobacco leaf symbolizes the family, living in the task of reading the delicate pirouettes that the leaf demands when it is being rolled and the notion of time is lost in its company. The novel merges into a single element within the symbolism of the cultivation of tobacco and the poetics of its description. With sugar, although the poetic flow exists in the feeling of the narrative, does not show with the same intensity its presence and emphasizes more in the difficulties of physical and mental effort.

Paradiso was built on the two foundations, the craftsmanship of tobacco and the hard work with which strength and talent are used to produce sugar. These highlight the duality of the feminine of the tobacco work and the masculine of the cane and the sugar, i.e., the grandmother, Eloísa, who is the Cuban Creole, and the Basque grandfather, who portrays the Spanish heritage. And José Eugenio, the son, is the complete Basque-Cuban fusion, the maturity of creole, sugar and tobacco.

Seasoning & Cooking

The dualities are maintained in the kitchen, the confrontation is not now caused by the physical nature of the protagonists but by their way of elaborating the elements, the confrontation of learning that each one considers indispensable, but that ends up negotiating what becomes the metaphor of the symbiosis that means the miscegenation, here seen not only in the human elements but in their cultural products.

As highlighted before, the detailed recipe for the *natilla* of the grandmother, Augusta; the *adobado*/a kind of "pickling" seasoning,[5] exacerbating the situation due to the complaints of the mulatto, Juan Izquierdo; the confrontation between Rialta, Doña Augusta and Juan Izquierdo that ends so badly in this first clash for the mulatto, is the inevitable struggle between the traditional and the new. The art of the grandmother, faced with the gastronomic symbiosis of the mulatto and, although Juan Izquierdo only appears in this first chapter of the novel, the insolence of his presence and the captivating and assertive character of the character which makes him persist in the atmosphere of the novel until the end. Given his necessary evocation in facts without needing to mention it, he himself, as a mulatto, represents the identity symbiosis of Cuban-ness and the metaphorical representation of poetic and culinary art. The rivals, grandmother and mulatto, show their pride and impetuousness—manifested more explicitly in Juan Izquierdo, who defines himself as the lineage that handles the style of cuisine of five countries: "noble I am as the one who is most relevant for Cuban-ness," is the discernable between the lines in such a speech.

Doña Augusta, honoring the suggestions of her name, obtained her knowledge by blood and, in that way, the knowledge she treasures is also beyond all doubt or controversy because this is certified by the canon of each. The first confrontation between the two occurs in relation to the preparation of the *double buds*,[6] the traditional way that Doña Augusta transmits to her daughter, opposed to the sophistication of the current that Juan Izquierdo proclaims, without secrets, violating the attitude of reserve among the ladies. The attitude of approval that the mulatto chef achieves for his culinary proposal is given in subtle attitudes of approval and adhesion. For the grandmother, the perfect selection of cinnamon, vanilla, eggs and milk and their careful mixture guarantees the perpetuation of her art, whether we believe it or not, it indicates an art that fuses, without ever having pretended to be "fusion food," in perfect symbiosis, the Chinese, French, American, Spanish and Cuban traditions learned from her master Leng, in its perfect symbiosis. Juan Izquierdo, without claiming nobility of blood, does have a wide knowledge of other worlds. Juan confirms the element of symbiosis and freshness by adding the traditional to please the local and foreign palate and slowly but surely conquers the national palate.

Lezama assumes his poetic gastronomic task, combining knowledge and skills of the classic and the modern. He understands that transforming the traditional into the new can produce forms pleasing to the eye but sometimes empty—or can become an attack that goes from exoticism to the extinction of the Creole. But the author seems to suggest that this symbiosis is absolutely essential, in the same way that it was in his family and in Cuban culture, as in that of tobacco and sugar. The chef then gives way, having been fired by the colonel because of his pride and rebelliousness, he returns when the family realizes the impossibility of finding someone who surpasses his art. Although José Eugenio warns that the modernization of art is needed, elements of the classical form must be maintained, thus, the preparation reflects the tension resulting from the hybridization process (Escobar-Trujillo 2012).

The Family Feast

Two family dinners introduce the gastronomic delights of *Paradiso*: the family reunion created by the Basque grandfather in the first chapter and Doña Augusta's dinner, which becomes the last moment of family reunion before moving into adulthood in chapter seven. At this end of the first part, the author condenses what belongs to childhood, the farewell to childhood and the prelude to a new life. The two meetings, *comilonas*/binges or banquets, are related to the process of transformation and they signify the acceptance of his new homeland by the Basque grandfather of what, until then, he had rejected, because he felt such acceptance culturally apocalyptic.

The grandfather suffers nightmares in which a fly attacks his stomach, which, in his words, is symbolically its root, and fills its mouth with seeds that are not its own, i.e., Spanish. The American is the other, emphasized through the *prieta*/black fly that invades the Spanish vine. Now the grandfather has lost his fear by virtue of the tasted and repeated introduction of the American seed, the *zapote*,[7] whose seed is the only food digested during the meal, candied only as narrative elements, the *zapote* is both named verbally with the word and digested by the Basque. American fruit is not only food, but a white wine that is mixed, unlike red wine from the Christian Eucharist. The two elements merge into one, symbolizing the Eucharist itself, no longer between the divine and human, but between the American and European: the phenomenon of transculturation produced through the tasting of the fruit.

This is how the American fruit and the European grape are finally part of the digestive system and cultural identity of the grandfather. The transculturation also occurs at Doña Augusta's dinner, with the variety and abundance of fruits and vegetables of the island, along with the traditional Cuban twist that the grandmother gives to her food, adding as symbolic the products chosen by her for the salad and the last dish of the banquet. For the salad, Doña Augusta selects the asparagus, introduced by the Arabs in Spain and Europe in the eighteenth century, and the beetroot, which has an African origin but, unlike cassava or banana, came to the island to satisfy the palate of the Spaniards—but not to feed the slaves.

As a seasonal fruit, the Spanish palate does not prefer *zapotes*, pineapples or soursop but products of foreign origin like apples, pears, tangerines and grapes. Therefore, not only has the Basque grandfather accepted and assimilated the American fruit but also the American has adopted the Spanish product and both have made it their own. Everything confirms that, although one cannot be solely American, even if one cannot be absolutely American, one cannot be solely European either. In *Paradiso*, it is not possible to be only American or European. The Cuban implies first the fear of losing one's identity, then a transformation and finally, a symbiosis that sums up the insular identity.

It is possible to contemplate the colors and shapes of the food from the story but it is not possible to sense the smell of them or to ingest them with the character, the delight, that lies in the evocation and in the images that the grandmother builds. At grandma's dinner, food is transformed into a cyclical process of life and death but, in turn, into a process of transforming the word into poetry. The dinner is both an omen of the death of the grandmother and of Alberto and a preamble of the passage of Cemí's childhood to his adulthood. The banquet also offers as a dish the word made image, poetry. Each element that the author mentions is a brushstroke, a message of taste for color, for the word and for the image finally achieved.

> We talk about the allegory of the prawn, the backwater rhythm that the food needs, not only because of the content of the conversation that refers to death and from which the allegorical content of the shrimp is formed, but also because of the backwater that, in the image, implies the freshness of the salad. The backwater is created through the contrast of colors, purple, green and yellow with the red, pink, "open" tones of the soufflé. (Escobar-Trujillo 2012)

When alluding to the discourse of identity from the theme of food in Lezama's novel, we also find ourselves in the circumstance of a story in which nature and identity define a national essence. The food in *Paradiso*

> se convierte en elemento fundacional de identidad cultural y familiar, y el proceso de transformación y presentación de los alimentos establece una equivalencia entre el proceso del alimento transformado en gastronomía y el de la palabra transformada en imagen poética/converts into a foundational element of cultural and family identity. The process of transformation and presentation of food establishes an equivalence between the process of food transformed into gastronomy and that of the word transformed into poetic image. (Escobar-Trujillo 2012).

Notes

1 García Márquez won the Novel Prize in 1975 largely as a result of this novel.
2 According to Wikipedia, "Onomastics or onomatology is the study of the etymology, history, and use of proper names [while] An anagram is a word or phrase formed by rearranging the letters of a different word or phrase, typically using all the original letters exactly once."
3 Also called quimbombó, and African-origin dish using okra, similar to the gumbo known as a creole dish in New Orleans in the U.S., according to Cuban Quimbombo—My Recipe Magic.
4 Though defined as *"bread roll . . . a feminine name" by Traducción de MOGOLLA al español por Oxford Dictionary* en Lexico.com y también el significado de MOGOLLA en, this presumably refers to the seeds ball in the center of an uncut/uncleaned melon and implies a similarity to female anatomy.
5 adobado—English Translation—Word Magic Spanish-English Dictionary (wordmagicsoft.com)
6 In Cuban vernacular, "double buds" refers to tastebuds, therefore, dishes which are especially delicious, according to Cuban American friends.
7 A fruit with a rind, which must be peeled away to reveal an orange flesh, with a sweet flavor characterized as a cross between fig and avocado, according to Zapote Information, Recipes and Facts .

Bibliography

adobado—English Translation—Word Magic Spanish-English Dictionary (wordmagicsoft.com)

Ainsa, Fernando. "Image and possibility of utopia in Paradiso by José Lezama Lima." *Magazine Iberoamericana,* (1983) 263–277 PDF revista-iberoamericana. pitt.edu WEB: Feb. 20, 2021.

Arrom José Juan. "The Cuban Tradition in the Novelistic World of José Lezama Lima." *Revista Iberoamericana* (1975) 469–477 PDF revista-iberoamericana.pitt.edu WEB: Feb. 20, 2021.

Chiampi, Irlemar. "On the reading interrupts of Paradiso." *Revista Iberoamericana.* (1991) 65–76 PDF revista-iberoamericana.pitt.edu: Feb. 20, 2021.

Cruz-Malave, Arnaldo. "The Fate of the Father. Phallocentrism in *Paradiso.* " *Ibero-American Magazine* (1991) 51–64 PDF revista-iberoamericana.pitt.edu WEB: Feb. 20, 2021.

Cuban Quimbombo—My Recipe Magic.

Escobar-Trujillo, Maria. "From Food to Poetry: The Cuban identity in *Paradiso* by José Lezama File." *Periphrases* 123 (2012), 65–80 PDF Revista Uniandes PDF uniandes.edu.co WEB Feb. 20, 2021.

Gimbernat, Ester. "Between Cuba and Spain. Some counterpoints of José Lezama Lima." *Confluence* (1990) 129–133 PDF jstor.org: Feb. 20, 2021.

Gómez, Santiago. "The Mockery of the Hook. *Paradiso* by José Lezama Lima." *University Magazine Antioquia* (2010), 63–68

PDF magazines.udea.edu.co WEB: Feb. 20, 2021.

Ingenschay, Dieter. "Neo-baroque Feasts. The Literary Menu Between Excess and Populism." *Journal of Romance Philology*, 2007. PDF: revistas.ucm.es WEB: Feb. 20, 2021.

Leo, Juliet. "The Unquestioned Symbols in *Paradiso* by José Lezama Lima." *Magazine of Technological Humanities of Monterrey*. 24 (2008), 13–31 PDF: Redalyc.org WEB: Feb. 20, 2021.

Teuber Bernardo. "Or Felix's Slip of the Tongue. Autobiography, Genetic Criticism and Genealogy of the Subject in *Paradiso* of José Lezama Lima." *MLN,* Mar. (108), 314–330 1993 PDF jstor.org WEB Feb. 20, 2021.

Traducción de MOGOLLA al español por *Oxford Dictionary* en Lexico.com y también el significado de MOGOLLA en . . .

Zapote Information, Recipes and Facts (specialtyproduce.com) (specialtyproduce.com)

Metamorphosis and Food: Adela Fernández and Leonora Carrington's Short Stories, A Comparative Reading

Eduardo Cerdán

To Adriana de Teresa Ochoa,
for motivating me to challenge canon.
To Fabián Espejel, for his contributions to this text.

Not many texts linked to Surrealism have entered the literary canon. Critics tend to analyze the surreal in relation to the visual arts and the cinema, which reduces the appreciation of the wide scope that last century's movement had. Canonical literature of the surreal? Maybe the novel, *Nadja* (1928), by André Breton. We could also think of certain works from the Generation of '27, with Federico García Lorca and his *Poet in New York* (1940) as the quintessential example, or the novel, *The Hearing Trumpet* (1977), by English author and painter Leonora Carrington (1917–2011). There are, however, more notable, and underserved, literary texts related to Surrealism. Carrington's just-mentioned novel is one of the dozens of narrative pieces she produced. It would be worth expanding the reading of those other written pieces of hers (the short stories, in particular); critical attention to Carrington as a writer does not compare with that which has been given to her as a painter.

On the other hand, it would not be an exaggeration to say that the narrow-mindedness in relation to Surrealism also operates in geographical terms. Since Paris was the center of the movement, European cities have come to the fore when it comes to Surrealism (New York is the exception, of course). In addition to well-known Latin American names like Julio Cortázar, Alejo Carpentier or Octavio Paz, all of whom published essays on Surrealism and even short stories; those in the book, *Arenas movedizas/Quicksand*, influenced by this movement. In addition to them, I was saying, there are some writers in whose work permeated surrealist ideas such as dreams' irrationality, the unconscious, childhood, etc. In Mexico there was a *sui generis* and marginal writer, Adela Fernández (1942–2013), who had an unusual link with the movement: "in 1958 [she writes] I approached the group of surrealist painters: Leonora Carrington, Remedios Varo, the Duchamps, the Hornas, Tichernon . . . It was there, with them, that I began to write professionally and publish . . . The influence and teachings of that group have been, for me, indissoluble" (Fernández 2009, 16–17). Adela Fernández, who wrote two books of short stories—and some more, in more than only one genre—published in prestigious magazines of her time. Despite her undeniable relevance, she has hardly been studied in the context of Mexican 20th century literature. I stress here the importance of promoting her presence in critical discussion.

When confronted with their short stories (none are extensive, by the way), it became evident to me that the domestic space, with all that it implies, the idea of "home," relationships, parents, children, and so on, has a leading role in the construction of their stories, most of which belong to the fantastic realm. Domestic space representation is configured as a disturbing element for the characters and the readers themselves in the stories of both. The kitchen plays a leading role in space construction and there are testimonies, both about Fernández and Carrington, that show their personal fondness for it. Fernández, who studied anthropology, even dedicated a book to kitchen: *Sabrosuras de la muerte. Comida para las ánimas/Savory Flavors of Death. Food For Souls*) (1999), in which she reflects on the importance of gastronomy in the worldview of the pre-Hispanic cultures of Mexico. About Carrington, on the other hand, Katharine Conley writes:

Everyone who has written about visiting Leonora Carrington in Mexico describes her kitchen . . . Carrington's kitchen was her living, talking, and thinking space. It was her intellectual hub, her equivalent of Breton's study in Paris, as Jonathan Eburne has persuasively argued . . . Carrington, like Breton, was intentional about the objects with which she surrounded herself and was interested in those she understood as having magical, animate qualities, even a 'quasi-animal life,' as Antonin Artaud once described objects seen close up and magnified by a camera . . . She takes a Bretonian abstraction [the so-called transformism] and concretizes it in an ordinary everyday fashion and she does so repeatedly with her hybrid, animal-human creatures who live in her paintings in a suspended synchronous time. We see this hybridity in *The House Opposite* with the central figure of the woman with the shadow of a horse or the tree with a human head upstairs in the same painting, and with *Tartar*, the speaking wooden rocking-horse in *The Oval Lady* and the various horse-guides for the human female narrators in *The House of Fear* and *Uncle Sam Carrington*, as well the half-human, half- horse protagonist stand-in for herself in the novella, *Little Francis*. This all-at-once hybridity is epitomized in Carrington's mythology in the kitchen environment—the domestic space, par excellence, literally at the heart of her house. (2013, 1–13)

I do not seek to do an exhaustive reading about Fernández and Carrington here but perhaps a few notes about a couple of their stories in which both food and the domestic articulate metamorphosis: *White Rabbits* by Leonora Carrington, published in 1941, and *La jaula de la tía Enedina/Aunt Enedina's Cage* by Adela Fernández, written in 1973. In the first, a woman asks her neighbor for bad meat that—later we find out—she uses to feed monstrous rabbits living in her house with her husband. In the second, a woman is left at the altar and goes mad, so much so that she is locked up by her family in the junk room, where she grows old and gives birth to two children—the result of an incestuous relationship with her nephew, who tells the story—who have the appearance of birds. In both texts, the allusion to female stereotypes and the creation of an uncanny atmosphere through space construction, with dislocated characters, are palpable.

In the roles that male (psychic, social and cultural) narratives have associated, and in which they have inscribed, women—and, there-fore, any character of this gender, they can be located, according to Sherry B. Ortner, at the lower and upper ends of the human scale of relationships with individuals. These can be understood—in the case of the lower end—as a perception that ignores and subverts or, in the opposite case, as one that transcends (1974, 85). Two archetypes established in the 19th century (*the angel in the house* and *the mad-woman in the attic*) are easy to identify on this scale: the upsetting relationship with the madwoman in the attic and the one that trans-cends the body, mind and spirit of the angelic being. The latter, the conception of *the angel in the house*, of the pure woman, was reinforced during the Victorian era (1837–1901), in which religious structures and terminology were central to the family ideal, with "the *paterfamilias* as the patriarchal authority and the wife as the innocent 'angel' dedicated to his service" (Moran 2006, 24). In Victorian prose, on the other hand, is where *the madwoman in the attic* appears with all her rebellion and transgression. The paradigm, and the novel that inspired the iconic Gilbert and Gubar's book entitled like that (*The Madwoman in the Attic*), is *Jane Eyre* (1847) by Charlotte Brontë. Even the most conservative and decorous authors, Gilbert and Gubar point out, created fiercely independent characters to destroy "all the patriarchal structures which both their authors and their authors' submissive heroines seem to accept as inevitable" and from this projection that was always punished (and with which they avoided rebellious impulses in heroines), "female authors dramatize their own self-division, their desire both to accept the structures of patriarchal society and to reject them" (2000, 78). Such is the case of Bertha Mason Rochester—a woman who goes insane, locked up by her husband in the attic, who, according to Madeleine Wood, "acts out the frustrated and repressed passion of the imprisoned woman" (2009, 108).

But let's go back to *White Rabbits* by Leonora Carrington. Ethel, the narrator's neighbor, seems to be the antipodes of the angel in the house. On the one hand, heralded by a spider corpse and an ominous raven on her balcony, her first appearance violates the image expected of a woman dedicated to the home: "She carried a large dish full of bones, which she emptied onto the floor" (2017, 109). The following sentence refers for the first time to her appearance and ends by describing an action that, although in a disconcerting, nightmarish way, seems to fulfill the tasks of an angel in the house: "The woman, who had very long black hair, used her hair to wipe out the dish" (109). The construction of Ethel plays with the reader, because for brief moments she makes us think of the angelic figure. The allusions to the care and responsibilities of the home and its inhabitants are clear, such as rabbits: "Won't my poor little rabbits *be pleased?*" (110. Italics mine). These animals postulate from the fantastic a force of oppression on Ethel that, although it does not come from her husband, is, by her implications, clearly masculine from her. These white rabbits, according to Annette Shandler, hide in their apparent innocence a predatory, carnivorous nature that takes over space by rapidly procreating (1996, 70). Likewise, one can glimpse Ethel's interest in being a good hostess, "for she tossed her head coquettishly and gave me a very elegant salute after the fashion of a queen" (Carrington 2017, 108) and gestures of delicacy. "We mounted the stairs and my companion walked so carefully that I thought she was frightened" (110); "She uttered a low, sweet whistle" (111) to call rabbits *like a lady*. It is, therefore, a way of increasing the tension of the sinister interventions of the story from the already-established pattern of a housewife character, apparently fragile.

Everything revolves around food: bad meat is what sets up the world erected by the author and those who are pleased by the meat are the rarefying force in Ethel's life. The hybridity, that is, the animal–human creatures of which Conley spoke, in reference to the *transformism* proposed by Breton and executed by Carrington, becomes clear.

Now, close to the monster is also, of course, Aunt Enedina from Adela Fernández's short story. The archetype of the monstrous woman passed from patristic antiquity to the 18th century English satirists, who populated their works with monstrous women, in which they affirmed that the language in the mouth of women was destroyed and lost its meaning, or that after an angelic woman was hiding, without a doubt, a totally opposite being: a demon (Gilbert and Gubar 2000, 31). In the Hebraic tradition, opposed to Eve, there is Lilith, similar to Adam: "in patriarchal culture, female speech and female 'presumption,' that is, angry revolt against male domination, are inextricably linked and inevitably daemonic" (35).

It is not unreasonable to think that, in Adela Fernández's story, that angry revolt that breaks the reality's parameter is triggered by the message delivered to Enedina by a dirty, ragged man, about whom we never know if he was "an envoy of God or of the Devil" (2009, 28). When he predicts that her fiancé will not arrive at the altar and gives her an empty cage for canaries, the character "goes mad with loneliness" (27). The transgression of the crazy woman in the attic is also related, as has been hinted previously, with the way in which she faces the spaces dominated by men. Hence the importance of this archetype possessing harmful and dangerous energy and powers, such as Bertha Mason: "She was a big woman, in stature almost equalling her husband, and corpulent besides: she showed virile force in the contest—more than once she almost throttled him, athletic as he was" (Brontë 2001, 250).

In the case of Enedina, there is no masculinization of the character but rather an *animalization*. According to Mexican author Magali Velasco, the fantastic in Adela Fernández's text is articulated through the character's zoomorphic qualities (2007, 105). The story's narrator states: "she [was] used to the dark . . . she looked like a gray rat . . . She was very similar to one of those spiders" (Fernández 2009, 29). That is why Enedina is similar to Bertha Mason, the double of Jane Eyre, according to the reading of Gilbert and Gubar. The madwoman in the attic is the transcript of Jane's autonomous character, who, according to her aunt and protector, had "sudden starts of temper, and her continual, unnatural watchings of one's movements! . . . [S]he talked to me once like something mad, or like a fiend" (Brontë 2001, 197), descriptions that fit the animalistic character of Enedina.

Although Enedina never tries to escape or transcend the space to which she has been relegated, via the incestuous relationship she maintains with her nephew, she breaks the cycle of loneliness destined for both her and him: "The incestuous relationship unleashed among them is summarized in the need for affection, in the fatality of their destinies" (Velasco 2007, 104). Both Enedina, the madwoman, and her nephew, a black character whose skin color has also caused him to be segregated by his own family, somehow vindicate their position in society through their union, which will produce, at the end of the story, another uncanny element: the monstrous children of both.

There is a popular saying in Spanish, "Eres lo que comes/You are what you eat," which Fernández makes hers in *La jaula de la tía Enedina* to create the text. The short story's narrator feeds Enedina with birdseed, and she, along with her children, ends up not being what she eats *per se* but the animal that usually eats it. In another of the author's stories, *Las gallinitas/The Little Chickens*, bird-women creatures reappear. This is the beginning of the text:

> In the central market, old and rotten heart of the city, a human, feminine and senile cackling erupts daily at dawn. In the warehouses where chickpea and wheat are stored, innumerable men receive merchandise, carry heavy sacks on their backs and, through their gaps, jets or drizzles. The grains escape, spreading on the slimy garbage. Attracted by these foods, the old women arrive to dedicate themselves to the harvest. They are skinny, almost blind, dressed in black or gray, and they are smelly. A crust of consuming grime darkens their faces. With their fingers like a bird's beak, the old early risers, hunched over, collect the seeds and store them in small, fetid bags. (Fernández 2009, 119)

If *magical realism* is about inserting the mythological vastness in Latin America into a day-to-day context, the tag could easily be applied to Adela Fernández' work. A popular saying is turned, more than once, into a twisted version of the world in which we live. In another of her short stories, *Cordelias*, a little girl, carried by an Arab, an exotic character, gets to upset the dynamics of a town, since she is a fantastic creature whose reflections, in the water or in the mirror, sprout *doppelgängers*. When she arrives, the townspeople start spreading rumors about her identity:

There were feelings of compassion, assumptions and making up stories about where she came from: that the Arab had stolen her and left her there by mistake; that if maybe he didn't know anything about her and that someone threw her into the box to get rid of her; that if perhaps the corn had been transformed into a girl, daughter of the deity of corn and that she should be worshiped as a goddess; that if she maybe she was the devil himself who, in an image of apparent innocence, had come to town to unleash evil and a chain of tragedies. (34)

In *Cordelias,* appears, in addition, what, according to Alicia Llarena González, is one of the essential characteristics of the magical realism: like *the real marvelous,* term of the Cuban writer Alejo Carpentier, it proposes "a universe marked by cultural syncretism (indigenous and ladinos, white and black) and, by its innumerable contradictions, among which the survival of magic, of the pre-logical mentality, in the face of rationality, is visible" (1994, 25).

So far I have elaborated on Adela Fernández because, compared to Leonora Carrington, she has been, as I said above, rather ignored. You can count on the fingers of one hand the serious investigations on her. It is convenient to bring into account the theses of Raúl Alcántara Vega and Clara Angélica Ureta Calderón, from UNAM and BUAP, respectively, who focused on ambiguity and horror, the first, and the masculine/feminine dichotomy; the second, within the stories of Adela Fernández. Ureta (2003) focuses on a particular story: *El montón/The Crowd*, and she comes to important findings about the configuration of two worlds within the story: a violent one and a violated one, both in the confines of a house populated by a miserable family. Alcántara (2008), on the other hand, reviews the stories included in *Duermevelas*/Flickering Candles (1986) by Fernández and elaborates about a valuable idea: her texts postulate horror, anchored many times in the unspoken, as a transgression of reality.

Things change when it comes to Leonora Carrington. Rachel Carroll's (1998) paper, in which she analyzes the spectacularization of the grotesque and the animalization of Carrington's characters, is an important reference. Carroll distinguishes that, although in Carrington's work in general there are "enchanted landscapes," in her writing, we find facts that, even though they do transgress the logical order, do not always resort to those landscapes but are installed in the home. It is also worth mentioning Ana Rosa Domenella's (1992) reading of two stories by Carrington, *The Oval Lady* and *La debutante*, in which she analyzes, based on theories of the fantastic and the uncanny, the two stories and comes to important conclusions about, for instance, the representations of the father in Carrington, in addition to pointing out a specific quality—humor—which also interested Giulia Ingarao, who titled her postgraduate thesis *El humor y lo macabro en la obra de Leonora Carrington y Kati Horna/Humor and the Macabre in the Work of Leonora Carrington and Kati Horna* (2005). Gabriel García Ochoa (2016), on the other hand, reads Carrington by taking into account the separation of Surrealism that, she herself stated at some point, traces a kind of personal poetics of hers and contrasts it with Alejo Carpentier 's and his idea of the real marvelous, which is absolutely related to Adela Fernández's esthetics, as I said earlier.

We see, then, that there have already been comparative exercises with Carrington's work (Ingarao's and García Ochoa's, for example), but none that brings it closer to the writing of Adela Fernández, an almost unknown author whose reading in dialogue with Carrington could generate interesting findings. Let this text be a first approach to such productive matter.

Bibliography

Alcántara Vega, R. *Ambigüedad y horror en los cuentos de Adela Fernández* (Tesina de licenciatura). Facultad de Filosofía y Letras, UNAM, 2008. Recuperada de <http://oreon.dgbiblio.unam.mx/>.

Brontë, C. *Jane Eyre.* (3ª ed.). Nueva York: W. W. Norton & Company, 2001.

Carrington, L. *The Complete Stories of Leonora Carrington.* Nueva York: The Dorothy Project, 2017.

Carroll, R. "'Something to See: Spectacle and Savagery in Leonora Carrington's Fiction." *Critique. Studies in Contemporary Fiction,* 39(2), 1998, 154–166.

Conley, K. "Carrington's Kitchen," *Papers of Surrealism,* 10, 2013, 1–18: <https://scholarworks.wm.edu/aspubs/290>.

Domenella, A. R. "Leonora Carrington, escritora surrealista." *Escritos. Revista del Centro de Ciencias del Lenguaje,* 8, 1992, 49–59.

Fernández, A. *Cuentos de Adela Fernández: Duermevelas y Vago espinazo de la noche.* Nueva York: Editorial Campana, 2009.

García Ochoa, G. "The Surrealist Parallels of Leonora Carrington and Alejo Carpentier." *Journal of Iberian and Latin American Research,* 22(3), 2016, 280–296.

Gilbert, S. M. y Gubar, S. *The Madwoman in the Attic. The Woman Writer and the Nineteenth-Century Literary Imagination.* New Haven: Yale University Press, 2000.

Ingarao, G. *El humor y lo macabro en la obra de Leonora Carrington y Kati Horna* (Tesis de especialidad). Facultad de Filosofía y Letras, UNAM, 2005. Recuperada de <http://oreon.dgbiblio.unam.mx/>.

Llarena González, A. "Claves para "El realismo mágico" y "Lo real maravilloso": Espacio y actitud en cuatro novelas latinoamericanas." *Vector Plus*, 2, 1994, 15–27.

Moran, M. *Victorian Literature and Culture*. Londres: Continuum, 2006.

Ortner, S. B. "Is Female to Male as Nature is to Culture?" *Woman, culture, and society*. M. Z. Rosaldo y L. Lamphere (Eds.), Stanford: Stanford University Press, 1974, 68–87.

Ureta Calderón, C. A. *Lo masculino y lo femenino en el cuento «El montón» de Adela Fernández* (Tesis de maestría). Instituto de Ciencias Sociales y Humanidades, BUAP, 2003. Recuperada de <https://repositorioinstitu-cional.buap.mx/>.ç

Velasco, M. *El cuento: la casa de lo fantástico*. Ciudad de México: Fondo Editorial Tierra Adentro, 2007.

Wood, M. "Enclosing Fantasies: *Jane Eyre*," *The Madwoman in the Attic: After Thirty Years*. A. R. Federico, Ed. Columbia: University of Missouri Press, 2009, 94–110.

Conclusions and Reflections

According to my upbringing and that, I suspect, of almost everyone who was fortunate enough to grow up with significant others and food-secure, s/he who prepares food and drink does so with love and to express love. Meals are not just nutrition but enjoyable social events per se with important socialization and relational imprinting aspects. Certain ethnicities may emphasize this aspect more than others in my experience. The idea that this phenomenon is reciprocal, that s/he who consumes also does so with love and/or to counter-demonstrate love, may well have something to do with the overconsumption and/or health-related results of same in modern food-secure settings. In certain groups, not-necessarily-food-secure ones, the conception of beauty as related to a more voluptuous physicality than in those societies obsessed with thinness, may well also factor in more than just admiration of fat-stores-for-survival in some early societies.

This collection could have contained ever so many more chapters in each of the parts and sub-parts—or added additional ones of each, hence passing references to other possibilities and studies, presented and/or published, abound through the introductions to the parts. As it is, there are an unprecedented 20 chapters in this collection, 15 new and five reprints; this, in spite of what several collaborators have characterized as "a hellish year" of health and socio-political challenges worldwide. I, myself, have been struck by the amazing number of rather specific connections, far beyond the general themes of food and drink and/or the parts and sub-parts I chose as a result of the connections, which run through the chapters, though the collaborators did not consult with each other as they researched and wrote nor were they aware of my decisions on parts and sub-parts either before or after they submitted their chapters. Those connections especially address cultural identity, as well as feminist critique, special interests of my own as a sociologist who most frequently examines fictitious societies in terms of literature by and about women. The cross-cultural references to, and similarities among, secular and/or ceremonial foodstuffs and drinks like wine and *pulque* and *mate* also abound. In any case, I'm not sure if these notable connections establish generalities in terms of the areas of study—or if they can be attributed to the facts that so many of us have known each other professionally and personally for years, during which we have shared conference and scholarly work over our careers and/or worked together on this particular series of seven books so far!

Focusing studies on food and drink in these contexts, Amerindian, Spanish and Latin American, and tying those studies together in a collection, has been something of a surprising source of "new" knowledge and insights for me as editor/collaborator. Though it's not culturally in keeping, as I finalize this manuscript, I repeatedly think of the Broadway musical based on Charles Dickens' *Oliver Twist* and the song, *Food, Glorious Food*, a bittersweet experience to see/hear. The semi-starving orphans who sing it remind me of those worldwide who are still not food-secure, as well as of those of us fortunate food-secure types privileged enough to have been able to buy tickets—and now who have been able to research and write about food and drink from a "disinterested" intellectual point-of-view. But, on a more upbeat theme-related note, if still not culturally in keeping or particularly empathetic, as of the first day of summer, 21 June 2021, The Smithsonian's National Museum of National History in the U.S. has announced that it is establishing a new position: the Winiarski Curator of Food and Wine History!

The overall key concept is that, though *what* is eaten/drunk, *how* it's eaten/drunk, *why* it's eaten/drunk, *by whom* it's eaten/drunk, *where* it's eaten/drunk or *when* it's eaten/drunk varies, eating and drinking are universal, whether for sustenance for the body or for the soul/spirit. The emotional and communicative aspects of those actions themselves tie us all together across cultures but the "question word" details give us insights into each—and, hopefully, some understanding of and appreciation for each.

The Editor and Contributors

Debra D. Andrist, PhD, Professor of Spanish, retired 9-1-2021, formerly founding Chair of Foreign Languages at Sam Houston State University, formerly Chair of Modern & Classical Languages/Cullen Professor of Spanish, University of St. Thomas/Houston and before that, Associate Professor of Spanish, Baylor University, holds the BA, Fort Hays Kansas State University; MA, University of Utah; PhD, SUNY/Buffalo; and a Mellon Post-Doctoral Fellow at Rice University. A sociologist of created societies (literature) in works by and about women, her scholarly works include international conference papers and other presentations, books of criticism and textbooks; translations, critical articles, reviews, interviews and movie study guides, plus current books in progress. She has received internal and external grants plus awards and honors for teaching (SUNY) and service (Baylor and UST). She has personally studied abroad in Mexico and Spain and taught in study abroad in Mexico, Spain, Ireland and Costa Rica, was an exchange professor in Chile and Canada and a Fulbright-Hays Scholar in Morocco. A member of many professional organizations, an officer in most, she was, e.g., president of SCMLA and of the Houston Area Teachers of Foreign Language and Senior Vocal of AILCHF. Active in service, e.g., she is a docent at Bayou Bend, has been secretary of Houston Hispanic Forum (a Board member for 17+ years), on the Montgomery County Arts Council Grants Committee and others.

John Francis Burke, PhD, teaches political theory, religion and politics, US Latinx politics, comparative politics and US American politics at Trinity University in San Antonio, Texas. He is an interdisciplinary scholar who has published articles especially on political theory, intercultural relations, social justice and religion & politics in several journals and periodicals, including *The Review of Politics and Commonweal*. He is the author of *Mestizo Democracy* (College Station, TX: Texas A&M Press, 2002), a text on democracy and multiculturalism in the U.S. Southwest and *Building Bridges Not Walls: Nourishing Diverse Cultures in Faith /Construyamos puentes, no muros: Alimentar a las diversas culturas en la fe* (Collegeville, MN:

Liturgical Press, 2016), a text on integrating diverse cultural spiritualties constructively in faith-based communities. He has also appeared as a political commentator on many Texas media outlets, both in English and Spanish. In addition to his scholarly work, he has coordinated social justice institutes and programs at the University of St. Thomas in Houston, TX and Cabrini University in Radnor, PA. He has also served on several committees and conducted workshops in Indiana, Pennsylvania and Texas dealing with social justice and intercultural issues. Finally, he has extensive experience in church liturgy and has earned a "reputation" for cultivating vibrant multilingual choirs.

Eduardo Cerdán, MA (Xalapa, México, 1995), adjunct professor of undergraduate studies in Letras Hispánicas de la Universidad Nacional Autónoma de México, is a writer of narrative and an essayist. He has won prizes in national story competitions, has collaborated on collected writings and on periodical publications like *Revista de la Universidad de México, La Jornada Semanal, Literal: Latin American Voices* y *La Palabra y el Hombre*. He studies sinister stories by writers of mid-century Mexico and is a columnist for *Cuadrivio Semanal*. Some of his stories have been translated to French.

Jorge Chavarro, MD, MA, ABD in Spanish, was born in Colombia in a village with jungle heat and sun. The natives called it Tora, it's now known as Barrancabermeja; however, he lived in Bogota from the age of ten months. He graduated from medical school in the turbulent Seventies, met and married his wife, Marthica. Their first child is now a physician in the U.S. Chavarro's medical degree came after his children, including a specialization in urology in the Eighties. His cherished daughter was a gift born during his urologist degree and is now a Spanish teacher in Texas. He practiced his specialty in Colombia and taught urology at his alma mater, the National University of Colombia. In early 2002, he was a victim of kidnapping by the Colombian Self-Defense, the reason for his immigration to the U.S., which led to starting over professionally in the surgery field in the U.S. His avocation and dream to become a writer and teach literature; in fact, his first poetry collection and first short story collection are to be published in 2021. His interest in literature led him to an MA in Spanish at Sam Houston State University in 2014. He is currently a PhD candidate at Texas A&M University in College Station whose dissertation projected for 2022 is entitled *History of Death in the Modern Period of Poetry*.

Elizabeth White Coscio, PhD, presently teaches Spanish language, literature, culture, clinical conversation and other Spanish applied language courses at the University of St. Thomas in Houston, Texas. She has been the Cullen Endowed Chair of Spanish and Chair of the Modern and Classical Languages Department since 2007 and has also led study abroad experiences. Although she has also worked in marketing and sales, an area that provided experience in budgeting, staff development, and influencing clients, she has always taught language courses at all levels. Past experience includes many years of teaching secondary level French, university Spanish courses including practical language application courses (translation, business, media, for the medical professions and English as a Second Language at Rice University, University of Houston, and other institutions. As collaborator on a Spanish middle school text, she wrote and edited games and projects and has produced critical articles on a variety of both Peninsular and Latin American topics, as well as books, translations, international presentations, reviews, interviews, and other. She is a past vice president and president of the South-Central Modern Language Association, Associate Professor of Spanish, Director of the Latin American and Latino Studies Program and Sponsor for Sigma Delta Pi Spanish Honor Society.

Lauren M. P. Derby holds an MA in English and American Literature with a certificate in Empire studies from the University of Houston. Her articles, book reviews, devotionals, and short stories have appeared in various non-academic publications. She has spoken at several conferences, including the South-Central Modern Language Association's 2012 conference on Death and Eros. Two of her articles—"Steel-Plated Petticoats: The Heroism of Woman in *Don Quixote*" and "Rudolfo Anaya's *Bless Me, Última*: A *Mestizaje* Education"—have been published in the University of Houston's journal, *Plaza: Dialogues in Language and Literature*. Her area of focus is postcolonial and Nineteenth-century British literatures. After living abroad in Suriname and China, among others, with her diplomat husband, she lives in Washington D.C. in 2021, awaiting another international assignment.

Jeanne Gillespie, PhD, exhibits a passion for finding fascinating stories and rendering them into accessible narratives for reflection and further investigation. She has taught courses at all levels of Spanish language and cultures. In addition, she teaches in the Women's and Gender Studies program and in Interdisciplinary Studies at Southern Mississippi University at Hattiesburg. Gillespie has published on

Spanish colonial literary and cultural studies as well as on innovative pedagogies and interdisciplinary inquiry. Her current research project is the documentation of plant materials and healing practices in indigenous Mexican documents, especially poetic and dramatic texts. In conjunction with that research, she is preparing an article on women's voices in the Iberian colonial record that examines Native American women whose words and accounts have been recorded in Spanish documents. Gillespie holds a Bachelor of Arts in Spanish from Purdue, a Master of Arts in Latin American Studies with concentrations in Anthropology and Art History from the University of Texas at Austin and a doctorate in Spanish American Literature from the Arizona State University. She is currently Associate Professor of Spanish and Associate Dean at Southern Mississippi. Gillespie is married to musician, John Palensky, and is the mother of three vivacious children. Her home is filled with good food, great music and much love.

Kimberly A. Habegger, PhD, is Professor of Spanish and outgoing chair of languages at Regis University in Denver, Colorado, where she teaches language, literature, culture and interdisciplinary courses. She graduated from Ohio State University with a doctorate in Romance Languages and Linguistics with an emphasis on historical theater from the Post-war period. Participation in several seminars and institutes such as an NEH Summer Teaching Institute have afforded her the opportunity to connect her research interests with the needs of the curriculum. In past years, her research has produced several presentations and publications that explore the iconography and semiotics of the traditional arts of the American Southwest and of Spain. Of late, she has been investigating the phenomenon of the contemporary iconic wineries of Spain designed by widely renowned architects. Recent professional and personal trips to Spain, the Dominican Republic, Costa Rica, and Peru have informed her awareness of the cultural aesthetics of the Hispanic world.

Enrique Mallén, PhD, is a Professor in the Department of Foreign Languages at Sam Houston State University. He completed his PhD at Cornell University. Dr. Mallen has published numerous articles and book chapters on linguistics, literature and art history. The titles of some of his books are *Con/figuración Sintáctica*, *The Visual Grammar of Pablo Picasso*, *La Sintaxis de la Carne: Pablo Picasso y Marie-Thérèse Walter*; *Poesía del Lenguaje: De T. S. Eliot a Eduardo Espina* and *A Concordance of Pablo Picasso's Spanish Writings*, *Antología Crítica de la Poesía del Lenguaje* and *A Concordance of Pablo Picasso's French Writings*, *La Muerte y la máscara en Pablo Picasso*.

Dr. Mallen is a recognized expert on Pablo Picasso. He is director and general editor of the *Online Picasso Project*, an encyclopedic digital archive and catalog of the works and life of the Spanish artist, which he created in 1997.

Stephen J. Miller, PhD, is Professor of Hispanic Studies at Texas A&M University. Among his research fields are nineteenth nentury through Contemporary Narrative with special emphasis on Spanish Peninsular and American narrative. He is the author of the following volumes: *El mundo de Galdós: teoría, tradición y evolución creativa del pensamiento socio-literario galdosiano (1983); Del realismo/naturalismo al modernismo: Galdós, Zola, Revilla y Clarín (1870–1901) (1993); Galdós gráfico (1861–1907): orígenes, técnicas y límites del socio-mimetismo (2001).* He is co-editor and contributor to *Critical Studies on Gonzalo Torrente Ballester* (1988; with Janet Pérez) and *Critical Studies on Armando Palacio Valdés* (1993; with Brian J. Dendle). In 2001, he did the introductions to his facsimile editions of three Galdosian graphic narratives: *Gran teatro de la pescadería, Las Canarias,* and *Atlas zoológico,* and to two of Galdós's sketchbooks: *Álbum arquitectónico and Álbum marítimo.* For the last decade, he has been doing short book reviews for *Choice* of critical studies, biographies and collected letters of Hemingway, Bellow and Updike. As contributor and co-editor with José Pablo Villalobos, he published Rolando Hinojosa's *'Klail City Death Trip Series': A Retrospective, New Directions* in 2013. He is presently working on an original book-length critical study of Hinojosa's *Klail City Death Trip* Series.

Rose Mary Salum Nemer, MFA, founder and director of the bilingual literary/art magazines, *Literal: Voces Latinoamericanas/Literal: Latin American Voices,* as well as the publishing house, Literal Press, and *Visible,* was born in Mexico of Lebanese descent. She holds the MFA from University of St. Thomas/Houston. She is the author of four books of short stories, *El agua que mece el silencio/The Water That Rocks the Silence* (Vaso Roto, 2015); *Delta de las arenas. Cuentos árabes, cuentos judíos/Delta of the Sands: Arabic & Jewish Stories* (International Latino Book Award; Literal Publishing, 2013; Vigía, 2015); *Entre los espacios/Spaces In-Between* (Tierra Firme, 2002) y *Vitrales/Stained Glass* (Edomex, 1994). In 2009, she edited the collection, *Almalafa y Caligrafía, Literatura de origen árabe en América Latina/Moorish Apparel and Calligraphy: Literature of Arabic Origen in Latin America,* for the magazine, *Hostos Review.* Her stories and essays have appeared in the anthologies, *Women Writers in the U.S.* (Hostos Review, 2014); *Cruce de fronteras:*

Antología de escritores iberoamericanos en Estados Unidos/Crossing Fronteras: An Anthology of Iberian-American Writers in the U.S. (SubUrbano, 2013); *Poéticas de los (dis)locamientos/Poetics of (Dis)Locations* (Literal Publishing, 2012); *Raíces latinas, narradores y poetas inmigrantes/Latin Roots, Immigrant Narrators and Poets* (Vagón azul, 2012); *América nuestra: antología de narrativa en español en Estados Unidos/Our America: An Anthology of the Narrative in Spanish in the U.S.* (Linkgua, 2011); *Professions* (MLA, 2009); among others. For her literary and editorial work, she has received the Author of the Year 2008 from the Hispanic Book Festival, the Hispanic Excellence Award, the International Latino Book Award, four Lone Star Awards, two CELJ Awards, the Classical Award from the University of St. Thomas, a recognition from the U.S. Congress, the Mujeres Destacadas/Outstanding Women Award, from the journalistic agency, ImpreMedia, three nominations for the Nora Magid Award from Pen America (2013), the Ana María Matute (Torremozas, 2008) y the Maggie Award (2005). She is a Fellow of the Academia Norteamericana de la Lengua/North American Academy of the Language.

Michelle Sharp, PhD, is the co-editor of the first critical edition of Carmen de Burgos scholarship in English, *Multiple Modernities: Carmen de Burgos, Author and Activist* (Routledge 2017). This collection was the fortuitous outcome of a series of panels dedicated to Carmen de Burgos's literacy legacy at the 23014 KFLC: The Languages, Literatures and Cultures Conference. Another featured recent publication is a chapter, "Carmen de Burgos: Teaching Women of the Modern Age" in *Kiosk Literature of Silver Age Spain*, Eds. Susan Laron and Jeffrey Zamostny (Intellect 2017). She defended her PhD dissertation titled "The Narrative of Carmen de Burgos: An Innovative Portrayal of the Family and Gender Roles in Spain," inspired by research at the Biblioteca Nacional in Madrid. Dr. Sharp now evaluates Burgos's domestic manuals and cookbooks for their contributions to Burgos's overreaching feminist mission. She was a visiting assistant professor at Macalester College (Satin Paul, MN). She was the editorial advisor and contributor for the entry on Carmen de Burgos in the *Twentieth-Century Literary Criticism (TCLC)* (Cengage 2016). The chapter, "Vitamin F: The Rise of First-Wave Feminist-Fueled Home Economics," was inspired by a presentation she gave at the inaugural Early Modern Food Studies Conference at the University of Minnesota/Twin Cities in the fall of 2019. An independent scholar, she works as the administrator for the Notre Dame Club of Minnesota and writes a local newspaper column titled "Meet the Minnesota Makers: Land of 10,000 Treats." You can follow her adventures with the makers and growers of the Land of 10,000 Lakes on social media @MeettheMNMakers.

Haiqing Sun, PhD, Texas Southern University, is Professor of Spanish, with research focus on Latin American narrative and comparative study of Latin American and Chinese film and literature. She has published research on Latin American detective fiction, on writers, Jorge Luis Borges, Mario Vargas Llosa, Roa Bastos, Rodolfo Walsh, encyclopedic entries, and Chinese translations of works by Octavio Paz, Gabriela Mistral, and Luis Buñuel. She currently serves as editor for journals, *Caribbean Vistas* and *Yangtze River Academic*, and is Invited Guest Professor of Pingdingshan University. She has also worked as principal investigator in literature and culture projects funded with grants of National Endowment for the Humanities (NEH), and Humanities Texas (HTx).

Index

Page numbers in italics refer to figures, plates or tables. Fictional characters are listed within single quotes, with the name of the book/story in brackets. In most cases the character is indexed under the first name e.g. 'Alberto' (Lezama's *Paradiso*).